Synopsis of Clinical Ophthalmology

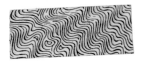

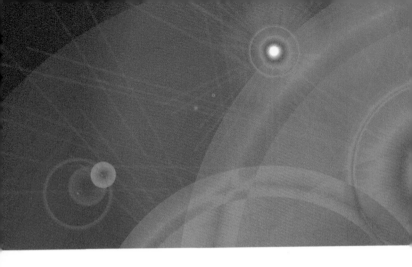

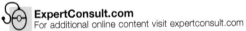 **ExpertConsult.com**
For additional online content visit expertconsult.com

Content Strategist: Russell Gabbedy
Content Development Specialist: Alexandra Mortimer
Project Manager: Caroline Jones
Design: Stewart Larking

THIRD EDITION

Synopsis of Clinical Ophthalmology

Jack J. Kanski
MD, MS, FRCS, FRCOphth
Honorary Consultant Ophthalmic
Surgeon
Prince Charles Eye Unit
King Edward VII Hospital
Windsor
UK

Brad Bowling
FRCSEd (Ophth), FRCOphth
Vision Eye Institute
Sydney
Australia

ELSEVIER
SAUNDERS

is an imprint of Elsevier Ltd

© 2013 Elsevier Ltd. All rights reserved.

First edition 2004
Second edition 2009

The right of Jack J. Kanski and Brad Bowling to be identified as authors of this work has been asserted by them in accordance with the Copyright, Designs and Patents Act 1988.

Notices
Knowledge and best practice in this field are constantly changing. As new research and experience broaden our understanding, changes in research methods, professional practices, or medical treatment may become necessary.

Practitioners and researchers must always rely on their own experience and knowledge in evaluating and using any information, methods, compounds, or experiments described herein. In using such information or methods they should be mindful of their own safety and the safety of others, including parties for whom they have a professional responsibility.

With respect to any drug or pharmaceutical products identified, readers are advised to check the most current information provided (i) on procedures featured or (ii) by the manufacturer of each product to be administered, to verify the recommended dose or formula, the method and duration of administration, and contraindications. It is the responsibility of practitioners, relying on their own experience and knowledge of their patients, to make diagnoses, to determine dosages and the best treatment for each individual patient, and to take all appropriate safety precautions.

To the fullest extent of the law, neither the Publisher nor the authors, contributors, or editors, assume any liability for any injury and/or damage to persons or property as a matter of products liability, negligence or otherwise, or from any use or operation of any methods, products, instructions, or ideas contained in the material herein.

ISBN: 978-0-7020-5021-3
International ISBN: 978-0-7020-5036-7
eBook ISBN: 978-0-7020-5037-4

Printed in Great Britain
Last digit is the print number: 9 8

Contents

Preface

The third edition of *Synopsis of Clinical Ophthalmology* is intended principally as a companion to the seventh edition of *Clinical Ophthalmology: A Systematic Approach*. It provides a précis of the larger book that can be used as a portable and rapidly searchable reference suitable for use in a busy clinic. It is also ideal as a basis for revision, formatted as a series of easily digested topic summaries that can be supplemented from the larger book as necessary to aid understanding. Practitioners, medical students and specialist nurses requiring a shorter but comprehensive review of ophthalmology may find *Synopsis* a more appropriate text than the lengthier consideration of *A Systematic Approach*.

Since the publication of the previous edition, there have been significant developments in the theory and practice of ophthalmology; examples include the transformation of the management of ocular neovascular processes by the widespread introduction of VEGF inhibitors, and substantial progression in the understanding and management of angle-closure glaucoma. More broadly, understanding of the genetic and molecular basis of ophthalmic disease continues to advance on an accelerating basis, with the promise of revolutionary therapeutic gains.

This edition has been enhanced and extended, facilitating its use as a stand-alone text where required. The illustrations have been comprehensively reviewed and updated, a majority differing from those in the seventh edition of *A Systematic Approach*.

The authors are possessed of a sense of excitement about the present and future of ophthalmology and hope to have communicated a little of their enthusiasm in the pages of this book.

JJK
BB

Acknowledgements

We are extremely grateful to **Dr. Irina Gout** of the Prince Charles Eye Unit and the following colleagues and medical photographic departments for supplying us with images without which this book could not have been written:

Barry C. 8.10, 9.20, 9.26, 11.46, 11.47, 12.37, 12.39, 13.16, 13.19, 13.21, 14.7, 14.17, 14.23, 14.26, 14.31, 14.34, 15.2, 15.15, 21.1. **Bates R.** 1.1, 1.23, 1.53, 2.9, 3.11, 5.37, 5.55, 6.30, 6.48, 6.61, 8.2, 9.31, 10.47, 12.4, 12.10, 18.2. **Bajwa R.** 14.22, 5.1, 15.3. **Curtis R.** 6.21, 12.5, 12.18, 12.54. **Damato B.** 12.26, 12.28, 12.29, 12.30, 12.32, 12.38, 12.47, 12.51, 12.52. **Fogla R.** 9.22, 21.26. **Gass JDM.** *Stereoscopic Atlas of Macular Disease; Diagnosis and Treatment,* Mosby, 1997. 11.26, 11.37, 12.49, 13.30, 13.39, 14.20, 15.13, 19.4, 20.10, 20.11. **Gili P.** 8.9, 9.21, 11.53b, 12.13, 14.6, 14.30, 19.6, 19.16, 21.11. **Hayreh S.** 19.8. **Jager M.** 1.12, 12.15. **Krachmer JH, Mannis MJ, Holland EJ.** *Cornea,* Mosby, 2005. 6.44, 6.65, 6.72. **Leyland M.** 7.8. **Link T.** 12.44. **Martinkova R.** 10.29. **Merin L.** 10.15, 14.24, 15.27. **Milenkov S.** 14.21, 15.8. **Moore A.** 15.5. **Moorfields Eye Hospital.** 15.17, 15.18. **Nischal K.** 3.34, 18.4. **Parluekar M.** 10.33, 19.47. **Pavesio C.** 11.11, 11.15, 11.30, 11.38. **Pearson A.** 3.12, 3.47, 3.48. **Rogers N.** 1.18, 1.85, 1.86, 6.14, 12.50. **Rosen ES, Eustace P, Thompson HS, Cumming WJK.** *Neuro-ophthalmology,* Mosby, 1998. 19.42. **Saine P.** 13.34, 16.20, 19.5. **Romanowska-Dixon B.** 12.40. **Salmon J.** 10.24. **Schepens CL, Hartnett ME, Hirose T.** *Retinal Detachment and Allied Diseases,* Butterworth-Heinemann, 2000. 13.14, 16.10. **Schuman JS, Christopoulos V, Dhaliwal DK, Kahook MY, Noecker RJ.** *Lens and Glaucoma, in Rapid Diagnosis in Ophthalmology,* Mosby, 2008. 9.7, 9.25, 9.28, 9.29, 10.4, 10.13, 14.43b. **Singh AD, Damato BE, Pe'er J, Murphree AL, Perry JD.** *Clinical Ophthalmic Oncology,* Saunders, 2007. 1.28. **Smit D.** 1.45, 1.55. **Talks J.** 15.23. **Tanner V.** 16.8. **Trobe JD.** *Neuro-ophthalmology, in Rapid Diagnosis in Ophthalmology,* Mosby, 2008. 19.7. **Tuft S.** 1.31, 1.40, 1.44, 1.76, 5.16, 5.17, 5.25, 5.27, 5.28, 5.29, 5.32, 5.33, 5.34, 5.36, 5.40, 5.44, 5.45, 5.54, 6.3, 6.10, 6.12, 6.24, 6.25, 6.26, 6.29, 6.35, 7.4, 7.10, 7.13. **Wykes W.** 13.38. **Zografos L.** 20.2, 20.3.

Abbreviations

AAION	arteritic anterior ischaemic optic neuropathy
AAU	acute anterior uveitis
AC/A ratio	accommodative convergence/accommodation ratio
AD	autosomal dominant
AHP	abnormal head posture
AI	accommodative insufficiency
AIDS	acquired immune deficiency syndrome
AION	anterior ischaemic optic neuropathy
AKC	atopic keratoconjunctivitis
ALT	argon laser trabeculoplasty
AMD	age-related macular degeneration
ANA	antinuclear antibody
APD	afferent pupillary defect
APMPPE	acute posterior multifocal placoid pigment epitheliopathy
AR	autosomal recessive
AREDS	Age-Related Eye Disease Study
ARN	acute retinal necrosis
BCC	basal cell carcinoma
BP	blood pressure
BRAO	branch retinal artery occlusion
BRVO	branch retinal vein occlusion
BSV	binocular single vision
BUT	breakup time
CAI	carbonic anhydrase inhibitor
CAU	chronic anterior uveitis
CCT	central corneal thickness
CDCR	canaliculodacryocystorhinostomy
CHED	congenital hereditary endothelial dystrophy
CHRPE	congenital hypertrophy of the retinal pigment epithelium
CI	convergence insufficiency
CMO	cystoid macular oedema
CNS	central nervous system
CNV	choroidal neovascularization
CPEO	chronic progressive external ophthalmoplegia
CRAO	central retinal artery occlusion
CRP	C-reactive protein
CRVO	central retinal vein occlusion
CSMO	clinically significant macular oedema
CSS	central suppression scotoma
CT	computed tomography
DALK	deep anterior lamellar keratoplasty
DCR	dacryocystorhinostomy
DR	diabetic retinopathy

DSEK	Descemet stripping endothelial keratoplasty
DVD	dissociated vertical deviation
ECG	electrocardiogram
EDTA	ethylenediaminetetraacetic acid
EKC	epidemic keratoconjunctivitis
EOG	electro-oculogram
ERG	electroretinogram
ESR	erythrocyte sedimentation rate
FA	fluorescein angiography
FAP	familial adenomatous polyposis
FAZ	foveal avascular zone
FBC	full blood count
FFM	fundus flavimaculatus
GCA	giant cell arteritis
GPC	giant papillary conjunctivitis
HAART	highly active antiretroviral therapy
HIV	human immunodeficiency virus
HRT	Heidelberg retinal tomograph
HSV-1	herpes simplex virus type 1
HSV-2	herpes simplex virus type 2
HZO	herpes zoster ophthalmicus
ICGA	indocyanine green angiography
Ig	immunoglobulin
IK	Interstitial keratitis
ILM	internal limiting membrane
INO	internuclear ophthalmoplegia
IOFB	intraocular foreign body
IOID	idiopathic orbital inflammatory disease
IOL	intraocular lens
IOP	intraocular pressure
IRMA	intraretinal microvascular abnormality
ITC	iridotrabecular contact
IU	intermediate uveitis
JIA	juvenile idiopathic arthritis
KCS	keratoconjunctivitis sicca
KP	keratic precipitate
LA	local anaesthesia
LASEK	laser epithelial keratomileusis
LASIK	laser *in situ* keratomileusis
LN	latent nystagmus
MLF	medial longitudinal fasciculus
MR	magnetic resonance imaging
MS	multiple sclerosis
MU	mega units
NF1	neurofibromatosis 1
NF2	neurofibromatosis 2

NRR	neuroretinal rim
NSAID	nonsteroidal anti-inflammatory drug
NSR	neurosensory retina
NVD	new vessels at the disc
NVE	new vessels elsewhere
OCT	optical coherence tomography
OHT	ocular hypertension
OKN	optokinetic nystagmus
PAC	primary angle-closure
PACG	primary angle-closure glaucoma
PACS	primary angle-closure suspect
PAM	primary acquired melanosis
PAS	peripheral anterior synechiae
PCF	pharyngoconjunctival fever
PCO	posterior capsular opacification
PCR	polymerase chain reaction
PCV	polypoidal choroidal vasculopathy
PDR	proliferative diabetic retinopathy
PDS	pigment dispersion syndrome
PDT	photodynamic therapy
PED	pigment epithelial detachment
PIOL	primary intraocular lymphoma
PION	posterior ischaemic optic neuropathy
PKP	penetrating kerotoplasty
POAG	primary open-angle glaucoma
POHS	presumed ocular histoplasmosis syndrome
PPCD	posterior polymorphous corneal dystrophy
PPRF	paramedian pontine reticular formation
PPV	pars plana vitrectomy
PRK	photorefractive keratectomy
PRP	panretinal photocoagulation
PVD	posterior vitreous detachment
PVR	proliferative vitreoretinopathy
PXF	pseudoexfoliation
RAPD	relative afferent pupillary defect
RD	retinal detachment
ROP	retinopathy of prematurity
RP	retinitis pigmentosa
RPE	retinal pigment epithelium
RRD	rhegmatogenous retinal detachment
SCC	squamous cell carcinoma
SF	short-term fluctuation
SJS	Stevens–Johnson syndrome
SLK	superior limbic keratoconjunctivitis
SLT	selective laser trabeculoplasty
SRF	subretinal fluid

TAL	total axial length
TB	tuberculosis
TEN	toxic epidermal necrolysis
TGF	transforming growth factor
TIA	transient ischaemic attack
TTT	transpupillary thermotherapy
UBM	ultrasonic biomicroscopy
US	ultrasonography
VA	visual acuity
VEGF	vascular endothelial growth factor
VHL	von Hippel–Lindau syndrome
VKC	vernal keratoconjunctivitis
VKH	Vogt–Koyanagi–Harada syndrome
VZV	varicella zoster virus
X-L	X-linked

To Amsler, Tom and Gerry.

Eyelids

Benign nodules and cysts

Chalazion (meibomian cyst)

Definition: very common chronic sterile inflammation of a meibomian gland that may resolve spontaneously.

Diagnosis

- *Signs:* (a) gradually enlarging tarsal nodule (*Fig. 1.1*); (b) conjunctival granulomatous extension is common, and (c) secondary infection (internal hordeolum; *Fig. 1.2*) may occur.

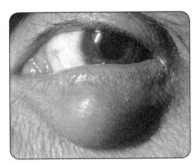

Fig 1.1

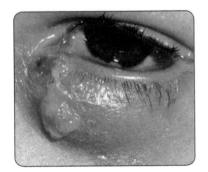

Fig 1.2

- *Associations:* (a) meibomian gland dysfunction, (b) acne rosacea, and (c) seborrhoeic dermatitis.

Treatment: (a) incision and curettage (*Fig. 1.3*), (b) local steroid injection (0.2–2 ml of 5 mg/ml triamcinolone diacetate), and (c) prophylactic systemic tetracycline in severe recurrent disease.

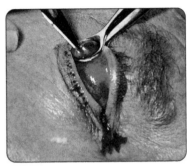

Fig 1.3

Miscellaneous

- *Cyst of Zeis:* nontranslucent cyst on the anterior lid margin arising from an obstructed sebaceous gland associated with a lash follicle (*Fig. 1.4*).

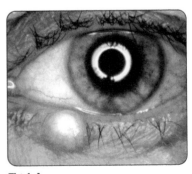

Fig 1.4

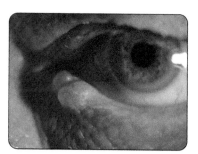

Fig 1.5

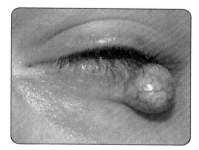

Fig 1.7

- **Cyst of Moll:** translucent, fluid-filled retention cyst on the anterior lid margin (*Fig. 1.5*) arising from an apocrine gland.
- **External hordeolum (stye):** tender, pointing swelling in the lid margin, usually with a lash at its apex (*Fig. 1.6*); caused by an acute staphylococcal infection of a lash follicle.
- **Epidermal inclusion cyst:** slow-growing, firm, round lesion containing keratin; located away from the lid margin (*Fig. 1.7*); caused by implantation of epidermis into dermis following trauma or surgery.

- **Sebaceous (pilar) cyst:** may occasionally occur at the medial canthus (*Fig. 1.8*).

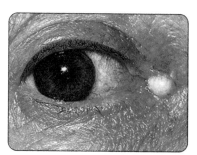

Fig 1.8

Benign tumours

Squamous cell papilloma

Pathogenesis: human papilloma virus.

Diagnosis: narrow-based pedunculated (skin tag; *Fig. 1.9*) or broad-based sessile lesion (*Fig. 1.10*).

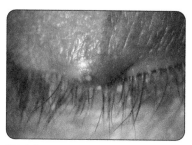

Fig 1.6

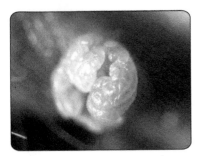

Fig 1.9

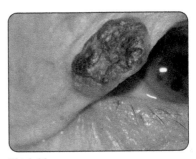

Fig 1.11

Treatment: curettage or excision.

Actinic (solar, senile) keratosis

Predisposition: elderly fair-skinned individuals with a history of chronic sun exposure; carries low/moderate malignant potential (squamous cell carcinoma).

Diagnosis: hyperkeratotic plaque with a scaly surface and well-defined borders (*Fig. 1.12*).

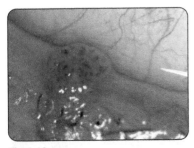

Fig 1.10

Treatment: simple excision.

Basal cell papilloma (seborrhoeic keratosis)

Diagnosis: discrete brown pedunculated or sessile lesion, often with a 'stuck on' appearance (*Fig. 1.11*), in an elderly individual.

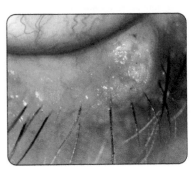

Fig 1.12

Treatment: cryotherapy, or excision biopsy if there is suspicion of malignancy.

Acquired melanocytic naevus

Diagnosis:

- *Intradermal naevus:* nonpigmented papilloma that may show protruding lashes (*Fig. 1.13*), in an elderly individual. The cells are confined to the dermis and have no malignant potential.

- *Compound naevus:* raised papule with variable pigmentation (*Fig. 1.15*), in a middle-aged individual. The cells extend from the epidermis into the dermis and have low malignant potential.

Treatment: excision for cosmesis or suspicion of malignancy.

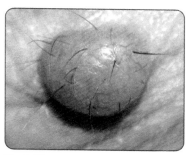

Fig 1.13

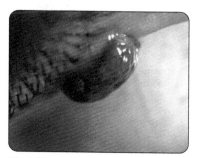

Fig 1.15

- *Junctional naevus:* flat brown lesion (*Fig. 1.14*) in a young individual. The cells are located at the junction of the dermis and epidermis, and they carry very low malignant potential.

Strawberry naevus (capillary haemangioma)

Definition: common tumour of childhood with a female-to-male ratio of 3:1. Visceral haemangiomas may be present in patients with multiple cutaneous lesions. The vast majority present soon after birth with a rapid growth phase during infancy followed by gradual involution.

Diagnosis: raised, bright red lesion (*Fig. 1.16*) that blanches on pressure and may swell on crying; orbital extension may be present (see Chapter 3).

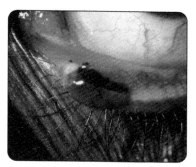

Fig 1.14

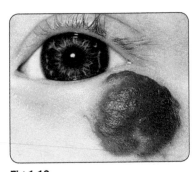

Fig 1.16

Port-wine stain (naevus flammeus)

Definition: congenital lesion that is usually unilateral/dermatomal and occasionally bilateral. In some cases, it forms a component of the Sturge–Weber syndrome.

Diagnosis: (a) sharply demarcated, soft pink patch that does not blanch with pressure (*Fig. 1.18*), (b) darkens with age but does not enlarge, (c) overlying skin may become hypertrophied, coarse, and nodular (*Fig. 1.19*).

Treatment

- *Indications:* (a) cosmesis, (b) severe ptosis (*Fig. 1.17*), and (c) corneal distortion that may give rise to amblyopia.
- *Options:* intralesional or systemic steroid, or systemic propranolol (2 mg/kg/day).

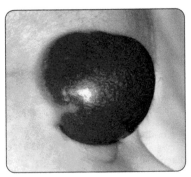

Fig 1.17

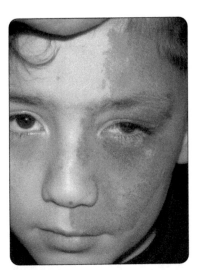

Fig 1.18

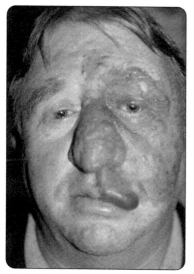

Fig 1.19

Treatment: erbium laser may decrease skin discoloration, if undertaken early; photodynamic therapy.

Diagnosis of Sturge–Weber syndrome (encepholotrigeminal angiomatosis)
- *Skin:* unilateral naevus flammeus in the distribution of one or more branches of the trigeminal nerve.
- *Brain:* ipsilateral parietal or occipital leptomeningeal haemangioma.
- *Ipsilateral ocular features:* (a) glaucoma, (b) episcleral haemangioma, and (c) diffuse choroidal haemangioma (see Chapter 12); heterochromia iridis is uncommon.
- *Classification:* (a) trisystem involves the face, leptomeninges, and eyes; (b) bisystem disease involves the face and eyes, or the face and leptomeninges.

Xanthelasma

Definition: common, typically bilateral lesion occurring in middle-aged and elderly individuals. It is associated with a higher risk of coronary heart disease, and in younger patients may indicate hypercholesterolaemia.

Diagnosis: white-yellow subcutaneous plaques often located medially (*Fig. 1.20*).

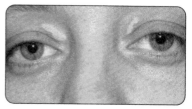

Fig 1.20

Treatment: (a) excision, (b) laser ablation, or (c) cryotherapy; systemic cholesterol abnormalities should be addressed to reduce risk of recurrence.

Neurofibroma

- *Plexiform:* affects children with neurofibromatosis type 1 (NF1).
- *Solitary:* occurs in adults, 25% of whom have NF1.

Diagnosis: upper lid involvement by a plexiform lesion gives rise to a characteristic S-shaped deformity (*Fig. 1.21*).

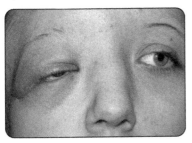

Fig 1.21

Treatment: solitary lesions can be excised, but removal of diffuse plexiform lesions may be difficult.

Malignant tumours

Basal cell carcinoma (BCC)

Table 1.1 Predisposing systemic conditions
• Xeroderma pigmentosum
• Gorlin–Goltz (naevoid basal cell carcinoma) syndrome
• Dysplastic naevus (atypical mole) syndrome
• Muir–Torre syndrome
• Bazex syndrome
• Albinism
• Immunosuppression

Definition: common, slow-growing, and locally invasive but nonmetastasizing tumour. 90% occur on the head and neck, and 10% of these involve the eyelids, most commonly the lower.

Diagnosis

- *Nodular:* shiny, pearly nodule with overlying fine irregular blood vessels (*Fig. 1.22*).

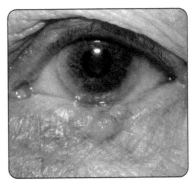

Fig 1.22

- *Noduloulcerative (rodent ulcer):* nodule with central ulceration and rolled telangiectatic edges (*Fig. 1.23*).
- *Sclerosing (morphoeic):* indurated plaque whose margins may be impossible to delineate clinically; often associated with loss of overlying lashes (*Fig. 1.24*).

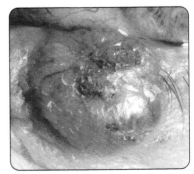

Fig 1.23

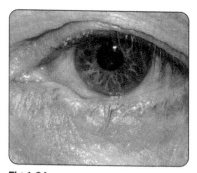

Fig 1.24

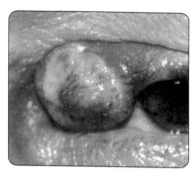

Fig 1.25

Treatment (see below).

Squamous cell carcinoma (SCC)

Introduction: SCC is much less common than BCC but is more aggressive, with metastasis to lymph nodes in about 20%.
- *Origin:* (a) *de novo,* (b) in pre-existing actinic keratosis, or (c) from carcinoma *in situ* (Bowen disease).
- *Risk factors:* (a) increasing age, (b) fair skin, (c) chronic sun exposure, and (d) immunosuppression (e.g. HIV, post-transplantation).

Diagnosis
- *Signs:* (a) nodular (*Fig. 1.25*), (b) noduloulcerative (*Fig. 1.26*), and (c) associated with a cutaneous horn (*Fig. 1.27*); it has a predilection for the lower eyelid and the lid margin.
- *Differentiation from BCC:* hyperkeratosis is frequent, telangiectasis is less common, and growth is usually more rapid.

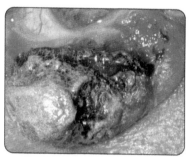

Fig 1.26

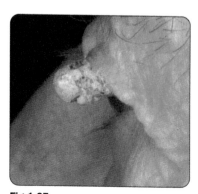

Fig 1.27

Treatment (see below).

Keratoacanthoma

Definition: often regarded as a well-differentiated form of SCC; risk factors include chronic sun exposure and immunosuppression.

Diagnosis

- *Presentation:* fast-growing, pink, dome-shaped hyperkeratotic lesion (*Fig. 1.28*).
- *Course:* (a) development of a keratin-filled crater (*Fig. 1.29*), (b) no change in size for 2 or 3 months, then (c) slow involution.

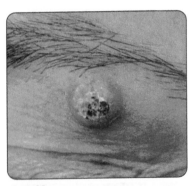

Fig 1.28

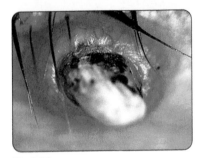

Fig 1.29

Treatment: excision biopsy, radiotherapy, or chemical cauterization.

Sebaceous gland carcinoma

Definition: rare, slow-growing but aggressive tumour that usually arises from the meibomian glands. It most commonly affects elderly females and has a mortality of 5–10%. In contrast to BCC and SCC, it occurs more commonly on the upper eyelid.

Diagnosis

- *Nodular:* beware mistaken diagnosis of chalazion (*Fig. 1.30*); biopsy should be performed on any atypical chalazion or suspicious persistent eyelid thickening, particularly in an older patient.

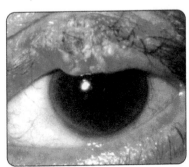

Fig 1.30

- *Spreading:* diffuse thickening of the lid margin (*Fig. 1.31*), which can be mistaken for chronic blepharitis.
- *Pagetoid spread:* extension of the tumour within the epithelium including the conjunctiva (*Fig. 1.32*), which may be mistaken for chronic inflammation.

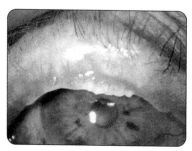

Fig 1.31

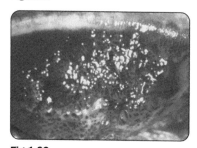

Fig 1.32

Treatment (see below).

Principles of surgical treatment

Biopsy

- *Incisional:* only part of the lesion is removed to allow histological diagnosis.
- *Excisional:* entire lesion is removed.

Excision

- *Shave excision:* for shallow epithelial tumours, such as papilloma and seborrhoeic keratosis.
- *Full-thickness skin excision:* most small BCCs can be excised with a 2 to 4 mm clearance margin.
- *Radical surgical excision:* for large BCCs and aggressive malignant tumours.

- *Mohs micrographic surgery:* allows maximal tumour detection and is particularly useful for lesions in which extension may not be clinically detectable such as sclerosing BCC, and in difficult anatomical sites such as the medial canthus.

Reconstruction

- *Skin defects:* closed directly or with a local flap or skin graft.
- *Small defects:* (less than one-third of lid) can be closed directly, with a lateral cantholysis if necessary (*Fig. 1.33*).
- *Moderate defects:* (up to half of lid) require a flap (e.g. Tenzel semicircular; *Fig. 1.34*).
- *Large defects:* (over half of lid) may require: (a) posterior lamellar

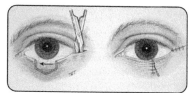

Fig 1.33

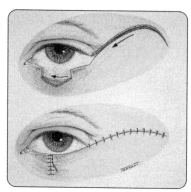

Fig 1.34

reconstruction using hard palate graft, buccal mucous membrane graft, or a Hughes flap, or (b) anterior lamellar reconstruction may involve skin advancement, a local skin flap, or a free skin graft.

- *Laissez-faire:* approximation of wound edges with residual defect left to heal spontaneously.

Disorders of eyelashes

Trichiasis

Definition: common acquired condition, which may occur in isolation or secondary to scarring of the lid margin.

Diagnosis

- *Presentation:* foreign body sensation worse on blinking; sometimes asymptomatic, particularly in long-standing cases.
- *Signs:* lashes are posteriorly misdirected but arise from normal sites; corresponding punctate corneal epithelial erosions are common.
- *Complications:* corneal ulceration and pannus, in severe cases (*Fig. 1.35*).

Treatment

- *Epilation:* with forceps for temporary control.
- *Ablation:* (a) argon laser for sparse lashes, (b) electrolysis (may cause scarring), or (c) cryotherapy for profuse lashes.
- *Surgery:* full-thickness wedge resection or anterior lamellar rotation in resistant cases.

Congenital distichiasis

Definition: very rare disorder which may be autosomal dominant (AD), and is frequently associated with lymphoedema of the legs (lymphoedema–distichiasis syndrome).

Diagnosis: partial or complete second row of lashes emerge at or behind the meibomian gland orifices (*Fig. 1.36*); usually well tolerated during infancy.

Treatment: cryotherapy for lower lid distichiasis, or lamellar lid splitting with cryotherapy to the posterior lamella for upper lid involvement.

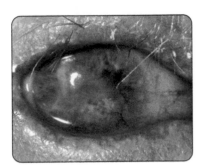

Fig 1.35

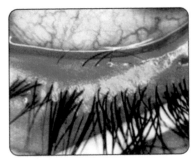

Fig 1.36

Acquired distichiasis (metaplastic lashes)

Pathogenesis: metaplasia and dedifferentiation of the meibomian glands to become hair follicles; typically associated with cicatrizing conjunctivitis (e.g. chemical injury, Stevens–Johnson syndrome, ocular cicatricial pemphigoid; see Chapter 5).

Diagnosis: nonpigmented, often stunted, lashes originating from meibomian gland orifices (*Fig. 1.37*).

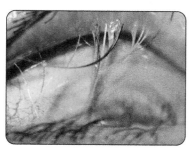

Fig 1.37

Treatment: mild cases as for trichiasis; severe cases require lamellar lid splitting and cryotherapy to the posterior lamella.

Eyelash ptosis

- *Definition:* downward sagging of upper lashes (*Fig. 1.38*).
- *Causes:* (a) involutional changes, (b) long-standing facial palsy, and (c) floppy eyelid syndrome (see below).

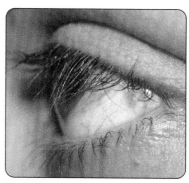

Fig 1.38

Trichomegaly

- *Definition:* excessive eyelash growth (*Fig. 1.39*).
- *Acquired causes:* (a) drug-induced (topical prostaglandin analogues, phenytoin, ciclosporin), (b) malnutrition, (c) AIDS, (d) porphyria, (e) hypothyroidism, and (f) familial.
- *Associated congenital syndromes:* (a) Oliver–McFarlane (pigmentary retinopathy, dwarfism, mental handicap), (b) Cornelia de Lange (mental and physical developmental abnormalities), (c) Goldstein–Hutt (cataract, hereditary spherocytosis), and (d) Hermansky–Pudlak (albinism, bleeding diathesis).

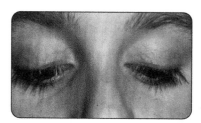

Fig 1.39

Madarosis

- **Definition:** absence or decreased number of lashes (*Fig. 1.40*).
- **Local causes:** (a) infiltrating lid tumours, (b) burns, and (c) iatrogenic following radiotherapy or cryotherapy to the lids.
- **Associated skin disorders:** (a) generalized alopecia, (b) psoriasis, and (c) atopic dermatitis.
- **Associated systemic diseases:** (a) myxoedema, (b) systemic lupus erythematosus, (c) acquired syphilis, and (d) lepromatous leprosy.
- **Following lash removal:** (a) iatrogenic for trichiasis and (b) trichotillomania (psychiatric disorder of hair removal).

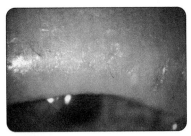

Fig 1.40

Poliosis

- **Definition:** premature localized whitening of hair, which may involve the lashes and eyebrows (*Fig. 1.41*).
- **Ocular causes:** (a) chronic anterior blepharitis, (b) sympathetic ophthalmitis, and (c) idiopathic uveitis.
- **Systemic associations:** (a) Vogt–Koyanagi–Harada syndrome, (b) Waardenburg syndrome, (c) vitiligo, (d) Marfan syndrome, and (e) tuberous sclerosis.

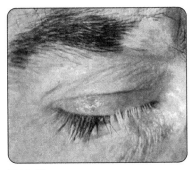

Fig 1.41

Allergic disorders

Acute allergic oedema

Pathogenesis: pollens that typically affect children during the spring/summer months.

Diagnosis: sudden onset of profuse bilateral periorbital oedema (*Fig. 1.42*), often accompanied by prominent jelly-like conjunctival swelling (chemosis).

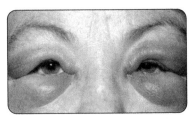

Fig 1.42

Treatment: usually unnecessary as spontaneous resolution occurs within a few hours, once exposure to the allergen is discontinued.

Contact dermatitis

Pathogenesis: inflammatory response following exposure to a causative substance, usually a medication or contained preservative, a cosmetic preparation, or a metal; type IV delayed hypersensitivity response with initial sensitizing exposure and reaction to subsequent exposure.

Diagnosis

- *Presentation:* itching and tearing.
- *Signs:* (a) eyelids show oedema, scaling, angular fissuring, and tightness (*Fig. 1.43*), (b) chemosis and papillary conjunctivitis, and (c) mild punctate corneal epithelial erosions.

Atopic dermatitis (eczema)

Definition: common idiopathic condition, typically associated with asthma and hay fever; eyelid involvement is infrequent.

Diagnosis

- *Presentation:* itching and irritability of eyelid skin.
- *Signs:* (a) eyelids show erythema, thickening, crusting, and fissuring, (b) staphylococcal blepharitis, (c) madarosis (*Fig. 1.44*), (d) keratinization of the lid margin, and (e) tightening of facial skin and lower lid ectropion.

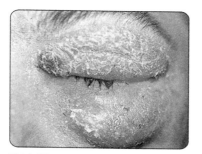

Fig 1.43

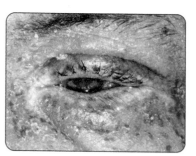

Fig 1.44

Treatment

- Avoidance of exposure to antigen, if identified.
- Change to preservative-free drops, if sensitivity to preservative is suspected.
- Topical steroids are rarely required.
- Oral antihistamines for severe cases.

Ocular associations

- *Common:* vernal disease in children and chronic atopic keratoconjunctivitis in adults.
- *Uncommon:* (a) keratoconus, (b) presenile cataract, and (c) retinal detachment.

Treatment: emollients and mild topical steroids (e.g. hydrocortisone 1% skin cream).

Viral infections

Molluscum contagiosum

Pathogenesis: skin infection typically affecting healthy children (peak 2–4 years) or immunocompromised individuals; transmission is by contact and subsequent autoinoculation.

Diagnosis
- (a) Single or multiple pale, waxy, umbilicated nodules (*Fig. 1.45*); (b) cheesy material can be expressed from the lesions, and (c) ipsilateral chronic follicular conjunctivitis may be present.
- The lid margins should be examined carefully in any patient with chronic conjunctivitis because a causative molluscum lesion may be overlooked (*Fig. 1.46*).

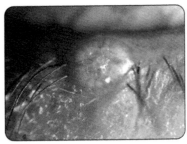

Fig 1.46

Treatment
- Spontaneous resolution is the rule in the immunocompetent, although autoinoculation may cause recurrences.
- Lid margin lesions with secondary conjunctivitis should be treated with (a) shave excision, (b) cauterization, (c) cryotherapy, or (d) laser.

Herpes zoster ophthalmicus

Pathogenesis: shingles affecting the first division of the trigeminal nerve. It is caused by varicella zoster virus (VZV) and typically affects the elderly; tends to be more severe in immunocompromised individuals.

Diagnosis
- *Presentation:* 3- to 5-day prodromal phase of tiredness, fever, malaise, and headache precedes the appearance of the rash; there may be pain in the affected dermatome.
- *Signs:* (a) erythematous maculopapular rash on the forehead, respecting the midline; (b) appearance of groups of vesicles (*Fig. 1.47*) within 24 h,

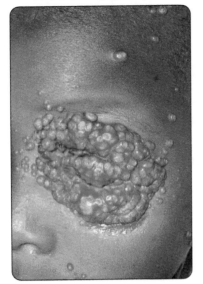

Fig 1.45

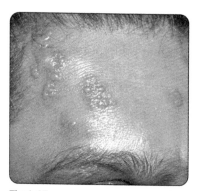

Fig 1.47

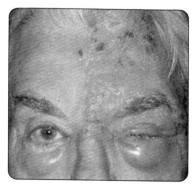

Fig 1.49

(c) confluent vesicles, which may become pustular before crusting (*Fig. 1.48*) and drying after 2–3 weeks; (d) periorbital oedema that may spread to the other side (*Fig. 1.49*); (e) depigmented scars may follow healing.
- *Ocular complications* (see Chapter 6).

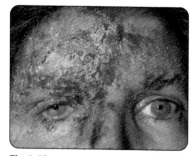

Fig 1.48

Treatment
- *Systemic antivirals:* (a) oral aciclovir 800 mg five times daily for 7–10 days, ideally commenced within 72 h of onset of symptoms may reduce the risk and severity of late complications, (b) alternatives (often better tolerated and may be more effective) include famciclovir, valaciclovir and brivudine, and (c) intravenous aciclovir may be required for severe complications (e.g. encephalitis).
- *Topical:* (a) skin should be kept clean to avoid secondary bacterial infection, and (b) an antibiotic (e.g. erythromycin) or steroid–antibiotic combination (e.g. Fucidin-H 1% and fusidic acid 2%).
- *Patients can transmit chickenpox:* avoid contact with the non-immune, pregnant, and immunodeficient individuals until crusting is complete.
- *Vaccination:* against VZV reduces the incidence of shingles.

Herpes simplex

Pathogenesis: primary infection, or rarely reactivation, of herpes simplex virus previously dormant in the trigeminal ganglion.

Diagnosis
- *Prodromal phase:* facial and lid tingling (24 h).
- *Signs:* (a) eyelid and periorbital vesicles (*Fig. 1.50*) which break down over 48 h, (b) boggy lid swelling, and (c) gradual resolution over a week.
- *Other ocular features:* papillary conjunctivitis and dendritic corneal ulceration.

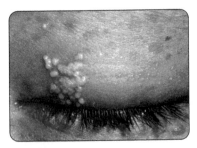

Fig 1.50

Treatment
- *Topical antiviral:* (aciclovir cream) 5 times daily for 5 days.
- *Oral antiviral:* aciclovir 400–800 mg 5 times daily for 3–5 days; famciclovir and valaciclovir are alternatives.
- *Oral antibiotic:* co-amoxiclav or erythromycin for secondary staphylococcal infection in patients with eczema herpeticum.

Chronic blepharitis

Chronic marginal blepharitis

Pathogenesis
- *Anterior blepharitis:* may be staphylococcal (partly immune-mediated) and/or seborrhoeic (often associated with seborrhoeic dermatitis).
- *Posterior blepharitis:* associated with meibomian gland dysfunction with alterations in meibomian gland secretions (often associated with acne rosacea).

Diagnosis
- *Presentation:* burning, grittiness, mild photophobia, and crusting and redness of the lid margins, usually worse in the mornings.
- *Staphylococcal blepharitis:* (a) scales and crusting around the base of lashes (collarettes; *Fig. 1.51*), (b) mild papillary conjunctivitis and chronic conjunctival hyperaemia, (c) long-standing cases may develop scarring and notching (tylosis) of the lid margin, as well as madarosis, trichiasis, and poliosis, and (d) secondary changes including styes, marginal

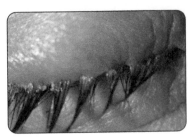

Fig 1.51

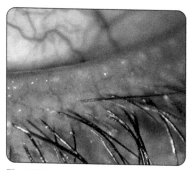

Fig 1.52

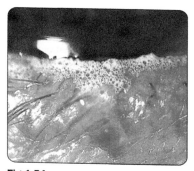

Fig 1.54

keratitis, and occasionally phlyctenulosis.

- *Seborrhoeic blepharitis:* (a) hyperaemic and greasy anterior lid margins (*Fig. 1.52*), and (b) adherence of lashes to each other.
- *Posterior blepharitis:* (a) meibomian gland orifices show pouting, recession, or plugging (*Fig. 1.53*), (b) hyperaemia and telangiectasis of the posterior lid margin, (c) oily and foamy tear film (*Fig. 1.54*), and (d) secondary changes including papillary

conjunctivitis and inferior corneal punctate epithelial erosions.

- *Associations:* tear film instability and dry eye syndrome.

Treatment

- *Lid hygiene:* (a) warm compresses to soften crusts, (b) lid cleaning to remove crusts mechanically and (c) massaging the lid to express accumulated meibum may be useful in posterior blepharitis.
- *Tear substitutes:* for associated tear dysfunction.
- *Topical antibiotics:* fusidic acid, bacitracin, or chloramphenicol ointment can be applied to the lid margin to treat acute folliculitis but are of limited value in long-standing cases.
- *Oral antibiotics:* (a) azithromycin (500 mg daily for 3 days) to control acute exacerbations in staphylococcal blepharitis, (b) oral tetracyclines are often highly effective (but should not be used in children younger than the age of 12 years, or in pregnant or breast feeding women): oxytetracycline 250 mg twice daily for 6–12 weeks or doxycycline

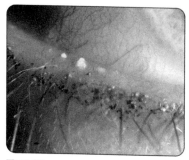

Fig 1.53

100 mg twice daily for 1 week and then daily for 6–12 weeks; (c) erythromycin 250 mg once or twice daily is an alternative to tetracycline.

- **Weak topical steroid:** fluorometholone 0.1% three or four times daily for 1 week in patients with severe papillary conjunctivitis or marginal keratitis.

Phthiriasis palpebrarum

Pathogenesis: the crab louse *Phthirus pubis* is principally adapted to living in pubic hair but can also infest the chest, axillae, or eyelids. Eyelash infestation, phthiriasis palpebrarum, typically affects children living in conditions of poor hygiene.

Diagnosis

- **Presentation:** chronic irritation and itching of the lids.
- **Signs:** (a) lice anchored to the lashes (*Fig. 1.55*), and (b) ova and empty shells appear as brownish, opalescent pearls adherent to the base of the cilia.

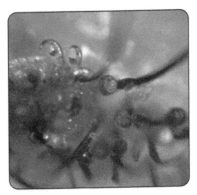

Fig 1.55

Treatment: mechanical removal of the lice with forceps, and topical yellow mercuric oxide 1% or petroleum jelly applied to the lashes and lids twice a day for 10 days.

Ptosis

Introduction

Definition: congenital or acquired abnormally low position of the upper eyelid.

Classification

- **Neurogenic:** innervational defect (e.g. 3rd nerve paresis, Horner syndrome; see Chapter 19).
- **Myogenic:** (a) myopathic (e.g. myotonic dystrophy), and (b) neuromyopathic (e.g. myasthenia gravis).
- **Aponeurotic:** defect in the levator aponeurosis, commonly involutional.
- **Mechanical:** (a) gravitational effect (e.g. tumour), or (b) contracted scar tissue.

Table 1.2 Causes of pseudoptosis

- Lack of support of the lids by the globe (e.g. phthisis bulbi, enophthalmos)
- Contralateral lid retraction
- Ipsilateral hypotropia
- Brow ptosis
- Dermatochalasis

Measurements

- Margin-corneal light reflex distance (*Fig. 1.56*): normal 4–4.5 mm.
- Palpebral fissure height (*Fig. 1.57*): normal in males is 7–10 mm and in females 8–12 mm.

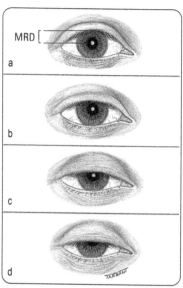

Fig 1.56

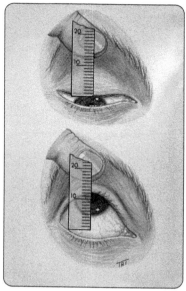

Fig 1.58

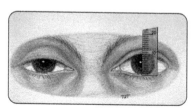

Fig 1.57

- Levator function (*Fig. 1.58*):
  normal > 15 mm.
- Upper lid crease: normal in males
  is 8 mm and in females 10 mm.

Simple congenital ptosis

Pathogenesis: developmental failure of
neuronal migration. Ptosis may be
associated with amblyopia due to
occlusion of the visual axis or from
coexisting refractive errors.

Diagnosis

- Unilateral or bilateral ptosis of
  variable severity with absent or
  diminished upper lid crease
  (*Fig. 1.59a*).

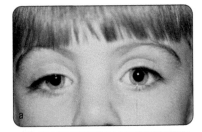

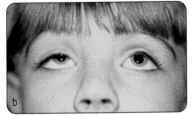

Fig 1.59

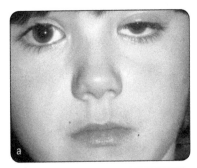

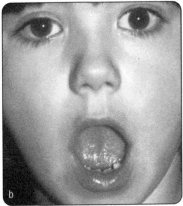

Fig 1.60

- Poor levator function (*Fig. 1.59b*).
- In downgaze the ptotic lid is higher than the normal because of poor relaxation of the levator muscle (contrast with acquired ptosis).
- Compensatory chin elevation in bilateral cases.
- 5% show Marcus Gunn jaw-winking phenomenon: retraction of the ptotic lid with stimulation of the ipsilateral pterygoid (e.g. chewing or opening the mouth; *Fig. 1.60*).

Treatment: levator resection (*Fig. 1.61*) during preschool years.

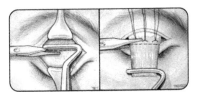

Fig 1.61

Involutional ptosis

Pathogenesis: age-related dysfunction of the levator aponeurosis.

Diagnosis: (a) typically bilateral and often asymmetrical ptosis, (b) high or absent upper lid crease with deep sulcus (*Fig. 1.62*), and (c) good levator function.

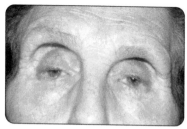

Fig 1.62

Treatment: levator advancement or resection.

Ectropion

Involutional ectropion

Diagnosis: (a) epiphora and (b) lower lid ectropion; (c) exposed tarsal conjunctiva may become thickened and keratinized (*Fig. 1.63*) in long-standing cases.

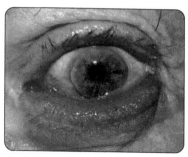

Fig 1.63

Treatment

- *Generalized ectropion:* horizontal lid shortening (lateral canthal sling or full-thickness wedge excision; *Fig. 1.64*).
- *Medial ectropion:* medial tarsoconjunctival diamond excision.

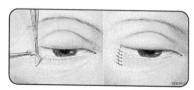

Fig 1.64

Cicatricial ectropion

Pathogenesis: contracture that pulls the lid away from the globe; causes include (a) trauma (*Fig. 1.65*), (b) chronic dermatitis, and (c) ichthyosis.

Diagnosis: (a) ectropion may be relieved by pushing the skin up over the orbital margin, and (b) opening the mouth may accentuate the ectropion.

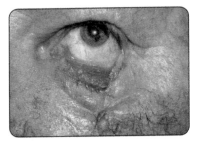

Fig 1.65

Treatment: scar tissue excision with lengthening procedure (e.g. Z-plasty; *Fig. 1.66*) in mild cases, and transposition flap or free skin graft in severe cases.

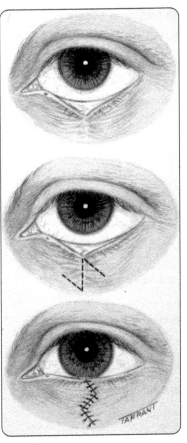

Fig 1.66

Paralytic ectropion

Pathogenesis: facial nerve palsy (e.g. Bell palsy, surgery for acoustic/parotid tumour; *Fig. 1.67*).

Diagnosis
- *Epiphora:* caused by a combination of punctual malposition, lacrimal pump failure,

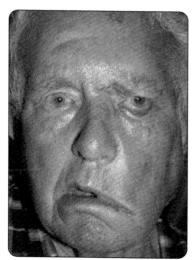

Fig 1.67

and increased tear production due to corneal exposure.

- *Associated features:* (a) retraction of upper and lower lids, (b) brow ptosis, and (c) exposure keratopathy.

Treatment

- *Temporizing measures:* (a) lubrication, (b) overnight lid taping, (c) botulinum toxin-induced ptosis, and (d) tarsorrhaphy (*Fig. 1.68*).
- *Definitive measures:* (a) medial canthoplasty, (b) lateral canthal sling, and (c) upper eyelid gold weight implantation.

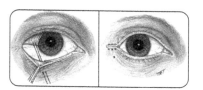

Fig 1.68

Entropion

Involutional entropion

Pathogenesis: the following age-related changes: (a) tissue laxity with stretching of the canthal tendons and tarsal plate, (b) dysfunction of the lower lid retractors, (c) overriding of the pretarsal orbicularis muscle by the preseptal component (*Fig. 1.69*), and (d) orbital septum laxity with prolapse of orbital fat into the lower lid.

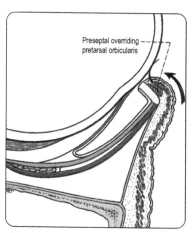

Preseptal overriding pretarsal orbicularis

Fig 1.69

Diagnosis: (a) grittiness from pseudotrichiasis and (b) intermittent or constant turning in of the lower lid (*Fig. 1.70*).

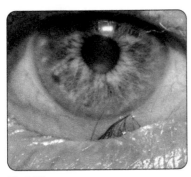

Fig 1.70

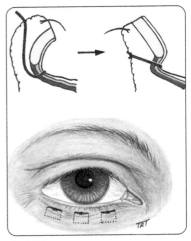

Fig 1.71

Treatment

- *Temporary:* (a) lubrication, (b) lid taping, (c) bandage contact lens, and (d) botulinum toxin orbicularis chemodenervation.
- *Transverse everting sutures (Fig. 1.71):* usually last several months.
- *For horizontal laxity:* lateral canthal sling or full-thickness wedge excision.
- *For overriding and disinsertion:* (a) Wies procedure (full-thickness horizontal lid splitting with insertion of everting sutures; *Fig. 1.72*), or (b) Jones procedure to tighten the lower lid retractors (*Fig. 1.73*).

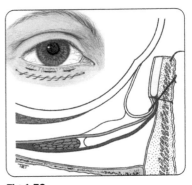

Fig 1.72

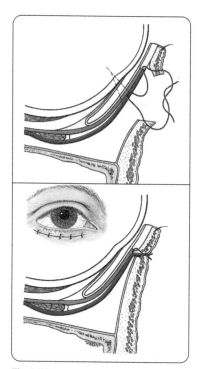

Fig 1.73

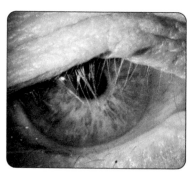

Fig 1.74

Treatment: (a) corneal protection (e.g. bandage contact lens), (b) transverse tarsotomy with anterior lid margin rotation for mild cases, and (c) tissue replacement with grafting for severe cases.

Miscellaneous acquired disorders

Blepharochalasis

Diagnosis

- *Presentation:* around puberty with episodic painless oedema of the upper lids lasting a few days, becoming less frequent over time.
- *Signs:* redundant wrinkled atrophic lid skin, with aponeurotic ptosis in severe cases (*Fig. 1.75*).
- *Differential diagnosis:* drug-induced urticaria, and angioedema.

Cicatricial entropion

Pathogenesis: scarring of the palpebral conjunctiva pulls the lid margin toward the globe (*Fig. 1.74*); causes include cicatrizing conjunctivitis (see Chapter 5) and trauma.

Diagnosis: in contrast to involutional entropion, both upper or lower lids may be affected; symptoms and findings may relate to the cause as well as the entropion itself.

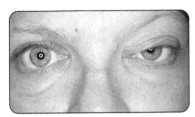

Fig 1.75

Treatment: blepharoplasty and correction of ptosis.

Floppy eyelid syndrome

Diagnosis
- *Presentation:* typically in an obese middle-aged man with chronic ocular irritation, usually worse on awaking.
- *Signs:* lax, rubbery, easily everted upper lids (*Fig. 1.76*).
- *Associated features:*
  (a) conjunctival hyperaemia and palpebral papillae, especially superior, caused by contact with the pillow during sleep,
  (b) punctate epithelial keratopathy,
  (c) filamentary keratitis, and
  (d) superior corneal vascularization in long-standing cases.

Treatment: lubrication, nocturnal eye shields or lid taping in mild cases; horizontal upper lid shortening in severe cases.

Cosmetic eyelid and periocular surgery

Nonsurgical cosmetic techniques

Table 1.3 Involutional changes
• Loose, wrinkled eyelid and periocular skin (*Fig. 1.77*)
• Orbital fat prolapse due to orbital septal weakness (*Fig. 1.78*)
• Generalized eyelid laxity with involutional ptosis, entropion and ectropion
• Enophthalmos due to orbital fat atrophy
• Brow ptosis

- *Periocular botulinum toxin injection:* for (a) lateral canthal 'crow's feet,' (b) glabellar frown lines, and (c) brow lift by depressor inhibition; complications include temporary lagophthalmos, ptosis, ectropion, and diplopia.

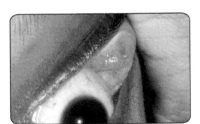

Fig 1.76

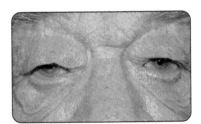

Fig 1.77

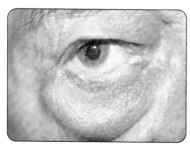

Fig 1.78

- *Hyaluronic acid tissue fillers:* to replace lost volume; generally last 6–12 months.
- *Fat transfer:* longer lasting, with 50–60% tissue survival.
- *Skin resurfacing:* removal of superficial skin layers by chemical peeling or laser to reduce wrinkling and remove blemishes.

Surgical cosmetic techniques

- *Upper eyelid blepharoplasty:* excess skin removal can be combined with reduction of superior orbital fat.
- *Lower eyelid blepharoplasty:* can be combined with reduction of the inferior orbital fat pads; complications include lower eyelid retraction, and contour abnormalities including ectropion.
- *Brow ptosis correction:* (a) direct, in which an incision is made above the eyebrows and an ellipse of skin removed, and (b) endoscopic via small incisions within the hairline.

Congenital malformations

Epicanthus

Definition: common bilateral condition in which vertical skin folds extend from the upper or lower lids toward the medial canthi; there are four main types (see below).

Diagnosis

- *Palpebralis:* folds are equally prominent between the upper and lower lids; most common type in Caucasians (*Fig. 1.79*).

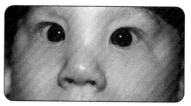

Fig 1.79

- *Tarsalis:* folds are most prominent superiorly; common in Orientals.
- *Inversus:* folds begin inferiorly and extend upwards to the medial canthal area; occurs in blepharophimosis syndrome (see below).
- *Superciliaris:* folds arise above the brow and extend downwards toward the lateral aspect of the nose.

Treatment: Y–V plasty for small folds; Mustardé Z-plasty if large.

Telecanthus

Definition: abnormally long medial canthal tendons; may occur in isolation or in association with blepharophimosis syndrome (see below), and other systemic syndromes.

Diagnosis: increased distance between the medial canthi (*Fig. 1.80*); should not be confused with hypertelorism (wide separation of the orbits).

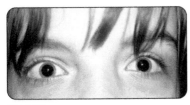

Fig 1.80

Treatment: shortening and refixation of the medial canthal tendons.

Blepharophimosis, ptosis and epicanthus inversus syndrome

Genetics: AD (FOXL2 gene); associated with premature ovarian failure in some patients.

Diagnosis: (a) symmetrical ptosis with poor levator function, (b) telecanthus and epicanthus inversus (*Fig. 1.81*),

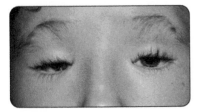

Fig 1.81

and (c) poorly developed nasal bridge with hypoplasia of the superior orbital rims; (d) amblyopia is common.

Treatment: initial correction of epicanthus and telecanthus; subsequent bilateral frontalis suspension.

Epiblepharon

Definition: excess lower lid tissue rotating the lower lid inwards; very common in Orientals and usually resolves spontaneously. Epiblepharon should not be confused with congenital entropion, which is much less common.

Diagnosis: (a) horizontal fold of skin stretched across the anterior lid margin, and (b) vertical direction of lashes, especially medially (*Fig. 1.82*).

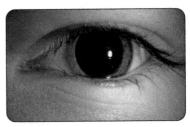

Fig 1.82

Treatment: excision of a strip of skin and muscle in persistent cases.

Coloboma

Associations: (a) upper lid coloboma is occasionally associated with Goldenhar syndrome; (b) lower lid coloboma is frequently associated

with systemic conditions, most
notably Treacher Collins syndrome
(see *Fig. 1.84*).

Diagnosis

- *Upper lid coloboma:* defect at the
  junction of middle and inner third
  of lid (*Fig. 1.83*).
- *Lower lid coloboma:* defect at the
  junction of middle and outer third
  (*Fig. 1.84*).

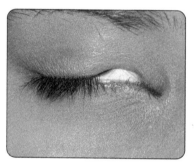

Fig 1.83

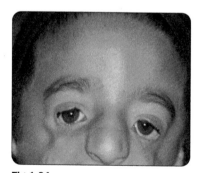

Fig 1.84

Treatment: primary closure of small
defects; skin flaps/grafts if large.

Cryptophthalmos

Pathogenesis: failure of neural crest
migration; may be associated with
Fraser syndrome.

Diagnosis

- *Complete:* lids are replaced by a
  layer of skin fused with a
  microphthalmic eye (*Fig. 1.85*).
- *Incomplete:* (a) microphthalmos,
  (b) rudimentary lids, and (c) a
  small conjunctival sac
  (*Fig. 1.86*).

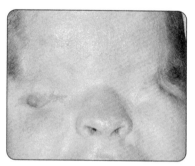

Fig 1.85

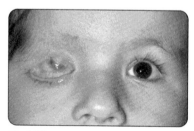

Fig 1.86

Chapter 2

Lacrimal drainage system

Acquired obstruction

Primary punctal stenosis

Causes: (a) idiopathic, (b) chronic marginal blepharitis, (c) herpetic (simplex, zoster) lid infection, and (d) conjunctival cicatrization.

Diagnosis: narrow inferior punctum in the absence of punctal malposition.

Treatment: dilatation alone (*Fig. 2.1*) rarely confers long-term improvement; surgical punctoplasty is usually necessary (*Figs. 2.2* and *2.3*).

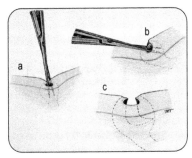

Fig 2.2

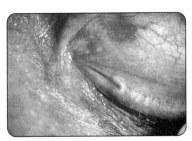

Fig 2.3

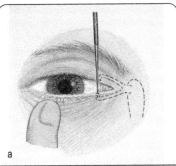

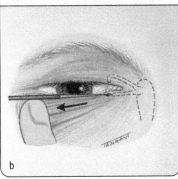

Fig 2.1

Secondary punctal stenosis

Diagnosis: narrow inferior punctum associated with punctal eversion (*Fig. 2.4*).

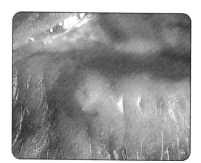

Fig 2.4

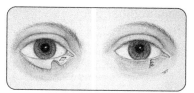

Fig 2.6

Treatment

- *Retropunctal cautery:* for pure punctal eversion.
- *Medial conjunctivoplasty:* for medial ectropion without lid laxity (*Fig. 2.5*).
- *Wider lid positional abnormalities:* addressed as appropriate (*Fig. 2.6*).

Canalicular obstruction

Causes: (a) congenital and (b) acquired (e.g. trauma, herpes simplex infection, drugs, irradiation, chronic dacryocystitis).

Diagnosis: site of obstruction will usually be evident on lacrimal irrigation as a 'soft stop' (*Fig. 2.7a*).

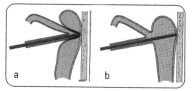

Fig 2.7

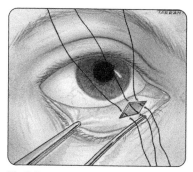

Fig 2.5

Treatment

- *Intubation:* silicone stents for partial obstruction.
- *Canaliculodacryocystorhinostomy* (**CDCR**): for total individual canalicular obstruction when there is 6–8 mm of patent normal canaliculus between the punctum and the obstruction.
- *Lester Jones tube insertion:* when it is not possible to anastomose the functional canaliculus to the sac (see below).

Nasolacrimal duct obstruction

Causes: (a) idiopathic age-related stenosis (most common), (b) trauma, (c) Wegener granulomatosis, and (d) nasopharyngeal tumours.

Diagnosis
- *Lacrimal irrigation:* 'hard stop' (*Fig. 2.7b*), without passage of irrigated fluid (complete obstruction), or sparse passage of fluid (partial obstruction).
- *Other investigations:* digital subtraction dacryocystography and nuclear lacrimal scintigraphy (*Fig. 2.8*).

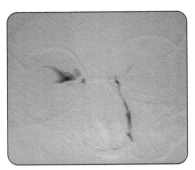

Fig 2.8

Treatment
- *Dacryocystorhinostomy (DCR):* (see below).
- *Other procedures:* stent insertion or balloon dilatation, usually in partial obstruction.

Dacryolithiasis

Pathogenesis: inflammatory obstruction with tear stagnation and lacrimal epithelial metaplasia.

Diagnosis: (a) intermittent epiphora and recurrent dacryocystitis usually in late adulthood, and (b) distended and firm lacrimal sac that may form a mucocele.

Treatment: DCR.

Congenital obstruction

Nasolacrimal duct obstruction

Pathogenesis: delayed canalization of the lower end of the nasolacrimal duct, affecting at least 20% of neonates.

Diagnosis
- *Presentation:* constant or intermittent epiphora, stickiness (*Fig. 2.9*), and sometimes frank bacterial conjunctivitis.
- *Signs:* reflux of purulent material from the puncta on pressure over the lacrimal sac.
- *Differential diagnosis:* should be considered congenital glaucoma in an infant with a watering eye.

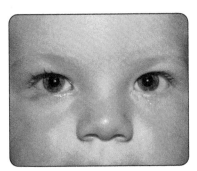

Fig 2.9

Treatment

- **Conservative:** spontaneous resolution occurs in approximately 95% of cases within 12 months.
- **Massage of the lacrimal sac** (*Fig. 2.10*): may rupture the membranous obstruction.
- **Probing** (*Fig. 2.11*): considered after 12–18 months (90% cure).

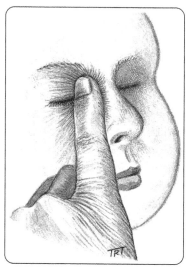

Fig 2.10

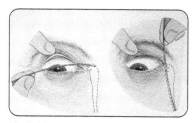

Fig 2.11

Congenital dacryocele (amniontocele)

Pathogenesis: collection of amniotic fluid or mucus in the lacrimal sac caused by an imperforate Hasner valve.

Diagnosis

- **Presentation:** perinatal epiphora and a bluish cystic swelling at or below the medial canthus (*Fig. 2.12*).
- **Differential diagnosis:** encephalocele, characterized by a pulsatile swelling above the medial canthal tendon.

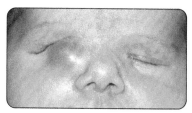

Fig 2.12

Treatment: probing in persistent cases.

Principles of adult lacrimal surgery

- **Conventional (open) DCR:** for obstruction beyond the medial opening of the common canaliculus. The skin is incised over the lacrimal sac, which is then anastomosed to the nasal mucosa (*Fig. 2.13*); success rate is approximately 90%.
- **Endoscopic approach (± laser):** has a lower success rate than open DCR.
- **Intubation (silicone stents):** option for partial obstruction.

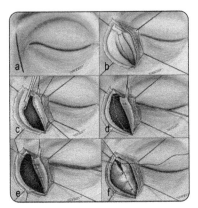

Fig 2.13

- *CDCR:* for total individual canalicular obstruction.
- *Lester Jones tube insertion (Fig. 2.14):* to bypass extensive canalicular obstruction.

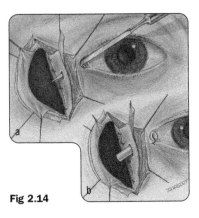

Fig 2.14

Infections

Chronic canaliculitis

Pathogenesis: infection with *Actinomyces israelii* without any identifiable predisposition.

Diagnosis
- *Presentation:* unilateral epiphora with refractory chronic mucopurulent conjunctivitis.
- *Signs:* (a) 'pouting' punctum with pericanalicular oedema (*Fig. 2.15*), (b) mucopurulent discharge (*Fig. 2.16*), and (c) concretions (*Fig. 2.17*) may appear on pressure over the canaliculus.

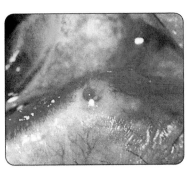

Fig 2.15

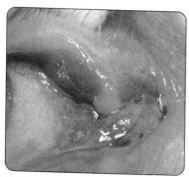

Fig 2.16

- *Differential diagnosis:* (a) herpes simplex infection (acute canaliculitis), (b) mucocele, (c) dacryolithiasis, (d) lacrimal diverticulum, and (e) giant fornix syndrome.

Treatment
- *Topical antibiotics:* (e.g. levofloxacin) may be tried.
- *Transconjunctival canaliculotomy with curettage:* necessary in most cases.

Dacryocystitis

Pathogenesis: secondary to nasolacrimal duct obstruction; may be acute or chronic.

Diagnosis
- *Acute:* (a) subacute onset of medial canthal pain and epiphora, and (b) tender tense red swelling (*Fig. 2.18*) that may progress to abscess formation and cellulitis.
- *Chronic:* (a) epiphora and chronic/recurrent unilateral conjunctivitis, and (b) reflux of mucopurulent material on pressure over medial canthus, with (*Fig. 2.19*) or without a mucocele.

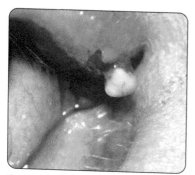

Fig 2.17

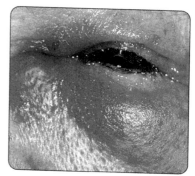

Fig 2.18

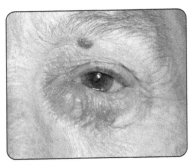

Fig 2.19

Treatment

- *Acute:* oral antibiotics (e.g. co-amoxiclav or erythromycin); incision and drainage may be considered for a pointing abscess (small risk of subsequent fistula); DCR considered once infection has settled.
- *Chronic:* DCR.

Orbit

Thyroid eye disease

Pathogenesis: organ-specific
autoimmune reaction in which
a humoral agent (IgG antibody)
produces inflammation and swelling
of orbital tissue, especially
extraocular muscles. It consists of
an active inflammatory stage (<3
years) followed by a quiescent/
fibrotic stage.

Diagnosis

- *Lid retraction:* (a) superior lid
  margin is either level with or
  above the superior limbus, with
  'scleral show' (*Fig. 3.1*), (b) Von
  Graefe sign ('lid lag') describes
  retarded descent of the upper lid
  on downgaze, and (c) inferior lid
  retraction.
- *Ocular surface involvement:*
  (a) grittiness, photophobia,
  lacrimation, and retrobulbar
  discomfort, (b) conjunctival
  hyperaemia, (c) chemosis and lid
  swelling (*Fig. 3.2*), and (d) superior
  limbic keratoconjunctivitis (SLK;
  see Chapter 5).
- *Axial proptosis:* if severe, along
  with lid retraction (*Fig. 3.3*) may
  compromise lid closure resulting
  in exposure keratopathy.

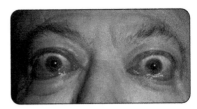

Fig 3.2

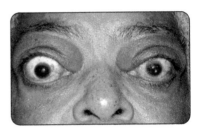

Fig 3.3

- *Restrictive myopathy:* motility
  defects in order of frequency are
  (a) elevation (*Fig. 3.4*), abduction,
  depression, and adduction;
  (b) intraocular pressure increase
  in upgaze (Braley sign).
- *Optic neuropathy:* compression
  of the optic nerve by enlarged
  muscles (*Fig. 3.5*); optic disc
  often appears normal.

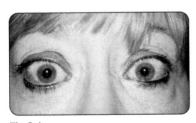

Fig 3.1

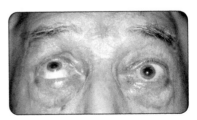

Fig 3.4

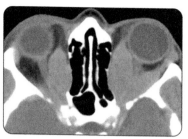

Fig 3.5

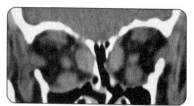

Fig 3.6

Treatment

- *Lid retraction:* (a) lid taping during sleep, (b) surgery (disinsertion of Müller muscle, levator recession, recession of the lower lid retractors) for stable retraction, but only after first addressing proptosis and strabismus, and (c) botulinum toxin chemodenervation for temporary effect.
- *Ocular surface involvement:* (a) lubricants, (b) topical anti-inflammatory agents (e.g. steroids, nonsteroidal anti-inflammatory drug [NSAIDs], ciclosporin), and (c) specific treatment of SLK.
- *Proptosis:* (a) systemic steroids (e.g. oral prednisolone, initially 60–80 mg with tapering on response) in acute sight-threatening cases, (b) radiotherapy (takes weeks–months for effect) in addition to steroids or when these are contraindicated, and (c) orbital decompression (*Fig. 3.6*) is sometimes used acutely, but more commonly is reserved for the quiescent phase.
- *Restrictive myopathy:* (a) initially prisms, (b) surgery (inferior and/or medial rectus recessions with adjustable sutures) for diplopia in the primary or reading positions of gaze once stable for at least 6 months, and (c) botulinum toxin injection.
- *Optic neuropathy:* (a) systemic steroids (oral prednisolone or intravenous methylprednisolone), and (b) surgical decompression if steroids are ineffective or inappropriate; vision, particularly colour, should be monitored carefully.

Infections

Preseptal cellulitis

Pathogenesis: infection of subcutaneous tissue anterior to the orbital septum. Causes include (a) skin trauma (*S. aureus, S. pyogenes*), and (b) spread from local or remote infection (e.g. stye, dacryocystitis, sinusitis).

Diagnosis

- *Presentation:* unilateral tender, red and swollen lid (*Fig. 3.7*).
- *Signs:* proptosis and chemosis are absent, and optic nerve function and ocular motility are unimpaired.
- *CT:* opacification anterior to the orbital septum (*Fig. 3.8*).

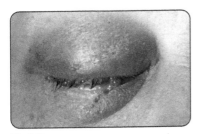

Fig 3.7

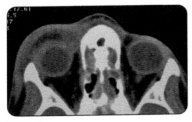

Fig 3.8

Treatment: oral antibiotics (e.g. co-amoxiclav) are usually adequate; severe infection/abscess may require intravenous administration.

Bacterial orbital cellulitis

Pathogenesis: life-threatening infection of the tissues behind the orbital septum, more common in children. Causes include; (a) secondary to sinusitis (most common), (b) spread from local or remote infection, (c) post-trauma, and (d) post-surgery; common isolates are *S. pneumoniae*, *S. aureus*, *S. pyogenes*, and *H. influenzae*.

Diagnosis

- *Presentation:* rapid onset of pain, visual impairment, malaise, and periocular swelling.
- *Signs:* (a) unilateral tender warm and red periorbital oedema,

(b) proptosis, (c) painful ophthalmoplegia (*Fig. 3.9*), and (d) optic nerve dysfunction.

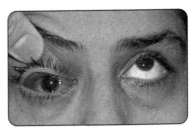

Fig 3.9

- *Ocular complications:* (a) exposure keratopathy, (b) optic atrophy, (c) retinal vascular occlusion, and (d) endophthalmitis.
- *Other serious complications:* (a) subperiosteal abscess, (b) meningitis, and (c) cavernous sinus thrombosis (bilateral rapidly progressive proptosis with abrupt general deterioration).
- *Investigations:* (a) CT of orbit (*Fig. 3.10*), sinuses, and brain, (b) white cell count, (c) blood culture, (d) nasal swab for culture, and (e) lumbar puncture if meningeal signs develop.

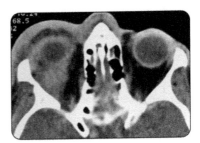

Fig 3.10

Treatment

- Hospital admission with otorhinolaryngological co-management.
- Urgent intravenous antibiotic therapy (e.g. cephalosporin or vancomycin, with metronidazole to cover anaerobes).
- Frequent ophthalmic review including optic nerve function.
- Surgical drainage of (a) infected sinuses and orbital collections if lack of response to antibiotics, or (b) subperiosteal/intracranial abscess.
- Orbital biopsy may be considered if atypical.

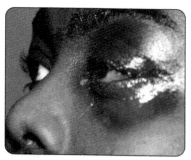

Fig 3.11

Non-infective inflammatory disease

Idiopathic orbital inflammatory disease (IOID)

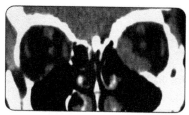

Fig 3.12

Pathogenesis: non-neoplastic and non-infective cellular infiltration that may involve any of the soft tissues of the orbit; previously referred to as 'orbital pseudotumour.'

Diagnosis

- *Presentation:* acute or subacute onset of periorbital redness, swelling (*Fig. 3.11*), and pain.
- *Signs:* (a) proptosis, (b) conjunctival hyperaemia and chemosis, (c) ophthalmoplegia, and (d) optic nerve dysfunction if the posterior orbit is involved.
- *CT:* ill-defined opacification (*Fig. 3.12*).
- *Course:* varies from spontaneous remission without sequelae to severe prolonged inflammation with fibrosis ('frozen orbit').

- *Differential diagnosis:* (a) bacterial orbital cellulitis, (b) acute thyroid eye disease, and (c) systemic inflammatory disorder (e.g. Wegener granulomatosis).

Treatment: observation for very mild disease; options in moderate-severe cases include NSAIDs, systemic steroids, radiotherapy, and antimetabolites.

Acute dacryoadenitis

Pathogenesis: usually idiopathic but occasionally infective (mumps, mononucleosis, rarely bacterial).

Diagnosis

- *Presentation:* acute discomfort with swelling of the lateral eyelid.
- *Signs:* (a) S-shaped ptosis and slight downward and inward

dystopia (*Fig. 3.13*), and (b) local tenderness, with conjunctival injection overlying the lacrimal gland (*Fig. 3.14*).

- *Imaging:* enlargement of the lacrimal gland.
- *Differential diagnosis:* ruptured dermoid cyst and malignant lacrimal gland tumour.

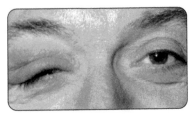

Fig 3.13

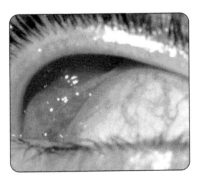

Fig 3.14

Treatment: spontaneous resolution is the rule; otherwise as for IOID.

Tolosa–Hunt syndrome

Definition: idiopathic condition characterized by granulomatous inflammation of the cavernous sinus, superior orbital fissure, and/or orbital apex.

Diagnosis
- *Presentation:* diplopia associated with unilateral periorbital or hemicranial pain.
- *Signs:* (a) proptosis is mild or absent, (b) ophthalmoplegia, often with pupillary involvement, and (c) sensory loss (first and second trigeminal divisions).
- *Course:* remissions and recurrences are common.

Treatment: systemic steroids.

Vascular abnormalities

Varices

Definition: weakened orbital venous segments, usually unilateral and involving the upper nasal orbit.

Diagnosis
- *Presentation:* from early childhood to late middle age.
- *Signs:* (a) intermittent nonpulsatile proptosis not associated with a bruit, precipitated by coughing, straining, or assuming a dependent position (*Fig. 3.15*),

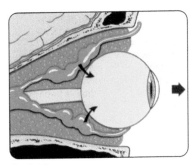

Fig 3.15

(b) often demonstrable with the Valsalva manoeuvre or jugular vein compression, and (c) coexisting varices of the eyelids (*Fig. 3.16*) and conjunctiva (*Fig. 3.17*) may be present.
- *Imaging:* may show phleboliths.
- *Complications:* acute haemorrhage and thrombosis, and orbital fat atrophy.

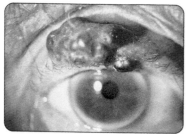

Fig 3.16

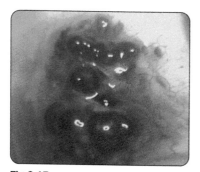

Fig 3.17

Treatment: indications include recurrent thrombosis, pain, severe proptosis and optic nerve compression; surgical excision is difficult as the lesions are friable.

Carotid–cavernous fistula

Introduction
- *Definition:* acquired communication between the carotid artery and the cavernous sinus resulting in increased episcleral venous pressure and decreased arterial blood flow. There are two types:
- *Direct fistula:* high-flow shunt with intracavernous carotid arterial blood passing directly into the sinus; trauma is responsible for 75%, spontaneous rupture of an aneurysm or atherosclerotic artery accounting for the remainder.
- *Indirect fistula:* low-flow shunt in which arterial blood flows indirectly into the cavernous sinus through the meningeal branches of the external or internal carotid arteries; frequently spontaneous or following straining.

Diagnosis of direct fistula
- *Presentation:* days or weeks after head injury with the classic triad of (a) pulsatile proptosis, (b) chemosis, and (c) whooshing noise in the head.
- *Signs:* (a) conjunctival injection and haemorrhagic chemosis (*Fig. 3.18*), (b) ophthalmoplegia and ptosis (3rd nerve involvement), (c) pulsatile proptosis associated with a thrill and a bruit; may be abolished by ipsilateral carotid compression (*Fig. 3.19*), (d) increased intraocular pressure, (e) anterior segment ischaemia (corneal epithelial oedema, aqueous cells and flare), (f) optic disc swelling, and (g) retinal venous dilatation.
- *CT (Fig. 3.20) and magnetic resonance (MR) imaging:* may

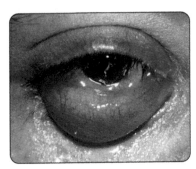

Fig 3.18

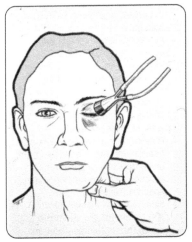

Fig 3.19

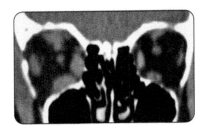

Fig 3.20

show an enlarged superior ophthalmic vein and extraocular muscles; definitive diagnosis involves CT or MR angiography.

Diagnosis of indirect fistula

- *Typical signs:* may be subtle and include (a) elevated intraocular pressure, (b) epibulbar vascular engorgement (classically corkscrew-like vessels; *Fig. 3.21*) with or without chemosis, and (c) exaggerated ocular pulsation.
- *Uncommon signs:* (a) mild proptosis, occasionally associated with a soft bruit, and (b) subtle retinal venous dilatation.

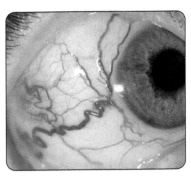

Fig 3.21

Treatment

- Most fistulae are not hazardous to life, with intervention usually indicated only when sight is threatened; spontaneous closure may occur, particularly in low-flow shunts.
- Endovascular embolization or balloon occlusion are options.
- Direct surgical repair is sometimes required.

Cystic lesions

Dacryops

Pathogenesis: ductal cyst of the lacrimal gland.

Diagnosis: frequently bilateral; round cystic lesion originating from the palpebral portion of the lacrimal gland, protruding into the superior fornix (*Fig. 3.22*).

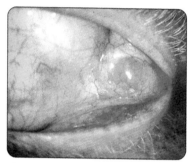

Fig 3.22

Treatment: excision or marsupialization.

Dermoid cyst

Pathogenesis: choristoma derived from displacement of ectoderm to a subcutaneous location; lined by skin-like epithelium, has a fibrous wall and contains dermal appendages; may be superficial or deep (i.e., anterior or posterior to the orbital septum).

Diagnosis

- *Superficial dermoid:* (a) presents in infancy with a firm, round, smooth, nontender 1–2 cm nodule, (b) usually tethered to the adjacent periosteum, (c) most commonly located in the superotemporal orbit (*Fig. 3.23*), and (d) with easily palpable posterior margins.

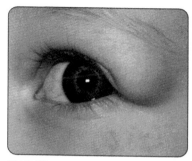

Fig 3.23

- *Deep dermoid:* presents in adolescence/adulthood with proptosis, dystopia, or a mass lesion with indistinct posterior margins; may extend into the inferotemporal fossa or intracranially; may enlarge and rupture spontaneously, inducing a substantial inflammatory reaction; imaging shows a well-circumscribed cystic lesion (*Fig. 3.24*).

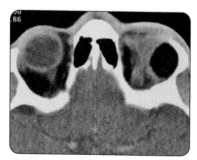

Fig 3.24

Treatment
- *Superficial dermoid:* excision, taking care not to rupture the lesion.
- *Deep dermoid:* excision is advisable to avoid spontaneous rupture.

Encephalocele

Pathogenesis: herniation of intracranial contents through a congenital defect of the base of the skull. A meningocele contains only dura (*Fig. 3.25*), and a meningoencephalocele also contains brain tissue; associations include other bony facial abnormalities, several developmental ocular anomalies, and NF1.

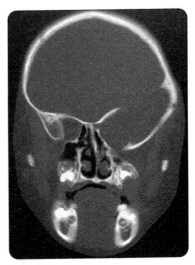

Fig 3.26

Treatment: surgical repair.

Tumours

Capillary haemangioma

Definition: vascular tumour composed of anastamosing small vascular channels without true encapsulation. It is the most common orbital tumour in childhood and affects girls more commonly than boys by a 3:1 ratio.

Diagnosis
- *Presentation:* first few weeks of life (30% at birth).
- *Signs:* (a) cutaneous lesions often coexist (see Chapter 1),
  (b) preseptal lesions appear blue/purple through the skin (*Fig. 3.27*),
  (c) deep orbital tumours give rise to proptosis without skin discoloration; (d) involvement of

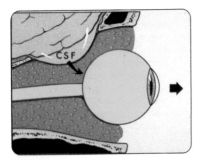

Fig 3.25

Diagnosis
- *Presentation:* during infancy.
- *Signs:* (a) proptosis and dystopia, increasing on crying;
  (b) pulsation may occur due to communication with the subarachnoid space but there is neither a thrill nor a bruit.
- *CT:* bony defect (*Fig. 3.26*).

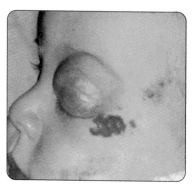

Fig 3.27

the forniceal conjunctiva may be an important diagnostic clue.
- *Imaging:* required when the diagnosis is not apparent on inspection.
- *Course:* rapid growth for 3–6 months after diagnosis, followed by a slower phase of natural resolution; 30% of lesions resolve by the age of 3 years and 70% by the age of 7 years.
- *Systemic associations:* (a) high-output heart failure (large lesions), (b) Kasabach–Merritt syndrome (thrombocytopenia, coagulation abnormalities, multiple haemangiomas), and (c) Maffucci syndrome (multiple haemangiomas, enchondromatosis).

Treatment
- *Indications:* (a) amblyopia (induced astigmatism, anisometropia, occlusion), (b) optic nerve compression, (c) exposure keratopathy, (d) severe cosmetic blemish, and (e) necrosis or infection.
- *Systemic steroids:* administered daily over several weeks.

- *Systemic propranolol (2 mg/kg/day):* novel effective treatment.

Cavernous haemangioma

Definition: vascular lesion that behaves like a low-flow arteriovenous malformation, typically located just behind the globe within the muscle cone; female preponderance of 70%.

Diagnosis
- *Presentation:* (a) 4th and 5th decades with slowly progressive unilateral axial proptosis; (b) gaze-evoked blurring of vision is typical.
- *Imaging:* well-circumscribed oval lesion with slow contrast enhancement (*Fig. 3.28*).

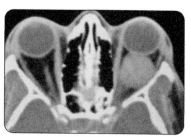

Fig 3.28

Treatment: symptomatic lesions require surgical excision.

Pleomorphic lacrimal gland adenoma (benign mixed cell tumour)

Definition: most common epithelial tumour of the lacrimal gland, derived from the ducts and secretory elements.

Diagnosis

- *Presentation:* in young to middle-aged adults with painless, slowly progressive proptosis or swelling in the superolateral orbit, usually of more than a year's duration.
- *Orbital lobe tumour:* (a) smooth, firm, nontender mass in the lacrimal gland fossa with inferonasal dystopia (*Fig. 3.29*); (b) posterior extension may cause proptosis, ophthalmoplegia, and choroidal folds.

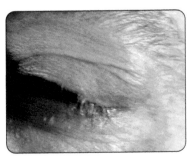

Fig 3.31

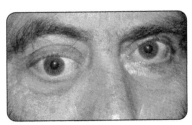

Fig 3.29

- *CT:* round or oval mass, with indentation but not destruction of the lacrimal gland fossa (*Fig. 3.30*).
- *Palpebral lobe tumour:* less common; tends to grow anteriorly causing upper lid swelling (*Fig. 3.31*) without dystopia; may be visible to inspection.

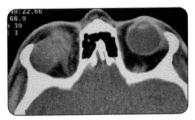

Fig 3.30

Treatment

- *Surgical excision:* (a) palpebral lobe tumours via an anterior (trans-septal) orbitotomy, and (b) orbital lobe lesions via a lateral orbitotomy; prior biopsy is avoided if possible in order to prevent tumour seeding into adjacent orbital tissue.
- *Prognosis:* excellent though incomplete excision or preliminary incisional biopsy with seeding is associated with recurrence and occasional malignant change.

Lacrimal gland carcinoma

Histological types: (a) adenoid cystic carcinoma, (b) pleomorphic adenocarcinoma, (c) mucoepidermoid carcinoma, and (d) squamous cell carcinoma.

Diagnosis

- *Presentation:* in early middle age with: (a) rapidly growing lacrimal gland mass of several months' duration, (b) long-standing swollen upper lid (*Fig. 3.32*) that suddenly starts to increase in size, and (c) following incomplete excision

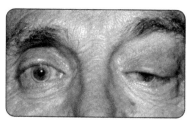

Fig 3.32

of a benign pleomorphic lacrimal gland adenoma.
- *Signs:* posterior extension, with involvement of the superior orbital fissure, may give rise to (a) periorbital oedema, (b) epibulbar hyperaemia, (c) proptosis, (d) ophthalmoplegia, (e) optic disc swelling and choroidal folds; (f) hypoaesthesia in the region supplied by the lacrimal nerve is common.
- *CT:* globular lesion with irregular edges, often with invasion of bone and calcification (*Fig. 3.33*).
- *Investigations:* (a) biopsy to establish the histology, and (b) neurological imaging because adenoid cystic carcinoma exhibits perineural spread and may extend into the cavernous sinus.

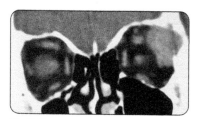

Fig 3.33

Treatment: (a) excision of the tumour and adjacent tissues; (b) extensive tumours may require orbital exenteration and carry a poor prognosis for life, when (c) radiotherapy may prolong life and reduce pain.

Optic nerve glioma

Definition: slow-growing pilocytic astrocytoma typically affecting children; approximately 30% have associated NF1 (see Chapter 19). Malignant gliomas are rare, almost always occur in adults, and have a very poor prognosis.

Diagnosis
- *Presentation:* slowly progressive visual loss followed by proptosis (*Fig. 3.34*).

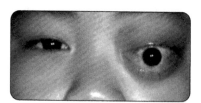

Fig 3.34

- *Signs:* (a) optic nerve head swelling followed by atrophy; (b) opticociliary collaterals and central retinal vein occlusion (uncommon); (c) intracranial spread to the chiasm and hypothalamus may occur.
- *Imaging:* (a) in patients with NF1, the tumour shows fusiform enlargement of the optic nerve with a clear-cut margin (*Fig. 3.35*) produced by the intact dural sheath; (b) in

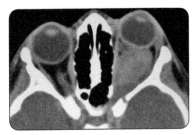

Fig 3.35

patients without NF1 the
lesion is more irregular; MR
may show intracranial extension
(*Fig. 3.36*).

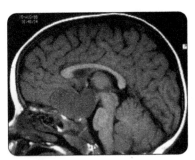

Fig 3.36

Treatment
- May not be required in patients
  with no evidence of growth and
  good vision.
- Surgical excision with preservation
  of the globe in those with large or
  growing tumours confined to the
  orbit, particularly if vision is poor.
- Radiotherapy/chemotherapy when
  intracranial extension precludes
  excision.
- Prognosis for life in childhood
  tumours is variable.

Optic nerve sheath meningioma

Definition: tumour arising from the
arachnoid villi surrounding the
intraorbital or, less commonly, the
intracanalicular portion of the optic
nerve. It typically affects women and
has a good prognosis for life.

Diagnosis
- *Presentation:* in middle-age with
  gradual unilateral visual
  impairment, and occasionally
  transient obscurations.
- *Subsequent course:* (a) optic nerve
  dysfunction and chronic disc
  swelling followed by atrophy, with
  opticociliary collaterals in 30%
  (*Fig. 3.37*), (b) ophthalmoplegia,
  and (c) proptosis caused by
  intraconal growth.

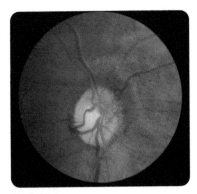

Fig 3.37

- *CT:* thickening and calcification of
  the optic nerve (*Fig. 3.38*).
- *MR:* more clearly delineates
  smaller tumours and those around
  the optic canal.

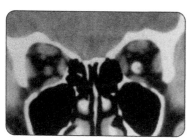

Fig 3.38

Treatment
- *May not be required:* in patients with slow-growing tumours.
- *Surgical excision:* in young patients with aggressive tumours, particularly if the eye is blind.
- *Fractionated stereotactic radiotherapy:* in selected cases.

Plexiform neurofibroma

Definition: most common peripheral neural tumour of the orbit, occurring almost exclusively in NF1.
Diagnosis
- *Presentation:* early childhood with periorbital swelling.
- *Signs:* (a) diffuse involvement of the orbit often causes disfiguring hypertrophy of periocular tissues (*Fig. 3.39*), (b) lid involvement causes mechanical ptosis with a characteristic S-shaped deformity, and (c) palpation of involved tissues is said to resemble a 'bag of worms.'
- *Imaging:* demonstrates extent of orbital involvement.
Treatment: often unsatisfactory; complete surgical removal is extremely difficult due to the intricate relationship between the tumour and important orbital structures.

Lymphoma

Pathogenesis: lymphomas represent one end of the spectrum of lymphoproliferative disorders, with benign reactive lymphoid hyperplasia at the other. The vast majority of orbital lymphomas are composed of 'small' B cells.
Diagnosis
- *Presentation:* in old age with an insidious onset that may occasionally be bilateral (*Fig. 3.40*).
- *Signs:* (a) proptosis with periocular swelling; (b) conjunctival involvement may be present.
- *Systemic assessment:* (a) chest X-ray, (b) serum immunoprotein electrophoresis, (c) thoraco-

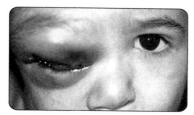

Fig 3.39

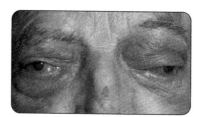

Fig 3.40

abdominal CT, and (d) bone marrow aspiration.

- *Course:* variable and often unpredictable.

Treatment: radiotherapy for localized lesions; chemotherapy for disseminated disease.

Embryonal sarcoma

Histology: (a) most common primary orbital malignancy of childhood; (b) derived from undifferentiated mesenchyme, and histologically varies from undifferentiated to differentiated, the latter often showing features of striated muscle (rhabdomyosarcoma).

Diagnosis

- *Presentation:* average age is 7 years with rapidly progressive, unilateral proptosis that may mimic inflammation (*Fig. 3.41*).
- *Signs:* (a) most common sites are upper nasal and retrobulbar; (b) overlying skin is swollen and red but not warm.
- *Imaging:* poorly defined mass (*Fig. 3.42*), often with bony destruction.

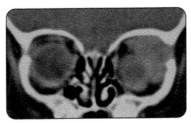

Fig 3.42

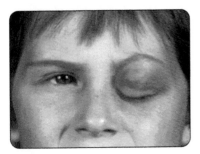

Fig 3.41

Treatment: radiotherapy and chemotherapy; surgical excision is reserved for recurrent or radio-resistant tumours.

Adult metastatic tumours

Primary sites: orbital metastases are an infrequent cause of proptosis and are much less common than metastases to the choroid. In order of frequency, the most common primary sites are breast, bronchus, prostate, and cutaneous melanoma. The prognosis is poor, most patients dying within 1 year.

Diagnosis

- *Presentation:* (a) sudden onset of proptosis with dystopia; (b) orbital apex lesions may cause only mild proptosis with predominance of cranial nerve involvement.
- *Signs:* (a) infiltration and inflammation of orbital tissues, (b) 'firm' orbit with resistance to globe retropulsion, or (c) enophthalmos with scirrhous tumours.
- *Imaging:* nonencapsulated mass.

Treatment: radiotherapy and occasionally surgery.

Childhood metastatic tumours

- *Neuroblastoma:* arises from primitive sympathetic neural cells, most commonly in the abdomen. Orbital metastases, sometimes bilateral, typically present with abrupt onset of proptosis with lid ecchymosis and a superior orbital mass (*Fig. 3.43*).

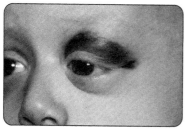

Fig 3.43

- *Myeloid sarcoma:* localized tumour composed of malignant cells of myeloid origin; may be associated with myeloid leukaemia. Orbital involvement usually presents at approximately age 7 years with rapid-onset proptosis, sometimes bilateral.
- *Langerhans cell histiocytosis*: proliferation of histiocytes. Presentation ranges from localized disease with bone destruction (eosinophilic granuloma) to fulminant systemic disease. Orbital involvement consists of unilateral or bilateral osteolytic lesions, typically in the superotemporal quadrant.

Orbital invasion from adjacent structures

- *Sinus tumours:* (a) maxillary carcinoma may cause facial pain and swelling, epistaxis and nasal discharge, epiphora, diplopia, and upward dystopia (*Fig. 3.44*), (b) ethmoidal carcinoma may present with lateral dystopia, and (c) nasopharyngeal carcinoma may spread to the orbit through the inferior orbital fissure—proptosis is a late finding.

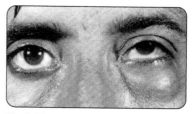

Fig 3.44

- *Bony invasion:* by intracranial meningiomas (sphenoidal ridge, tuberculum sellae, olfactory groove).
- *Fibrous dysplasia:* benign developmental disorder leading to slowly-developing irregular expansion of bone with a mass effect on adjacent structures; may cause facial asymmetry, proptosis, dystopia and visual loss. Most orbital disease is 'monostotic'; polyostotic is associated with endocrine disorders and cutaneous pigmentation (McCune–Albright syndrome).
- *Orbital invasion:* from (a) eyelid malignancies (e.g. squamous cell carcinoma), (b) conjunctival tumours (e.g. melanoma), and (c) intraocular

tumours (e.g. choroidal melanoma, retinoblastoma).

Anophthalmic socket

Surgical procedures for removal of an eye or the contents of the orbit

- *Enucleation:* removal of the globe is indicated for the following:
  (a) primary intraocular malignancies where other treatment modalities are not appropriate, (b) after severe trauma where the eye is either unsalvageable or the risk of sympathetic ophthalmitis may outweigh any prospect of visual recovery (see Chapter 11), and (c) when the eye is blind and painful or unsightly, although evisceration is generally preferred.
- *Evisceration:* removal of the cornea and the contents of the globe, leaving the sclera and extraocular muscles intact, provides better postoperative motility than enucleation; not suitable for suspected malignancy.
- *Exenteration:* removal of the globe and the soft tissues of the orbit (*Fig. 3.45*) is indicated for the following: (a) orbital malignancies where other forms of treatment are unlikely to be effective, and (b) rarely for nonmalignant disease such as orbital mucormycosis. Anteriorly-sited tumours may allow sparing of posterior orbital tissue, and posterior tumours may allow sparing of eyelid skin to line the socket.

Rehabilitation of the anophthalmic socket

- A cosmetic shell is a prosthesis used to cover a phthisical or unsightly eye; it can restore volume and often provides a good cosmetic appearance and motility.
- Orbital implants are used to counteract orbital volume deficit following enucleation or evisceration. A ball implant is usually placed at the time of eye removal; secondary placement can also be performed. Materials used may be solid (e.g. silicone) or porous (hydroxyapatite).
- Post-enucleation socket syndrome (PESS) is caused by failure to correct the volume deficit adequately. It is characterized by a deep upper lid sulcus, ptosis, enophthalmos, and backwards rotation of the top of the prosthesis (*Fig. 3.46*).

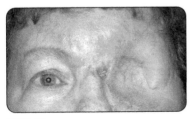

Fig 3.45

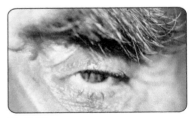

Fig 3.46

- After enucleation or evisceration, a conformer is placed to support the conjunctival fornices until the socket is fitted with an artificial eye (*Fig. 3.47*). Initial impression moulds are taken at 6–8 weeks for a prosthesis shaped to fit the individual socket and matched to the fellow eye.

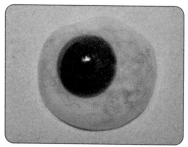

Fig 3.47

- Prostheses following exenteration can be stuck onto the surrounding skin, mounted on glasses (*Fig. 3.48*), or secured with osseo-integrated magnets mounted on the orbital rim bones.

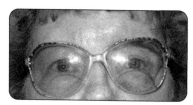

Fig 3.48

Craniosynostoses

Crouzon syndrome

Pathogenesis: premature fusion of the coronal and sagittal sutures; majority are AD, with a fresh mutation in 25%.

Diagnosis

- *General signs:* (a) short anteroposterior head distance but wide cranium, (b) 'frog-like' facies, and (c) mandibular prognathism.
- *Ocular signs:* (a) proptosis due to shallow orbits (can lead to exposure keratopathy), (b) hypertelorism, (c) 'V' exotropia (*Fig. 3.49*), (d) refractive errors and amblyopia, and (e) optic atrophy in 10–20%.
- *Uncommon ocular associations:* (a) blue sclera, (b) cataract, (c) ectopia lentis, (d) congenital glaucoma, (e) coloboma, (f) megalocornea, and (g) optic nerve hypoplasia.

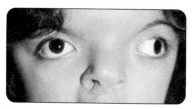

Fig 3.49

Apert syndrome

Pathogenesis: most severe of the
   craniosynostoses which may involve
   all the cranial sutures. The majority
   are sporadic but can be AD.

Diagnosis
  - *General signs:* (a) oxycephaly,
    (b) midfacial hypoplasia with a
    beak-like nose, (c) low-set ears,
    (d) horizontal groove above the
    supraorbital ridge (*Fig. 3.50*),
    (e) high-arched palate, cleft palate,
    and bifid uvula, (f) syndactyly of
    the hands and feet, and (g)
    anomalies of the heart, lungs,
    and kidneys.
  - *Ocular signs:* (a) shallow orbits
    (proptosis and hypertelorism
    are generally less pronounced
    than in Crouzon syndrome),
    and (b) exotropia and extorted

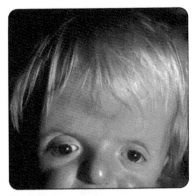

Fig 3.50

   slanting of the palpebral
   apertures.
  - *Uncommon ocular associations:*
    (a) keratoconus, (b) ectopia lentis,
    and (c) congenital glaucoma.

Dry eye

Definitions

- *Keratoconjunctivitis sicca (KCS):* eye with some degree of dryness.
- *Xerophthalmia:* dry eye associated with vitamin A deficiency.
- *Xerosis:* extreme dryness with keratinization occurring secondary to severe conjunctival cicatrization.
- *Sjögren syndrome:* autoimmune inflammatory disease of which KCS is a typical feature (see below).

Classification of keratoconjunctivitis sicca

- *Aqueous layer deficiency:* (a) Sjögren syndrome, (b) non-Sjögren age-related hyposecretion, (c) absence or damage to lacrimal tissue, (d) conjunctival scarring with obstruction of lacrimal gland ductules, (e) neurological lesions with sensory or motor reflex loss, and (f) vitamin A deficiency.
- *Evaporative:* (a) meibomian gland disease, (b) exposure keratopathy, (c) defective blinking, (d) contact lens-associated, and (e) environmental factors.

Sjögren syndrome

Pathogenesis: autoimmune inflammation and destruction of lacrimal and salivary glands occurring in isolation (primary) or in association with other diseases such as rheumatoid arthritis and systemic lupus erythematosus (secondary); affects females more commonly than males.

Diagnosis

- *Presentation:* adult life with grittiness of the eyes and dryness of the mouth (xerostomia).
- *Signs:* (a) enlarged salivary and occasionally lacrimal glands, (b) xerostomia with a fissured tongue, (c) dry nasal passages, (d) diminished vaginal secretions, (e) Raynaud phenomenon, and (f) arthralgia, myalgia, and fatigue.
- *Complications:* (a) dental caries, (b) reflux oesophagitis and gastritis, (c) malabsorption due to pancreatic failure, and (d) pulmonary disease.
- *Investigations:* (a) serum autoantibodies, (b) Schirmer test (*Fig. 4.1*), and (c) biopsy of minor salivary glands.

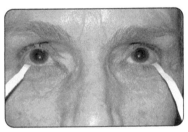

Fig 4.1

Treatment: symptomatic (see below), salivary stimulants, and immunosuppression.

Diagnosis

Symptoms

- Dryness, grittiness, and burning, characteristically worse during the day.

- Stringy discharge, transient blurring of vision, redness and crusting of the lids are common.

Signs

- Marginal tear meniscus is thinned (*Fig. 4.2*) or absent (normal height 1 mm).
- Mucous debris in the tear film (*Fig. 4.3*).
- Conjunctival injection and mild keratinization.
- Interpalpebral corneal punctate epithelial erosions.
- Corneal filaments (mucus/ epithelial debris strands; *Fig. 4.4*).

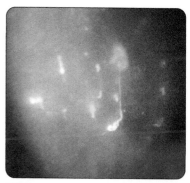

Fig 4.4

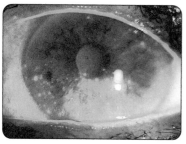

Fig 4.2

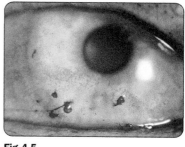

Fig 4.5

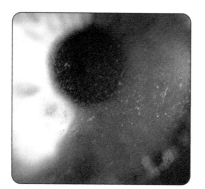

Fig 4.3

- Mucous plaques attached to the corneal surface staining with rose Bengal (*Fig. 4.5*).
- Complications in severe cases: (a) peripheral superficial corneal neovascularization, (b) epithelial breakdown, (c) corneal melting (*Fig. 4.6*), (d) corneal perforation (*Fig. 4.7*), and (e) secondary bacterial keratitis.

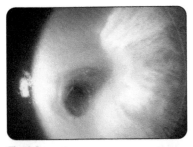

Fig 4.6

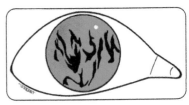

Fig 4.8

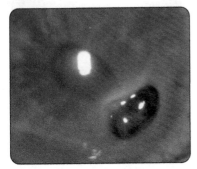

Fig 4.7

Special investigations

- **Tear film breakup time (BUT):** abnormal in aqueous tear deficiency and meibomian gland disorders. (a) Fluorescein is instilled into the lower fornix and the tear film is examined at the slit lamp using the cobalt blue filter; (b) after an interval, black spots or lines appear in the stained film, indicating the formation of dry areas (*Fig. 4.8*); (c) BUT is the interval between the last blink and the appearance of the first randomly distributed dry spot; BUT of less than 10 sec is abnormal.
- **Schirmer test:** amount of wetting of a special (No. 41 Whatman) filter paper 5 mm wide and 35 mm long is measured (see *Fig. 4.1*). (a) When performed with an anaesthetic (Schirmer 2), it is said to measure basic secretion; (b) when performed without anaesthetic (Schirmer 1), it measures maximum basic and reflex secretion; less than 10 mm of wetting after 5 min without anaesthesia and less than 6 mm with anaesthesia are considered abnormal.
- **Ocular surface staining:** (a) fluorescein stains corneal and conjunctival epithelium where there is sufficient damage to allow the dye to enter the tissues; (b) rose Bengal has an affinity for dead or devitalized epithelial cells that have a lost or altered mucous layer, and also stains corneal filaments and plaques (*Fig. 4.9*).
- **Staining pattern:** (a) interpalpebral staining of the cornea and conjunctiva is common in aqueous tear deficiency; (b) inferior corneal and conjunctival stain is often seen in blepharitis or exposure.
- **Other tests:** (a) tear lactoferrin (decreased in Sjögren syndrome and other lacrimal gland diseases), (b) fluorescein clearance test/tear function index, (c) phenol red thread test, (d) tear

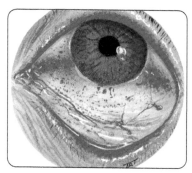

Fig 4.9

film meniscometry, (e) tear film osmolarity measurement, and (f) impression cytology to determine goblet cell population.

Treatment

Dry eye is generally not curable, and management is therefore structured around the control of symptoms and prevention of surface damage.

- *Patient education:* establishment of realistic expectations, emphasis on compliance, instruction on importance of blinking while reading/using a visual display unit, and review of work environment.
- *Conservation of existing tears:* (a) reduction of room temperature to minimize evaporation, (b) room humidifiers may be tried but are frequently disappointing, and (c) moist chamber goggles or side shields to glasses can be helpful but may be cosmetically unacceptable.
- *Tear substitutes:* (a) cellulose derivatives (e.g. hypromellose) for mild cases, (b) carbomers (e.g. Viscotears, GelTears) are longer lasting, (c) polyvinyl alcohol (e.g.

Hypotears, Liquifilm) in mucin deficiency, and (d) sodium hyaluronate (e.g. Vismed) may promote epithelial healing. Preservative-free drops should be used for frequent instillation.
- *Mucolytics:* acetylcysteine 5% drops (Ilube) for corneal filaments.
- *Ointments:* at bedtime.
- *Autologous serum:* in very severe cases.
- *Punctal occlusion:* in moderate to severe KCS if there is inadequate response to frequent topical treatment; (a) temporary (1–2 weeks) occlusion can be achieved by inserting dissolvable collagen plugs to exclude epiphora; (b) prolonged (silicone plugs) or permanent (cautery) occlusion can then be carried out but all four puncta should not be permanently occluded at the same time.
- *Anti-inflammatory agents:* low-dose topical steroids for acute exacerbations.
- *Topical ciclosporin (0.05%, 0.1%):* reduces T cell-mediated inflammation of lacrimal tissue and increase the number of goblet cells.
- *Systemic tetracycline:* for associated chronic blepharitis and reduction of lacrimal inflammatory mediators.
- *Contact lenses:* long-term contact lens wear may increase tear film evaporation, reduce tear flow, and increase the risk of infection, but these effects can be outweighed by the reservoir effect of fluid trapped behind the lens.
- *Other options:* (a) tarsorrhaphy, (b) oral cholinergic agonists (e.g. pilocarpine), (c) zidovudine in primary Sjögren syndrome, and (d) botulinum toxin to the medial canthus to reduce tear drainage.

Conjunctiva

Bacterial conjunctivitis

Acute bacterial conjunctivitis

Pathogenesis: direct eye contact with infected secretions; most common isolates are *S. pneumoniae*, *S. aureus*, *H. influenza*, and *Moraxella catarrhalis*; uncommon but serious are gonococci and meningococci.

Diagnosis

- *Presentation:* acute onset of redness, grittiness, burning and sticky discharge affecting first one then both eyes.
- *Conjunctival injection:* maximal toward the fornices (*Fig. 5.1*).
- *Discharge:* (a) typically mucopurulent (*Fig. 5.2*); (b) hyperacute purulent (*Fig. 5.3*) in gonococcal or meningococcal infection.
- *Eyelids:* oedema and erythema (*Fig. 5.4*) in severe infection.
- *Cornea:* (a) mild punctate epithelial erosions; (b) ulceration (*Fig. 5.5*) may occur in gonococcal and meningococcal infection.
- *Investigations:* not performed routinely but may be indicated in

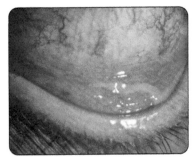

Fig 5.2

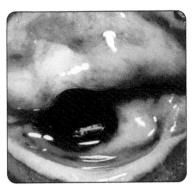

Fig 5.3

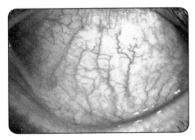

Fig 5.1

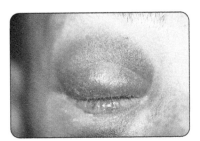

Fig 5.4

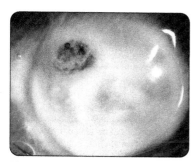

Fig 5.5

severe or atypical cases (e.g. urgent Gram staining to exclude gonococcal or meningococcal infection), and polymerase chain reaction (PCR) for *Chlamydia*.

Treatment

- *Topical antibiotics:* options include (a) chloramphenicol, (b) aminoglycosides (gentamicin, neomycin), (c) quinolones (ciprofloxacin, ofloxacin, levofloxacin, lomefloxacin, gatifloxacin, moxifloxacin), and (d) polymyxin B, fusidic acid, or bacitracin. Some practitioners believe that chloramphenicol should not be used for routine treatment because of a possible link with aplastic anaemia. Gonococcal and meningococcal conjunctivitis require a quinolone, gentamicin, chloramphenicol, or bacitracin 1–2 hourly as well as systemic therapy.
- *Systemic antibiotics:* (a) gonococcal infection is treated with a third-generation cephalosporin, (b) *H. influenzae*, particularly in children, requires oral amoxicillin with clavulanic acid, and (c) meningococcal

infection with intramuscular benzylpenicillin.
- *Topical steroids:* may reduce scarring in severe conjunctivitis.

Adult chlamydial conjunctivitis

Pathogenesis: oculogenital infection usually caused by serovars (serological variants) D–K of *Chlamydia trachomatis*. Transmission is usually by autoinoculation from genital secretions. In males, chlamydial infection is the most common cause of nongonococcal urethritis, and is frequently asymptomatic; in females, chlamydial urethritis typically causes dysuria and discharge.

Diagnosis

- *Presentation:* subacute onset of unilateral or bilateral redness, watering and discharge.
- *Discharge:* watery or mucopurulent.
- *Conjunctiva:* (a) large follicles are typical (*Fig.* 5.6); (b) chronic cases have less prominent follicles and may develop mild conjunctival

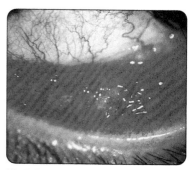

Fig 5.6

scarring and superior corneal pannus (*Fig. 5.7*).
- *Cornea:* superficial punctate keratitis is common, and peripheral subepithelial corneal infiltrates (*Fig. 5.8*) may appear 2–3 weeks after onset.
- *Tender preauricular lymphadenopathy:* very common.
- *Investigations:* (a) conjunctival scraping with Giemsa staining for basophilic intracytoplasmic bodies, (b) PCR, (c) immunoassay, and (d) cell culture and serology in selected cases.

Treatment
- *Systemic antibiotics:* options include (a) azithromycin 1 g repeated after 1 week (second or third course required in 30%), (b) doxycycline 100 mg twice daily for 10 days (avoid in pregnancy/ breast-feeding and children), and (c) erythromycin, amoxicillin, and ciprofloxacin as alternatives.
- *Topical antibiotics:* supplementary erythromycin or tetracycline for rapid relief of ocular symptoms.

Trachoma

Pathogenesis: recurrent infection occurring in individuals living in poor overcrowded communities eliciting a chronic immune response, particularly in vulnerable young children. Trachoma is associated principally with infection by serovars A, B, Ba, and C of *C. trachomatis*; the fly is an important vector.

Diagnosis
- *Active stage:* (a) mixed follicular/ papillary conjunctivitis (*Fig. 5.9*), (b) mucopurulent discharge, and (c) superior epithelial keratitis and pannus formation.

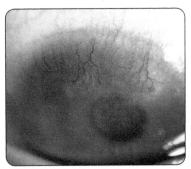

Fig 5.7

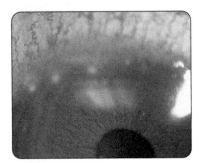

Fig 5.8

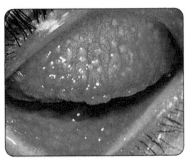

Fig 5.9

- *Cicatricial disease:* (a) conjunctival scars, most prominent on the upper tarsus (linear/stellate (*Fig. 5.10*), or broad and confluent [Arlt lines; *Fig. 5.11*]), (b) superior limbal follicles which may leave a row of depressions (Herbert pits; *Fig. 5.12*), (c) trichiasis, distichiasis, and cicatricial entropion, (d) dry eye (goblet cells and lacrimal gland ductule destruction), and (e) eventual severe corneal vascularization and opacification (*Fig. 5.13*).

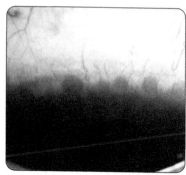

Fig 5.12

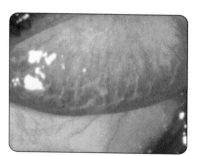

Fig 5.10

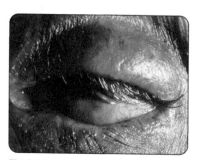

Fig 5.13

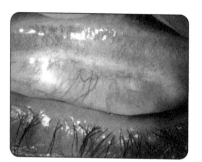

Fig 5.11

World Health Organization grading of trachoma

- **TF** = trachomatous inflammation (follicular): five or more follicles (>0.5 mm) on the superior tarsus.
- **TI** = trachomatous inflammation (intense): diffuse involvement of the tarsal conjunctiva, obscuring 50% or more of the normal deep tarsal vessels; papillae are evident.
- **TS** = trachomatous conjunctival scarring: easily visible fibrous white tarsal bands.
- **TT** = trachomatous trichiasis: at least one lash touching the globe.

- **CO** = corneal opacity sufficient to blur details of at least part of the pupillary margin.

Treatment

- *SAFE strategy:* (a) surgery for trichiasis, (b) antibiotics for active disease, (c) facial hygiene, and (d) environmental improvement.
- *Antibiotics:* (a) systemic azithromycin (single dose of 20 mg/kg up to 1 g) or erythromycin 500 mg twice daily for 14 days; (b) tetracycline ointment is less effective than oral treatment and should be given for 6 weeks. More than one antibiotic may be required, and communities may need to receive annual treatment to suppress infection.
- *Hygiene:* personal and environmental.
- *Surgery:* for entropion and trichiasis; bilamellar tarsal rotation is commonly performed.

Neonatal conjunctivitis (ophthalmia neonatorum)

Pathogenesis: conjunctival inflammation developing within the first month of life, usually as the result of infection transmitted from mother to baby during delivery. Staphylococci are usually responsible for mild conjunctivitis, but severe systemic involvement can result from infection with *C. trachomatis*, *N. gonorrhoeae*, and herpes simplex virus (HSV); chemical conjunctival irritation from infection prophylaxis may also occur.

Diagnosis

- *Presentation:* (a) chemical irritation—first few days, (b) gonococcal—first week,

(c) staphylococci and other bacteria—end of the first week, (d) herpes simplex—1–2 weeks, and (e) chlamydia—1–3 weeks.

- *Discharge:* depends on cause.
- *Eyelids:* (a) severe oedema may denote gonococcal infection (*Fig. 5.14*); (b) vesicles in HSV infection.
- *Investigations in moderate to severe cases:* (a) conjunctival scrapings for Gram and Giemsa staining, (b) conjunctival swabs for bacterial culture (chocolate agar if *N. gonorrhoeae* suspected), (c) Papanicolaou smear, (d) separate scrapings for PCR if indicated, and (e) viral culture for HSV of conjunctival scrapings or skin vesicle fluid.

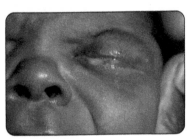

Fig 5.14

Treatment

- *Prophylaxis:* single instillation of povidone–iodine 2.5%, erythromycin 0.5%, tetracycline 1% ointment, or silver nitrate 1% is utilized in areas where gonococcal infection is common; a single intramuscular dose of benzylpenicillin is given when maternal infection is present.
- *Chemical conjunctivitis:* no treatment apart from artificial tears.

- *Mild conjunctivitis (sticky eye):* may require a broad-spectrum topical antibiotic (e.g. fusidic acid, chloramphenicol).
- *Chlamydial conjunctivitis:* oral (± topical) erythromycin for 2 weeks.
- *Gonococcal conjunctivitis:* hospital admission and systemic third-generation cephalosporin; co-treatment for chlamydia is prudent.
- *Herpes simplex infection:* should always be regarded as a systemic condition and treated with high-dose intravenous and topical aciclovir; early diagnosis and treatment of encephalitis may be life-saving or prevent serious disability.
- *Co-management:* paediatrician, microbiologist, and genitourinary specialist.

Viral conjunctivitis

Adenoviral conjunctivitis

Pathogenesis: highly contagious disease that may be sporadic or epidemic. Transmission is by contact with respiratory or ocular secretions, including fomites such as contaminated towels.

Diagnosis

- *Nonspecific acute follicular conjunctivitis:* most common form, usually mild; sore throat may be present.
- *Pharyngoconjunctival fever (PCF):* spread by droplets from patients with associated upper respiratory tract infection; keratitis (usually mild) occurs in approximately 30%.

- *Epidemic keratoconjunctivitis (EKC):* most severe type, associated with keratitis in approximately 80% of cases; (a) eyelid oedema, (b) tender pre-auricular lymphadenopathy, (c) petechial conjunctival haemorrhages (*Fig. 5.15*), (d) chemosis, and (e) pseudomembranes (*Fig. 5.16*).
- *Chronic/relapsing conjunctivitis:* nonspecific follicular/papillary lesions; can rarely persist for years.
- *Keratitis:* (a) nonstaining epithelial microcysts (early), (b) punctate epithelial keratitis (resolves within 2 weeks), and (c) focal white

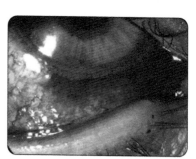

Fig 5.15

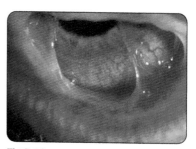

Fig 5.16

subepithelial infiltrates (*Fig. 5.17*) that may persist or recur over months or years.

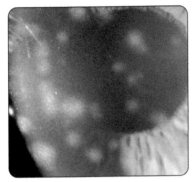

Fig 5.17

- *Differential diagnosis:* (a) acute haemorrhagic conjunctivitis (tropical areas, enterovirus or coxsackievirus), (b) herpes simplex infection (usually unilateral, may have skin vesicles), (c) systemic viral infections (varicella, measles, mumps), and (d) molluscum contagiosum (see below).
- *Investigations:* usually unnecessary but may include the following: (a) Giemsa stain shows mononuclear cells in adenoviral and multinucleated giant cells in herpetic disease, (b) PCR is sensitive and specific for viral DNA, (c) viral culture is expensive and slow but highly specific, and (d) 'point-of-care' immunochromatography test is rapid and accurate.

Treatment
- *Reduction of transmission risk:* meticulous hygiene and avoidance of towel sharing.

- *Topical steroids:* for symptomatic keratitis do not speed resolution, and the lesions commonly recur after early discontinuation; may extend the infectious period.
- *Other measures:* (a) artificial tears for symptomatic relief, (b) discontinuation of contact lens wear, (c) removal of symptomatic pseudomembranes, (d) topical antibiotics for secondary bacterial infection, (e) povidone–iodine is effective against free adenovirus, (f) ganciclovir shows some activity against adenovirus.

Molluscum contagiosum conjunctivitis

Pathogenesis: skin infection caused by a DNA poxvirus that typically affects children. Transmission is by contact with subsequent autoinoculation. Virus shedding from a lesion on the lid margin may be associated with conjunctivitis.

Diagnosis
- *Presentation:* chronic unilateral ocular irritation and mild mucoid discharge.
- *Signs:* (a) waxy umbilicated nodule on the lid margin, and (b) follicular conjunctivitis (*Fig. 5.18*).

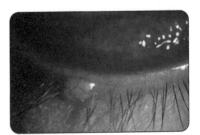

Fig 5.18

Treatment: expression, facilitated by a small nick at the lesion apex.

Allergic conjunctivitis

Acute allergic conjunctivitis

Pathogenesis: acute conjunctival reaction to an environmental allergen, usually pollen, typically occurring in younger children after playing outside in spring or summer.

Diagnosis: acute itching and watering associated with severe chemosis (*Fig. 5.19*) settling within a few hours.

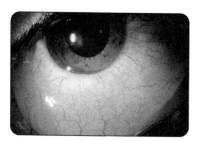

Fig 5.19

Treatment: not usually required; cool compresses can improve comfort, and a drop of adrenaline 0.1% may reduce extreme chemosis.

Seasonal and perennial allergic conjunctivitis

Classification
- *Seasonal allergic conjunctivitis ('hay fever eyes'):* worse during the spring and summer, is the more common and involves allergy to pollen.

- *Perennial allergic conjunctivitis:* causes symptoms throughout the year, allergens including house dust mites and animal fur.

Diagnosis
- *Presentation:* episodes of redness, watering and itching, with sneezing and nasal discharge.
- *Signs:* (a) conjunctival hyperaemia, (b) mild papillary reaction (*Fig. 5.20*), (c) chemosis, and (d) lid oedema.

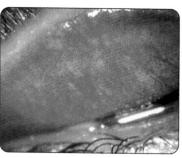

Fig 5.20

Treatment
- *Artificial tears:* for mild symptoms.
- *Mast cell stabilizers:* (e.g. sodium cromoglicate, nedocromil sodium, lodoxamide).
- *Antihistamines:* (e.g. emedastine, epinastine, levocabastine, bepotastine).
- *Combined antihistamine/ vasoconstrictor:* (e.g. Otrivin-Antistin).
- *Dual-action antihistamine and mast cell stabilizers:* (e.g. azelastine, ketotifen, olopatadine).
- *Topical steroids:* rarely necessary.
- *Oral antihistamines:* for severe symptoms.

Vernal keratoconjunctivitis (VKC)

Pathogenesis: recurrent bilateral disease involving IgE and cell-mediated immune mechanisms. It primarily affects boys (mean age 7 years), 95% remitting by the late teens. It is particularly common in warm dry climates such as the Mediterranean and the Middle East.

Classification

- *Palpebral:* primarily involves the upper tarsal conjunctiva often with significant corneal disease.
- *Limbal:* typically affects black and Asian patients.
- *Mixed:* features of both.

Diagnosis

- *Presentation:* intense itching, lacrimation, photophobia, grittiness, burning, and mucoid discharge.
- *Palpebral:* conjunctival hyperaemia, diffuse superior tarsal papillary hypertrophy (*Fig. 5.21*), sometimes giant (*Fig. 5.22*).
- *Limbal:* gelatinous papillae (*Fig. 5.23*) and transient apically-located white cellular collections (Horner–Trantas dots; *Fig. 5.24*).

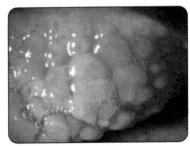

Fig 5.22

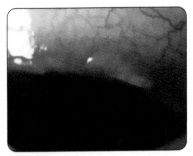

Fig 5.23

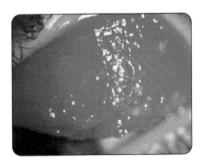

Fig 5.21

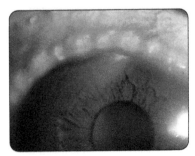

Fig 5.24

- **Keratopathy:** (a) superior punctate epithelial erosions associated with sheets of mucus (*Fig. 5.25*), (b) epithelial macroerosions, (c) plaques and 'shield' ulcers (*Fig. 5.26*), (d) subepithelial scarring, (e) pseudogerontoxon (*Fig. 5.27*), and (f) mild superior superficial vessel ingrowth; keratoconus and herpes simplex keratitis are more common than average.

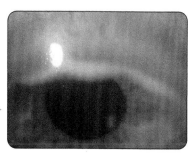

Fig 5.27

Treatment: see below.

Atopic keratoconjunctivitis (AKC)

Pathogenesis: chronic condition with a peak onset at age 30–50 years occurring in atopic patients (eczema, asthma). It tends to be perennial and unremitting with significant visual morbidity; distinction between AKC and VKC is clinical.

Diagnosis

- **Presentation:** similar to VKC but usually more severe and unremitting; discharge is generally more watery than in VKC.
- **Lids:** (a) erythema, (b) thickening, crusting and fissuring, (c) madarosis, (d) staphylococcal blepharitis, (e) keratinization of the lid margin, and (f) tight facial skin with lower lid ectropion.
- **Conjunctiva:** (a) papillae but smaller than VKC, (b) diffuse infiltration and cicatrization may give a whitish, featureless appearance (*Fig. 5.28*), (c) symblepharon formation and forniceal shortening (*Fig. 5.29*), and (d) keratinization of the caruncle.
- **Limbitis:** similar to limbal VKC.

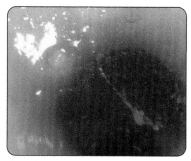

Fig 5.25

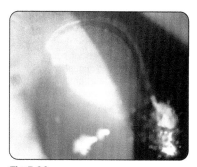

Fig 5.26

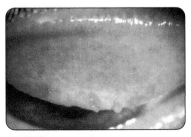

Fig 5.28

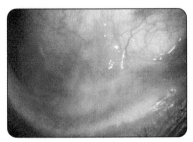

Fig 5.29

- *Keratopathy:* (a) punctate epithelial erosions (inferior third), (b) persistent epithelial defects, sometimes with focal thinning (*Fig. 5.30*), (c) plaques, (d) peripheral

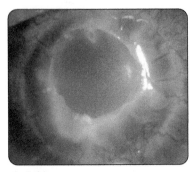

Fig 5.30

vascularization (*Fig. 5.31*), and (e) stromal scarring.
- *Ocular associations:* (a) infective keratitis, including aggressive herpes simplex, (b) keratoconus (15%), (c) presenile cataract (common), and (d) retinal detachment (rare).

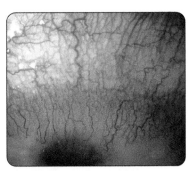

Fig 5.31

Treatment of VKC and AKC

- *General:* allergen avoidance, cool compresses, lid hygiene (blepharitis), and moisturizing cream (e.g. E45) for dry fissured skin.
- *Topical:* (a) mast cell stabilizers may be needed long term, (b) antihistamines for acute exacerbations, (c) dual-action preparations (e.g. antihistamine/ mast cell stabilizers), (d) topical steroids for severe exacerbations, particularly with keratopathy (e.g. fluorometholone 0.1%, rimexolone 1%, prednisolone 0.5%, loteprednol etabonate 0.2% or 0.5%), (e) immune modulators

(e.g. ciclosporin 0.05%, tacrolimus 0.03%), and (f) acetylcysteine for mucolysis.

- **Supratarsal steroid injection:** for severe palpebral VKC or noncompliance.
- **Systemic:** (a) antihistamines help itching, promote sleep, and reduce nocturnal eye rubbing, (b) antibiotics (doxycycline 50–100 mg daily for 6 weeks or azithromycin 500 mg once daily for 3 days) to reduce blepharitis-aggravated inflammation, and (c) immunosuppressive agents (e.g. steroids, ciclosporin, tacrolimus, azathioprine) may be effective at low doses in AKC unresponsive to other measures.
- **Surgery:** (a) superficial keratectomy for plaques/shield ulcers, and (b) surface maintenance/restoration procedures for severe persistent epithelial defects, ulceration, or perforation (e.g. gluing, amniotic membrane grafting, lamellar keratoplasty, botulinum toxin to induce ptosis, lateral tarsorrhaphy).

Giant papillary conjunctivitis

Pathogenesis: mechanically induced inflammation of the tarsal conjunctiva (e.g. contact lenses, ocular prostheses (*Fig. 5.32*), exposed sutures).

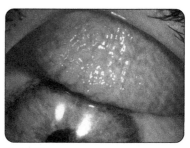

Fig 5.32

Diagnosis
- **Presentation:** foreign body sensation, redness, itching, increased mucus production, blurring, and loss of contact lens tolerance.
- **Signs:** (a) mucous discharge, (b) superior tarsal hyperaemia, and (c) superior tarsal papillae, initially fine-medium then larger.

Treatment
- **Removal of stimulus:** (e.g. contact lens replacement/change of solution type, and assessment of ocular prosthesis fit).
- **Topical:** Preservation-free with soft contact lenses, or instilled when the lenses are not in the eye; (a) mast cell stabilizers, (b) antihistamines, (c) NSAIDs, (d) combined antihistamines/mast cell stabilizers, and (e) steroids for the acute phase of severe cases.

Conjunctivitis in blistering mucocutaneous disease

Mucous membrane (cicatricial) pemphigoid

Pathogenesis: group of chronic autoimmune mucocutaneous blistering diseases characterized by a type II hypersensitivity response with antibody and complement deposition at epithelial basement membranes. A wide range of epithelial tissues can be involved. Particular clinical forms have a predilection for specific tissues (e.g. bullous pemphigoid for the skin and ocular cicatricial pemphigoid for the conjunctiva).

Diagnosis

- *Presentation:* in old age with insidious onset of nonspecific bilateral conjunctivitis.
- *Conjunctiva:* (a) papillary conjunctivitis, (b) diffuse hyperaemia and oedema, with necrosis in severe cases (*Fig. 5.33*), (c) subconjunctival fibrosis with shortening of the inferior fornices, (d) flattening of the plica and keratinization of the caruncle (*Fig. 5.34*),

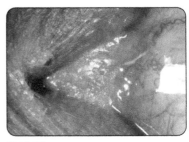

Fig 5.34

- (e) symblepharon formation (*Fig. 5.35*), and (f) dry eye.
- *Keratopathy:* (a) epithelial defects, (b) peripheral vascularization, (c) keratinization, and (d) 'conjunctivalization' of the cornea.
- *End-stage disease:* total symblepharon and corneal opacification (*Fig. 5.36*).

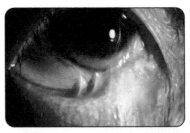

Fig 5.35

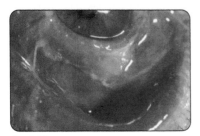

Fig 5.33

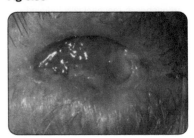

Fig 5.36

- **Eyelids:** (a) aberrant lashes, (b) chronic blepharitis, (c) keratinization of the lid margin, and (d) ankyloblepharon (adhesions between the upper and lower lids).
- **Systemic:** (a) subepidermal mucosal (e.g. oral) blisters (*Fig. 5.37*), (b) oesophageal stricture, (c) laryngeal and tracheal stenosis, and (d) skin blisters (*Fig. 5.38*) and erosions.

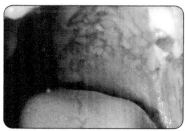

Fig 5.37

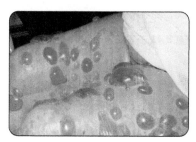

Fig 5.38

Treatment
- **Systemic:** dapsone, antimetabolites (azathioprine, methotrexate, and mycophenolate), prednisolone, intravenous immunoglobulin, and ciclosporin.

- **Local:** (a) lid hygiene for blepharitis, (b) punctal occlusion for dry eyes, (c) subconjunctival mitomycin C and/or steroid, (d) laser or surgery for aberrant lashes, and (e) lateral tarsorrhaphy or botulinum toxin-induced ptosis to promote corneal healing.
- **Topical:** (a) lubricants, (b) steroids, and (c) retinoic acid.
- **Reconstructive surgery:** (a) entropion repair, (b) mucous membrane autografting or amniotic membrane transplantation, (c) limbal stem cell transfer, (d) keratoplasty, and (e) keratoprosthesis in end-stage disease.

Stevens–Johnson syndrome/toxic epidermal necrolysis

Pathogenesis: Stevens–Johnson syndrome (SJS) is now believed to be a condition distinct from erythema multiforme. Toxic epidermal necrolysis (TEN), also known as Lyell syndrome, is a severe variant of SJS. It is thought that a cell-mediated hypersensitivity immune reaction is responsible, with precipitating agents including a very wide range of drugs such as antibiotics (especially sulfonamides and trimethoprim), NSAIDs, anticonvulsants, and microorganisms such as *Mycoplasma pneumoniae* and herpes simplex virus. In more than 50% of cases, the cause is uncertain.

Diagnosis
- **Presentation:** flu-like symptoms for up to 14 days.

- **Acute signs:** (a) papillary conjunctivitis, (b) conjunctival membranes, pseudomembranes (*Fig. 5.39*), haemorrhages, blisters, and patchy infarction, and (c) punctate corneal epithelial erosions progressing to larger epithelial defects.
- **Late signs:** (a) keratinization of the conjunctiva and lid margin (*Fig. 5.40*), (b) forniceal shortening and symblepharon formation, (c) cicatricial entropion and ectropion, (d) trichiasis, (e) ankyloblepharon, (f) keratopathy including scarring and keratinization, and (g) watery eyes due to fibrosis of the lacrimal puncta; dry eyes may also occur.
- **Systemic features:** (a) blistering and haemorrhagic crusting of the lips and sometimes the tongue (*Fig. 5.41*), oropharynx, and elsewhere, and (b) small purpuric, vesicular, or necrotic skin lesions involving the extremities (*Fig. 5.42*), face, and trunk—usually heal within weeks, leaving a scar.

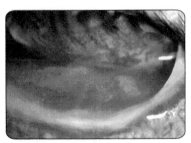

Fig 5.39

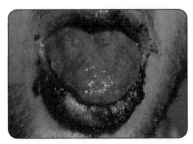

Fig 5.41

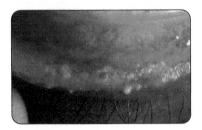

Fig 5.40

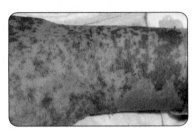

Fig 5.42

Treatment

- *Systemic:* (a) removal of the precipitant if possible, (b) general supportive measures (e.g. hydration), (c) immunosuppressive agents, including steroids in selected cases, (d) antibiotics, when indicated, (e) intravenous immunoglobulin may be effective and (f) anticoagulation with heparin.
- *Acute ocular:* (a) lubricants, (b) topical steroids, (c) lysis of developing symblepharon with a sterile glass rod or damp cotton bud, and (d) peeling of pseudomembranes or true membrane.
- *Later ocular:* (a) lubrication and punctal occlusion, (b) topical transretinoic acid to reverse keratinization, (c) treatment of aberrant lashes, (d) contact lenses (gas permeable scleral) for protection, and (e) mucous membrane grafting (e.g. buccal mucosa autograft) for forniceal reconstruction.
- *Corneal rehabilitation:* (a) superficial keratectomy for keratinization, (b) lamellar keratoplasty for superficial scarring (provided limbal stem cell population is adequate), (c) amniotic membrane grafting, (d) limbal stem cell transplantation (cadaveric or living relative), and (e) keratoprosthesis in end-stage disease.

Miscellaneous conjunctivitis

Superior limbic keratoconjunctivitis

Pathogenesis: chronic disease of the superior limbus and superior conjunctiva; typically affects both eyes of middle-aged women, approximately 50% of whom have abnormal thyroid function. It is believed to be the result of a self-perpetuating cycle of blink-related trauma between the upper lid and bulbar conjunctiva, exacerbated by tear insufficiency.

Diagnosis

- *Presentations:* foreign body sensation, burning, mild photophobia, and mucoid discharge, often intermittent and typically more marked than the signs.
- *Cornea:* (a) velvety papillary hypertrophy and hyperaemia of the superior tarsus (*Fig. 5.43*) and

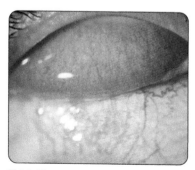

Fig 5.43

limbus (*Fig. 5.44*); (b) light downward pressure on the upper lid results in a fold of redundant conjunctiva crossing the upper limbus (*Fig. 5.45*).

- *Cornea:* (a) superior punctate epithelial erosions, (b) superior filamentary keratitis (*Fig. 5.46*), and (c) keratoconjunctivitis sicca in approximately 50%.

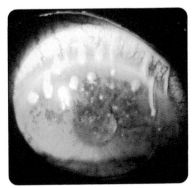

Fig 5.46

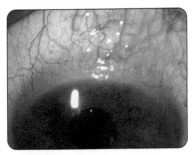

Fig 5.44

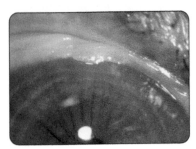

Fig 5.45

Treatment

- *Topical:* (a) lubricants, (b) mucolytics (e.g. acetylcysteine 5% or 10%) to break down filaments, (c) mast cell stabilizers and steroids to address the inflammatory component, (d) ciclosporin 0.05% twice daily, and (e) retinoic acid to retard keratinization.
- *Soft contact lenses:* may help by intervening between the lid and the superior conjunctiva.
- *Supratarsal steroid injection:* (0.1 ml of triamcinolone acetonide 40 mg/ml).
- *Other measures:* (a) temporary punctal occlusion, (b) resection of the superior limbal conjunctiva, (c) conjunctival ablation with silver nitrate 0.5% or thermocautery, and (d) treatment of associated thyroid dysfunction.

Ligneous conjunctivitis

Pathogenesis: systemic disease in which deficiency in plasmin-mediated fibrinolysis may be a key factor; death can occasionally occur from pulmonary involvement.

Diagnosis

- *Presentation:* nonspecific conjunctivitis in childhood, although may be at any age.
- *Signs:* (a) red-white conjunctival masses of wood-like consistency (*Fig. 5.47*), (b) thick yellow-white mucoid discharge (*Fig. 5.48*), and (c) corneal scarring and vascularization, with melting in advanced disease.

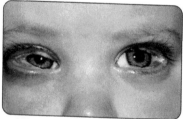

Fig 5.47

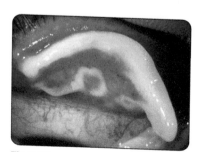

Fig 5.48

Treatment

- Discontinue any antifibrinolytic drugs.
- Surgical removal with diathermy of the base of the lesion.
- Following removal, hourly heparin and steroids are continued until the wound has re-epithelialized.
- Recurrence may be retarded by long-term topical ciclosporin and steroids.
- Intravenous and/or topical plasminogen may be helpful.

Parinaud oculoglandular syndrome

Pathogenesis: cat-scratch disease (*Bartonella henselae*) is by far the most common cause; others include various infective agents, and insect hairs (ophthalmia nodosum).

Diagnosis: (a) chronic low-grade fever, (b) unilateral granulomatous conjunctivitis (*Fig. 5.49*), and (c) ipsilateral preauricular lymphadenopathy.

Treatment: (see Chapter 11 for cat-scratch disease).

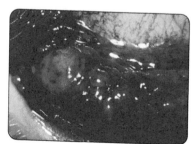

Fig 5.49

Factitious conjunctivitis

Pathogenesis: self-injury, usually intentional although can also occur inadvertently (e.g. mucus fishing syndrome and removal of contact lenses). Instillation of readily accessible irritant substances, such as soap, can also be responsible.

Diagnosis

- The patient may have sought multiple opinions over an extended period for a range of conditions.
- Affected site is usually inferior conjunctiva, with hyperaemia and staining (*Fig. 5.50*).
- Linear corneal abrasions, persistent epithelial defects, and occasionally corneal perforation.
- Secondary infection may occur, particularly fungal with *Candida* spp.

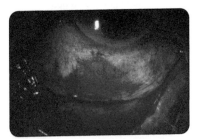

Fig 5.50

Management: (a) exclusion of other diagnoses, (b) confrontation (often leads to failure to return for review), and (c) psychiatric opinion may be appropriate.

Degenerations

Pingueculum

Pathogenesis: degeneration of the collagen fibres of the conjunctival stroma resulting from actinic damage, similar to the aetiology of pterygium (see below).

Diagnosis

- Usually asymptomatic yellow-white mound on the bulbar conjunctiva adjacent to the limbus (*Fig. 5.51*), more frequently nasal than temporal.
- Calcification is occasionally visible.
- Acute inflammation (pingueculitis) may occasionally occur.

Treatment: usually unnecessary; short course of a weak topical steroid for pingueculitis; excision occasionally required.

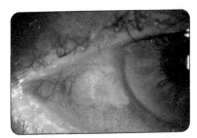

Fig 5.51

Pterygium

Pathogenesis: actinic damage in people living in hot, sunny climates. Pseudopterygium broadly resembles pterygium but is caused by a band of conjunctiva adhering to cornea at its apex as a response to an acute inflammatory episode.

Diagnosis

- *Presentation:* (a) often asymptomatic but sometimes irritation or (b) inflammation, and (c) occasionally visual interference (obstruction of the visual axis or induced astigmatism).
- *Signs:* triangular fibrovascular ingrowth, usually located medially, consisting of (a) a 'cap' (avascular zone at the advancing edge), (b) head, and (c) body (*Fig. 5.52*).

Concretions

Pathogenesis: deposits of epithelial debris, usually age-related although can also form in patients with chronic conjunctivitis.

Diagnosis: multiple tiny yellowish-white subepithelial cysts in the inferior tarsal and forniceal conjunctiva (*Fig. 5.53*); can become calcified and may erode the overlying epithelium to cause irritation.

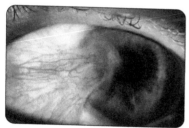

Fig 5.52

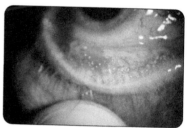

Fig 5.53

Treatment

- Lubricants and topical steroids for inflammatory episodes.
- Sunglasses may decrease the growth stimulus.
- Simple excision (80% recurrence); adjunctive treatment with mitomycin C or beta irradiation to prevent recurrence (risk of late scleral necrosis).
- Conjunctival autografting is commonly performed (donor patch from superior paralimbal area).
- Amniotic membrane patch grafting or peripheral lamellar keratoplasty is occasionally indicated.

Treatment: if symptomatic can be removed at the slit lamp with a needle.

Conjunctivochalasis

Pathogenesis: normal ageing change exacerbated by chronic blepharitis or dry eye.

Diagnosis: fold of redundant conjunctiva protruding over the lower eyelid margin (*Fig. 5.54*); may cause watering by mechanically obstructing the inferior punctum.

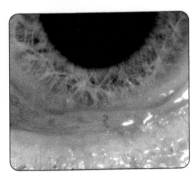

Fig 5.54

Treatment: (a) treatment of blepharitis, (b) lubricants, (c) short course of topical steroids, and (d) conjunctival resection in severe cases.

Retention (epithelial inclusion) cyst

Pathogenesis: fluid-filled cyst lined by a double epithelial layer that may be primary or secondary (e.g. post-surgical).

Diagnosis
- **Signs:** clear-walled lesion containing clear (*Fig. 5.55*) or occasionally turbid fluid.
- **Differential diagnosis:** lymphangiectasia, characterized by strings of cystic or sausage-shaped clear-walled channels that may fill with blood (haemorrhagic lymphangiectasia).

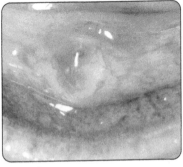

Fig 5.55

Treatment: needle puncture, with bleeding encouraged to promote adhesion; excision if puncture fails.

Cornea

Bacterial keratitis

Pathogenesis
- *Pathogens:* most common are
  (a) *Pseudomonas aeruginosa*,
  (b) *S. aureus*, and (c) streptococci.
- *Risk factors:* (a) contact lens wear,
  (b) trauma, and (c) ocular surface
  disease.

Diagnosis
- *Presentation:* subacute onset of
  pain, photophobia, blurred vision,
  and discharge.
- *Signs:* (a) epithelial defect
  with larger infiltrate (*Fig. 6.1*),
  (b) stromal oedema, (c) anterior
  uveitis, often with hypopyon
  (*Fig. 6.2*), and (d) severe
  ulceration may lead to
  descemetocele formation and
  perforation (*Fig. 6.3*).
- *Differential diagnosis:*
  (a) alternative microorganisms
  (fungi, acanthamoeba, stromal
  herpes simplex keratitis,
  mycobacteria), (b) severe marginal
  keratitis, and (c) sterile infiltrates
  associated with contact lens wear.
- *Investigations:* (a) corneal scraping
  for microscopy, (b) culture (blood,

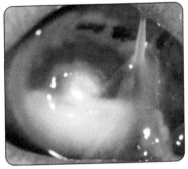

Fig 6.2

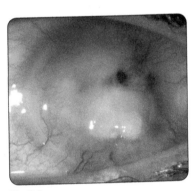

Fig 6.3

chocolate, and Sabouraud agar)
with antibiotic sensitivity
determination, (c) conjunctival
swabs, and (d) culture of contact
lenses and lens cases.

Treatment
- *Indications for hospital admission:*
  (a) patients unlikely to comply
  or unable to self-administer
  treatment, and (b) aggressive
  disease/only eye.
- *Topical antibiotics:* instillation at
  hourly intervals for 24–48 h, and
  then tapered according to clinical

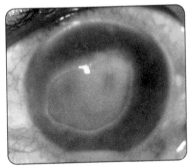

Fig 6.1

progress; options include (a) monotherapy with a fluoroquinolone (e.g. ciprofloxacin, ofloxacin, moxifloxacin, gatifloxacin); (b) duotherapy (e.g. cefuroxime 5%, gentamicin 1.5%) may be preferred as first-line empirical treatment in aggressive disease or if streptococci suspected; (c) if no improvement is evident after 24–48 hr, the regimen should be reviewed; and (d) if there is still no improvement after a further 48 hr, suspension of treatment should be considered for 24 hr and then re-scraping performed, with investigation for nonbacterial infection (additional stains and culture media). Corneal biopsy for histology and culture may be necessary in difficult cases.

- *Topical steroids:* may be commenced once clinical improvement is seen, but early discontinuation may lead to recurrence of sterile inflammation.
- *Indications for systemic antibiotics:* (a) potential for systemic involvement (*N. meningitidis*, *H. influenzae*, *N. gonorrhoeae*), (b) severe corneal thinning with threatened perforation (ciprofloxacin for antibacterial activity and a tetracycline for anticollagenase effect), and (c) scleral involvement.
- *Surgery:* excisional keratoplasty, (penetrating or deep lamellar), may be considered in resistant cases or for incipient or actual perforation.

Fungal keratitis

Predisposing factors: (a) chronic ocular surface disease, (b) long-term use of topical steroids, often with prior corneal transplantation, (c) contact lens wear, (d) systemic immunosuppression, (e) diabetes, and (f) trauma often involving plant matter or gardening/agricultural tools, (filamentous keratitis).

Diagnosis

- *Presentation:* gradual onset of pain, grittiness, photophobia, blurred vision, and watery or mucopurulent discharge; diagnosis is often delayed unless there is a high index of suspicion.
- *Candida keratitis:* (a) yellow-white densely suppurative infiltrate (*Fig. 6.4*); (b) a collar-stud morphology may be seen.
- *Filamentous keratitis:* (a) grey or yellow-white stromal infiltrate with indistinct fluffy margins, satellite lesions (*Fig. 6.5*), (b) feathery extensions, and/or (c) ring-shaped infiltrate.
- *Other features:* (a) anterior uveitis, (b) endothelial plaque, (c) scleritis, and (d) sterile or infective

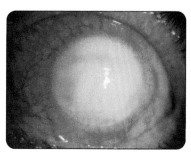

Fig 6.4

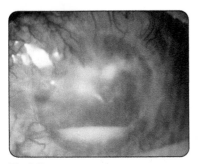

Fig 6.5

endophthalmitis; an epithelial defect is not always present.

- **Differential diagnosis:** bacterial, herpetic, and acanthamoebal keratitis; co-infection can occur.
- **Investigations:** (a) scraping for Gram and Giemsa staining (both approximately 50% sensitive), (b) silver stains (more commonly performed on histological sections), (c) culture on Sabouraud agar (most fungi will also grow on blood agar and enrichment media), (d) culture of contact lenses and lens cases, (e) corneal biopsy; (f) confocal microscopy may permit *in vivo* identification.

Treatment

- **Topical:** initially hourly for 48 h and then reduced as signs permit; most antifungals are only fungistatic, so treatment should be continued for at least 12 weeks. Improvement may be slower than in bacterial infection; removal of epithelium over the lesion may enhance drug penetration.
- **Candida infection:** amphotericin B 0.15% or econazole 1%; alternatives include natamycin 5%,

fluconazole 2%, and clotrimazole 1%.

- **Filamentous infection:** atamycin 5% or econazole 1%; alternatives include amphotericin B 0.15% and miconazole 1%.
- **Systemic antifungals:** (voriconazole, itraconazole, fluconazole) should be considered in (a) severe cases, (b) lesions near the limbus, or (c) suspected endophthalmitis.
- **Other measures:** (a) systemic tetracycline for significant thinning, (b) superficial keratectomy can be effective for de-bulking, and (c) therapeutic keratoplasty (penetrating or deep anterior lamellar) when medical therapy is ineffective or following perforation.

Herpes simplex keratitis

Pathogenesis

Herpes simplex keratitis is the most common infectious cause of corneal blindness in developed countries. Herpes simplex virus (HSV) has two subtypes:

- **HSV-1:** causes disease principally above the waist.
- **HSV-2:** causes venereally acquired infection (genital herpes).
- **Primary infection:** usually occurs subclinically in childhood; subclinical reactivation can occur, during which patients are contagious.
- **Clinical reactivation:** can occur in response to a variety of stressors (e.g. fever, hormonal change, ultraviolet radiation); the virus replicates and is transported in the sensory axons to the periphery, the

pattern of disease depending on the site of reactivation.

- *Epithelial (dendritic or geographic) keratitis:* caused by active viral replication.
- *Disciform keratitis:* caused by hypersensitivity reaction to viral antigen.
- *Necrotizing stromal keratitis:* caused by active viral replication within the stroma, although immune-mediated inflammation plays a significant role.

Epithelial keratitis

Diagnosis
- *Presentation:* mild discomfort, redness, photophobia, watering, and blurred vision.
- *Signs:* (a) swollen opaque epithelial cells arranged in a coarse punctate or stellate pattern, (b) formation of a branching 'dendritic' ulcer with characteristic terminal buds (*Fig. 6.6*), and (c) reduced corneal sensation; inadvertent use of topical steroids may promote enlargement of the ulcer to a geographic configuration (*Fig. 6.7*).

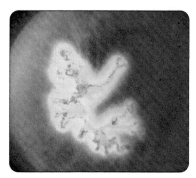

Fig 6.6

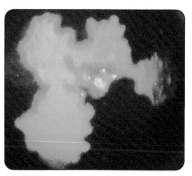

Fig 6.7

Treatment
- *Topical antivirals:* (aciclovir ointment, ganciclovir gel, trifluridine solution) have approximately equivalent effect, with vidarabine an alternative; most cases resolve within 2 weeks on treatment.
- *Debridement:* 2 mm beyond the ulcer edge with a sterile cellulose sponge may be used as an adjunct; this protects adjacent epithelium from infection and reduces the antigenic stimulus to inflammation.
- *Oral antivirals:* (aciclovir, famciclovir, valaciclovir) are an effective alternative to topical therapy, when the latter is poorly tolerated, or in resistant cases; combination of two topical agents with oral valaciclovir or famciclovir may be effective.

Disciform keratitis

Diagnosis
- *Presentation:* blurred vision, mild discomfort, and redness.
- *Signs:* (a) central zone of stromal oedema with overlying epithelial

oedema, underlying keratic precipitates, and folds in Descemet membrane (*Fig. 6.8*), (b) surrounding (Wessely) immune ring of stromal haze (*Fig. 6.9*), and (c) reduced corneal sensation.

- *Course:* consecutive episodes may be associated with gradually worsening scarring and superficial or deep vascularization; mid-stromal scarring can appear as interstitial keratitis.

Treatment

- *Initial:* topical steroids (prednisolone 1%, dexamethasone 0.1%) with antiviral cover, both four times daily.
- *Subsequent:* as improvement occurs, both are tapered. Some patients require a weaker steroid (fluorometholone 0.1%, loteprednol 0.2%) on alternate days for many months; topical ciclosporin 0.05% may be useful as a steroid-sparing agent.

Necrotizing stromal keratitis

Diagnosis: (a) stromal necrosis and melting; may be associated with an epithelial defect (*Fig. 6.10*), (b) progression to scarring, vascularization, and lipid deposition (*Fig. 6.11*).

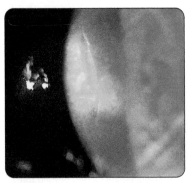

Fig 6.8

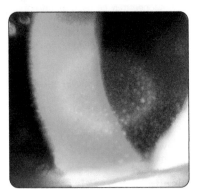

Fig 6.9

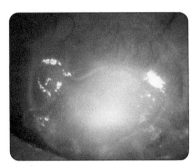

Fig 6.10

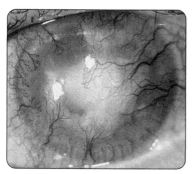

Fig 6.11

Treatment: similar to aggressive disciform keratitis (see above), but oral antivirals are required; restoration of epithelial integrity is vital.

Neurotrophic ulceration

Pathogenesis: failure of epithelial integrity resulting principally from corneal anaesthesia.

Diagnosis: (a) nonhealing epithelial defect; (b) underlying stroma is grey and opaque, and may become progressively thin (*Fig. 6.12*).

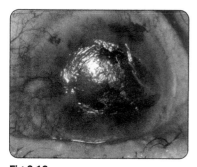

Fig 6.12

Treatment: as for any persistent epithelial defect; topical steroid to control any inflammatory component should be kept to a minimum.

Other considerations

- *Prophylaxis:* long-term daily oral aciclovir reduces the rate of recurrence of epithelial and stromal keratitis by approximately 50%. It should be considered in patients with frequent recurrences, particularly if bilateral or involving an only eye.
- *Major complications:* (a) secondary microbial infection, (b) glaucoma secondary to inflammation or prolonged topical steroids, (c) cataract secondary to inflammation or prolonged topical steroids, and (d) patchy iris atrophy following keratouveitis.
- *Keratoplasty:* carries a high risk of recurrence of active infection and rejection; prophylactic oral antivirals may improve the prognosis.

Herpes zoster ophthalmicus

Pathogenesis: VZV causes both chickenpox (varicella) and shingles (herpes zoster). After an episode of chickenpox, the virus travels to sensory ganglia and remains dormant, with reactivation thought to occur after specific immunity has faded. Herpes zoster ophthalmicus (HZO) is shingles involving a dermatome of the ophthalmic division of the trigeminal nerve. HZO occurs most frequently in the elderly, and immunocompromised patients tend to have more severe disease. Hutchinson's sign refers to the rash of HZO affecting the skin on the tip and side of the nose (*Fig. 6.13*), and correlates strongly with involvement of the eye.

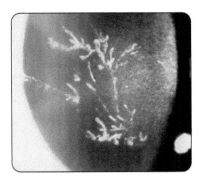

Fig 6.14

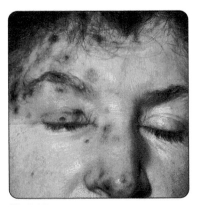

Fig 6.13

Diagnosis and treatment of cutaneous lesions (see Chapter 1).
Ocular manifestations
- *Acute epithelial keratitis:* small fine dendritiform lesions (*Fig. 6.14*); resolve spontaneously within a few days.
- *Conjunctivitis:* follicular and/or papillary is common; treatment is not required.
- *Episcleritis:* NSAIDs may be used if necessary.
- *Scleritis and sclerokeratitis:* treatment is with oral flurbiprofen.
- *Nummular keratitis (Fig. 6.15):* may develop at the site of epithelial lesions; treatment is with topical steroids if symptomatic, with slow tapering.

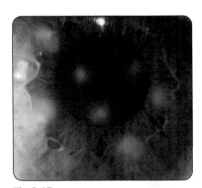

Fig 6.15

- *Stromal keratitis:* responds to topical steroids but can become chronic and requires slow tapering.
- *Disciform keratitis:* less common than with herpes simplex infection; treatment is with topical steroids.
- *Anterior uveitis:* affects at least one-third of patients and can be associated with sectoral iris atrophy (*Fig. 6.16*).
- *Intraocular pressure (IOP) elevation:* inflammatory or

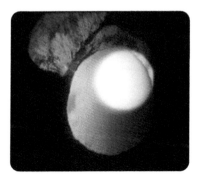

Fig 6.16

steroid-induced; prostaglandin derivatives should be avoided.
- **Neuro-ophthalmological complications:** may require intravenous antivirals and systemic steroids.
- **Neurotrophic keratitis:** common but usually mild and settles over months.
- **Mucous plaque keratitis:** uncommon; treatment involves topical steroids and acetylcysteine.
- **Eyelids:** cicatricial ptosis, entropion, and trichiasis.
- **Reactivation:** keratitis, episcleritis, scleritis, or iritis may occur years after an acute episode.
- **Post-herpetic neuralgia:** pain that persists for more than 1 month after the rash has healed develops in up to 75% of patients older than 70 years of age.

Interstitial keratitis

Pathogenesis

Interstitial keratitis (IK) is inflammation of the corneal stroma without primary involvement of the epithelium or endothelium; usually an immune-mediated process. Congenital syphilis is the classic cause but is now rare in developed countries. IK is less common in acquired than in congenital disease. Other causes include herpetic and other viral infections, tuberculosis, sarcoidosis, and Cogan syndrome (see below).

Syphilitic

Diagnosis
- **Systemic features of congenital syphilis:** (a) early features include rhinitis, failure to thrive, rash, mucosal ulcers, fissures around the lips (rhagades), pneumonia, and neurological and cardiovascular problems; (b) late features include deafness, 'saddle' nose (Fig. 6.17), 'sabre' tibiae, 'bulldog' jaw, Hutchinson's teeth (Fig. 6.18), and Clutton joints (painless effusions).
- **Ocular features of congenital syphilis:** (a) anterior uveitis, (b) IK, (c) subluxated lens, (d) 'salt-and-pepper' pigmentary retinopathy, and (e) Argyll Robertson pupils.

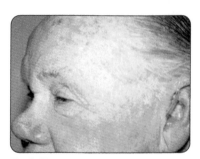

Fig 6.17

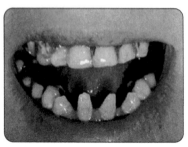

Fig 6.18

- *Progression of IK in congenital
  syphilis:* presents between the
  ages of 5 and 25 years with
  (a) deep stromal vascularization
  associated with clouding ('salmon
  patch'); (b) the cornea clears over
  months and the vessels become
  nonperfused ('ghost' vessels; *Fig.
  6.19*); (c) the healed stage is
  characterized by feathery deep
  stromal scarring (*Fig. 6.20*).
- *Ocular features of acquired
  syphilis:* (a) anterior uveitis, (b) IK,
  (c) madarosis, (d) optic neuritis,

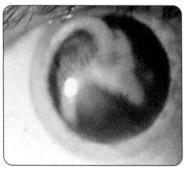

Fig 6.20

    (e) ocular motor nerve palsies,
    and (f) Argyll Robertson pupils.

Treatment

- *Acquired syphilis:* penicillin, or
  alternatives if penicillin-allergic.
- *Congenital syphilis:* all patients
  with positive treponemal serology
  should be referred to a
  genitourinary medicine specialist
  for evaluation.
- *Treatment of active syphilitic IK:*
  systemic antibiotics, topical
  steroids and cycloplegics.

Cogan syndrome

Pathogenesis: rare autoimmune
systemic vasculitis, typically affecting
young adults; characterized
by intraocular inflammation and
vestibuloauditory dysfunction.

Diagnosis

- *Presentation:* hearing loss and
  vertigo that may be separated by
  months.
- *Signs:* faint bilateral peripheral
  anterior stromal corneal
  opacities progressing to
  deeper opacification and
  neovascularization (*Fig. 6.21*).

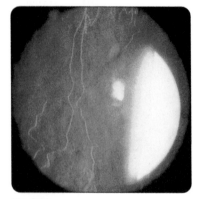

Fig 6.19

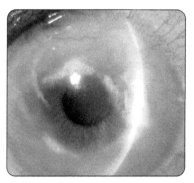

Fig 6.21

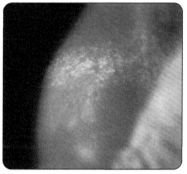

Fig 6.22

- *Associated features:* uveitis, scleritis and retinal vasculitis.

Treatment

- *Topical steroids:* for keratitis.
- *Systemic steroids:* for scleritis, retinal vasculitis and vestibuloauditory symptoms.
- *Immunosuppressive therapy:* may be required.

Protozoan keratitis

Acanthamoeba

Pathogenesis: *Acanthamoeba* spp. are commonly found in soil, water, and the upper respiratory tract. The cystic form is highly resilient. In developed countries, keratitis is most frequently associated with contact lens wear, especially if tap water is used for rinsing.

Diagnosis

- *Presentation:* blurred vision and pain, which may be severe and disproportionate to the clinical signs.
- *Keratitis:* (a) irregular and greyish epithelium (*Fig. 6.22*),

(b) pseudodendrites, (c) perineural infiltrates (radial keratoneuritis; *Fig. 6.23*) are pathognomonic, (d) diffuse or focal anterior stromal infiltrates may coalesce to a ring abscess (*Fig. 6.24*) which may progress to melting (*Fig. 6.25*), and to (e) slowly progressive stromal opacification and vascularization.

- *Limbitis:* progressing to scleritis.
- *Differential diagnosis:* herpes simplex keratitis.

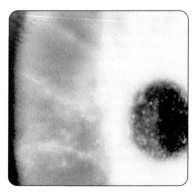

Fig 6.23

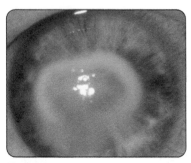

Fig 6.24

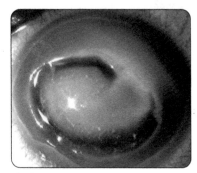

Fig 6.25

- **Investigations:** (a) staining of
  corneal scrapings using periodic
  acid–Schiff or calcofluor white
  stains (Gram and Giemsa may
  also demonstrate cysts);
  (b) culture on non-nutrient agar
  seeded with dead *Escherichia coli*;
  30% culture negative;
  (c) immunohistochemistry;
  (d) PCR; (e) *in vivo* confocal
  microscopy; and (f) corneal biopsy.

Treatment
- **Debridement** of infected
  epithelium.
- **Topical amoebicides:** (e.g.
  polyhexamethylene biguanide,

chlorhexidine digluconate), hourly
at first and gradually reduced;
relapses are common and
treatment may be required for
many months.
- **Topical steroids:** avoided if
  possible.
- **Pain control:** oral NSAIDs (e.g.
  flurbiprofen).
- **Keratoplasty:** for residual scarring.

Onchocerciasis

Pathogenesis: onchocerciasis ('river
blindness') is caused by infestation
with the parasitic helminth
Onchocerca volvulus. It is the second
most common infectious cause of
blindness in the world and is
endemic in areas of Africa.

Diagnosis
- **Systemic features:** (see
  Chapter 11).
- **Signs:** (a) anterior uveitis and
  pear-shaped pupillary dilatation,
  (b) sclerosing keratitis which
  starts at 3 and 9 o'clock
  and progresses (*Fig. 6.26*) to
  involve the entire cornea, and

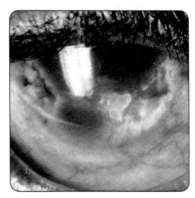

Fig 6.26

(c) chorioretinitis (see *Fig. 11.28*); live microfilariae may be seen in the anterior chamber.

Treatment: systemic ivermectin and topical steroids.

Bacterial hypersensitivity-mediated corneal disease

Marginal keratitis

Pathogenesis: hypersensitivity reaction to staphylococcal exotoxins and cell wall proteins.

Diagnosis
- *Presentation:* mild discomfort, redness, and lacrimation.
- *Signs:* (a) marginal subepithelial infiltrates separated from the limbus by a clear zone (*Fig. 6.27*); (b) epithelial defects, characteristically smaller than the underlying infiltrate; (c) superficial scarring, slight thinning, and mild pannus; associated chronic anterior blepharitis is common.

Treatment
- Spontaneous resolution generally occurs in 3–4 weeks, unless secondary infection occurs.
- Treat associated chronic blepharitis if necessary.
- Weak topical steroid three times daily for 1 week, sometimes in combination with an antibiotic.
- Oral tetracycline (erythromycin in children) may rarely be required.

Phlyctenulosis

Pathogenesis: delayed hypersensitivity reaction to staphylococcal antigen.

Diagnosis
- *Presentation:* in a child or young adult with photophobia, lacrimation, and blepharospasm.
- *Signs:* (a) small white nodule on the conjunctiva (*Fig. 6.28*) or limbus, associated with intense local hyperaemia; (b) a limbal phlycten which may extend onto the cornea (*Fig. 6.29*) and leave a scar; (c) spontaneous resolution

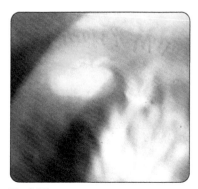

Fig 6.27

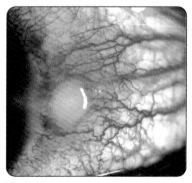

Fig 6.28

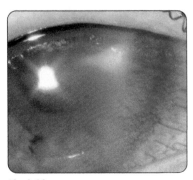

Fig 6.29

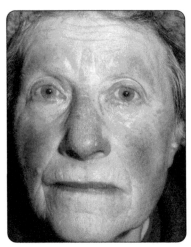

Fig 6.30

within 2–3 weeks; and (d) rarely thinning and perforation.

Treatment: topical steroids accelerate healing; oral tetracycline for recurrent disease.

Rosacea

Pathogenesis: uncertain, with interaction of different factors likely.

Diagnosis

- *Presentation:* in adult life with (a) facial flushing principally involving the forehead, nose, cheeks, and chin (*Fig. 6.30*), (b) papulopustular rash and focal skin thickening (e.g. rhinophyma), and (c) nonspecific ocular irritation, burning, and lacrimation.
- *Eyelids:* (a) telangiectasia, (b) chronic posterior blepharitis, and (c) recurrent chalazia.
- *Conjunctiva:* hyperaemia and occasionally phlyctenulosis.

- *Cornea:* (a) inferior punctate epithelial erosions, (b) peripheral vascularization (*Fig. 6.31*), (c) marginal keratitis, (d) corneal thinning, and (e) melting/ perforation and scarring (*Fig. 6.32*).

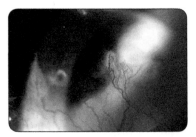

Fig 6.31

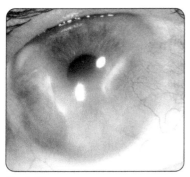

Fig 6.32

Treatment

- *General:* (a) avoidance of trigger factors (e.g. alcohol, spicy food), (b) topical metronidazole gel, azelaic acid cream, (c) oral isotretinoin (not in pregnancy), and (d) oral tetracycline (not in children or in pregnant or breast-feeding women); alternatives include clarithromycin and metronidazole.
- *Ocular:* (a) lubricants for mild symptoms, (b) hot compresses and lid hygiene, (c) topical antibiotics such as fusidic acid ointment to the lid margins at bedtime for 4 weeks, and (d) weak topical steroids for exacerbations.

Severe peripheral corneal ulceration

Mooren ulcer

Pathogenesis: probably an autoimmune disease, characterized by progressive peripheral stromal ulceration. One form affects predominantly older patients, whereas the second tends to occur in younger individuals, is more aggressive, more likely to be bilateral, and less responsive to treatment.

Diagnosis

- *Cornea:* (a) peripheral ulceration involving the superficial stroma, with variable epithelial loss, (b) circumferential (*Fig. 6.33*) and then central thinning with an undermined infiltrated leading edge, (c) vascularization involving the bed of the ulcer up to its leading edge but not beyond (*Fig. 6.34*), and (d) healing characterized by thinning, vascularization, and scarring.

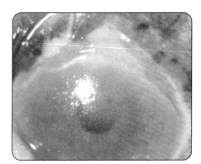

Fig 6.33

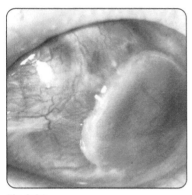

Fig 6.34

- *Complications:* (a) severe astigmatism, (b) perforation following minor trauma (spontaneous perforation is rare), (c) secondary bacterial infection, (d) cataract, and (e) glaucoma.
- *Differential diagnosis:* ulceration associated with systemic autoimmune disease (see below).

Treatment

- *Topical:* lubricants, steroids, ciclosporin, and acetylcysteine 10%.
- *Conjunctival resection:* if no response to topical therapy.
- *Systemic:* immunosuppressives for bilateral or advanced disease (e.g. ciclosporin, prednisolone, methotrexate, azathioprine).
- *Lamellar keratectomy:* dissection of the residual central island in advanced disease may remove the stimulus for further inflammation.

Peripheral ulcerative keratitis associated with systemic autoimmune disease

Systemic associations: rheumatoid arthritis is the most common, followed by Wegener granulomatosis, and occasionally relapsing polychondritis and systemic lupus erythematosus.

Diagnosis

- Crescentic ulceration and stromal infiltration at the limbus (*Fig. 6.35*).
- Limbitis, episcleritis, or scleritis is usually present.
- Circumferential and occasionally central spread; in contrast to Mooren ulcer, the process may also extend into the sclera.
- End-stage disease may result in a 'contact lens' cornea.

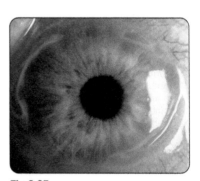

Fig 6.35

Treatment

- *Systemic:* (a) high dose steroids to control acute disease, (b) cytotoxic therapy for long-term management, and (c) tetracycline to retard thinning.

- **Topical:** lubricants; steroids are generally avoided because they may worsen thinning.
- **Other:** conjunctival excision if medical treatment is ineffective.

Terrien marginal degeneration

Definition: uncommon idiopathic thinning of the peripheral cornea. It is bilateral in 75% of patients, the majority of whom are older males.

Diagnosis

- **Presentation:** asymptomatic.
- **Signs:** (a) fine yellow-white punctate peripheral stromal opacities, frequently associated with mild superficial vascularization; start superiorly, spread circumferentially (*Fig. 6.36*), and are separated from the limbus by a clear zone; (b) peripheral guttering (*Fig. 6.37*), and rarely perforation either spontaneously or following blunt trauma; (c) gradual visual deterioration mainly due to astigmatism; and (d) formation of pseudopterygia in long-standing cases (*Fig. 6.38*).

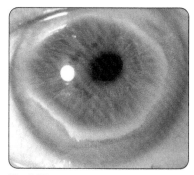

Fig 6.37

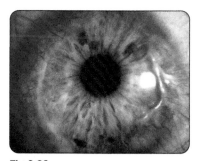

Fig 6.38

Treatment

- **General:** safety spectacle lenses if thinning is significant; contact lenses for astigmatism.
- **Topical:** lubricants or weak steroids (with caution) for inflammatory episodes.
- **Surgery:** crescent-shaped excision of the gutter with suturing of the margins, or peripheral lamellar transplantation; keratoplasty for actual or threatened perforation.

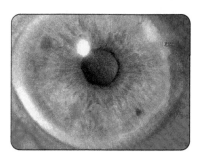

Fig 6.36

Neurotrophic keratopathy

Pathogenesis: loss of trigeminal innervation to the cornea resulting in partial or complete anaesthesia. Causes include (a) ocular disease (e.g. herpes zoster keratitis), (b) focal neurological disease (e.g. acoustic neuroma), and (c) generalized conditions (e.g. diabetes, leprosy).

Diagnosis

- Corneal sensation is tested with a wisp of cotton or an anaesthesiometer.
- Interpalpebral punctate keratopathy; mild epithelial opacification, oedema, and small epithelial defects.
- Persistent epithelial defect in which the epithelium at the edge of the lesion appears rolled and thickened (see *Fig. 6.12*).
- Stromal oedema, infiltration, melting, and occasionally perforation (*Fig. 6.39*).

Treatment

- *Protection of the ocular surface:* (a) taping of the lids, particularly at night, (b) botulinum toxin-induced ptosis, (c) tarsorrhaphy (temporary or permanent), and (d) contact lens (with careful monitoring).
- *Topical lubricants (nonpreserved).*
- *Amniotic membrane patching.*

Exposure keratopathy

Pathogenesis: inadequate lid closure (lagophthalmos), resulting in inadequate corneal wetting. Causes include facial nerve palsy, reduced muscle tone as in coma or parkinsonism, mechanical (e.g. eyelid scarring), and severe proptosis.

Diagnosis

- *Presentation:* symptoms are those of dry eye.
- *Signs:* (a) mild inferior third punctate epithelial changes, often progressing to breakdown (*Fig. 6.40*), (b) stromal melting (*Fig. 6.41*), sometimes with

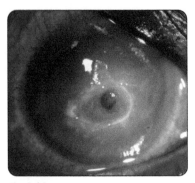

Fig 6.39

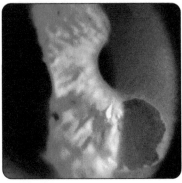

Fig 6.40

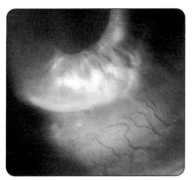

Fig 6.41

perforation, (c) secondary infection (*Fig. 6.42*), and (d) inferior fibrovascular change.

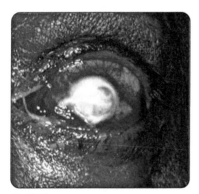

Fig 6.42

Treatment
- *Reversible exposure:* (a) daytime artificial tears, (b) ointment or lid taping at night, (c) bandage contact lens, and (d) temporary tarsorrhaphy.
- *Permanent exposure:* (a) permanent lateral tarsorrhaphy,

(b) upper lid gold weight insertion, and (c) permanent central tarsorrhaphy and/or conjunctival flap in extreme cases.

Miscellaneous keratopathies

Infectious crystalline keratopathy

Pathogenesis: indolent condition usually seen after long-term topical steroid therapy when an epithelial defect has previously been present, especially following penetrating keratoplasty. *Streptococcus viridans* is most commonly isolated.

Diagnosis: (a) slowly progressive grey-white branching stromal opacities (*Fig. 6.43*), (b) minimal inflammation, and (c) intact overlying epithelium.

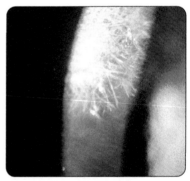

Fig 6.43

Treatment: topical antibiotics for several weeks; stopping steroid without adequate antibiotic cover can precipitate a rapid increase in inflammation.

Thygeson superficial punctate keratitis

Definition: uncommon, usually bilateral, idiopathic condition characterized by exacerbations and remissions; recurrences can continue for decades.

Diagnosis

- *Presentation:* typically in young adult life with recurrent attacks of irritation, photophobia, blurred vision, and watering.
- *Signs:* (a) central, coarse, distinct, granular, greyish, slightly elevated epithelial lesions (*Fig. 6.44*) which stain with fluorescein, and (b) mild subepithelial haze if topical antivirals have been used; the conjunctiva is uninvolved, and the eye is not hyperaemic.
- *Differential diagnosis:* adenoviral keratitis.

Treatment

- *Topical:* (a) lubricants in mild cases, (b) steroids (e.g. fluorometholone 0.1% or loteprednol 0.2%) twice daily, (c) ciclosporin 0.05% is a good alternative to steroids, particularly long term, and (d) bandage contact lenses.
- *Phototherapeutic keratectomy:* confers short-term relief but recurrence is likely.

Filamentary keratopathy

Pathogenesis: focal deposition of mucus and cellular debris at loose areas of epithelium. Causes include (a) dry eye, (b) excessive contact lens wear, (c) recurrent erosions, (d) superior limbic kerato-conjunctivitis, (e) neurotrophic keratopathy, and (f) prolonged eye closure.

Diagnosis

- *Presentation:* discomfort with foreign body sensation and redness.
- *Signs:* (a) strands of degenerated epithelial cells and mucus (*Fig. 6.45*), which move with blinking and are attached at one end to the cornea; (b) filaments stain better with rose Bengal than with

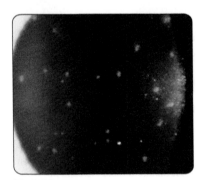

Fig 6.44

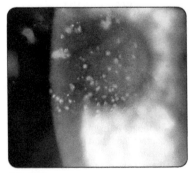

Fig 6.45

fluorescein; (c) chronic filaments may form plaques.

Treatment

- An underlying cause such as dry eye should be addressed.
- Mechanical removal of filaments provides short-term relief.
- Mucolytic drops (e.g. acetylcysteine 5% or 10%).
- NSAIDs (e.g. diclofenac).
- Hypertonic (5%) saline may encourage adhesion of loose epithelium.
- Bandage contact lenses of high oxygen permeability.

Recurrent corneal epithelial erosion

Pathogenesis: tendency for minor trauma to precipitate significant corneal epithelial disturbance, due to an abnormally weak attachment between the epithelium and its basement membrane. Eyelid–corneal interaction during sleep is a typical precipitant. May be associated with previous trauma and with certain corneal dystrophies (see below).

Diagnosis

- *Presentation:* severe pain, photophobia, redness, blepharospasm, and watering, often waking the patient during the night or present on awaking in the morning. There is often a prior history of corneal abrasion.
- *Signs:* a frank epithelial defect (see *Fig.* 6.40) may not be present because healing can be very rapid (hours), but the extent of loose epithelium may be highlighted by areas of pooling of fluorescein and rapid tear film breakup.

Treatment

- *Acute lesions:* (a) antibiotic ointment and a cycloplegic, (b) topical diclofenac 0.1% reduces pain; (topical anaesthetic dramatically relieves pain but should not be dispensed for patient use), (c) bandage contact lens, (d) debridement of heaped/ scrolled areas of epithelium with a cellulose sponge, (e) hypertonic sodium chloride drops and ointment may improve epithelial adhesion, and (f) following resolution, prophylactic topical lubricant such as carbomer gel four times daily for several months.
- *Prophylaxis for recurrent episodes:* (a) long-term gel or ointment instilled at bedtime, (b) debridement of the epithelium of involved areas (may be followed by smoothing of Bowman layer with a diamond burr or excimer laser), (c) long-term extended-wear bandage contact lens, and (d) anterior stromal puncture for localized areas not involving the visual axis.

Xerophthalmia

Pathogenesis: severe deficiency of vitamin A.

Diagnosis

- *Presentation:* night blindness (nyctalopia), ocular discomfort, and impairment of vision.
- *Conjunctiva:* (a) xerosis (dryness of the interpalpebral conjunctiva with loss of goblet cells and squamous metaplasia/ keratinization), and (b) Bitot spots (triangular patches of

foamy keratinized epithelium; *Fig. 6.46*).
- *Cornea:* (a) lack of lustre, (b) interpalpebral punctate corneal epithelial erosions which can progress to epithelial defects, (c) keratinization, and (d) corneal melting by liquefactive necrosis (keratomalacia; *Fig. 6.47*).

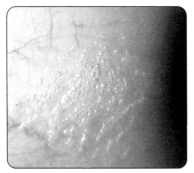

Fig 6.46

- *Retinopathy:* yellowish peripheral dots in advanced cases.

Treatment
- *Systemic:* oral vitamin A (intramuscular for keratomalacia, an indicator of very severe deficiency with risk of death), multivitamin supplements, and dietary sources of vitamin A.
- *Topical:* intense lubrication and retinoic acid to promote healing, but is insufficient without systemic supplements.

Corneal ectasias

Keratoconus

Introduction
- *Definition:* progressive disorder in which the cornea assumes a conical protruding shape (*Fig. 6.48*). Both eyes are affected in almost all cases, although asymmetrically.

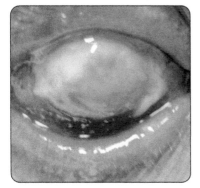

Fig 6.47

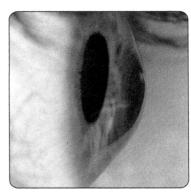

Fig 6.48

- **Systemic associations:** (a) Down, Turner, Ehlers–Danlos, and Marfan syndromes, (b) atopy, and (c) osteogenesis imperfecta.
- **Ocular associations:** (a) vernal keratoconjunctivitis, (b) aniridia, (c) retinitis pigmentosa, and (d) persistent eye rubbing.

Diagnosis

- **Presentation:** during adolescence with unilateral progressive myopia and irregular astigmatism.
- **Signs:** (a) central or paracentral stromal thinning, accompanied by apical protrusion, (b) red reflex shows a fairly well-delineated 'oil droplet' (*Fig. 6.49*), (c) retinoscopy shows an irregular 'scissoring' reflex, (d) fine vertical deep stromal stress lines (Vogt striae; *Fig. 6.50*), (e) epithelial iron

deposits may surround the base of the cone (Fleischer ring), and (f) bulging of the lower lid in downgaze (Munson sign; *Fig. 6.51*).

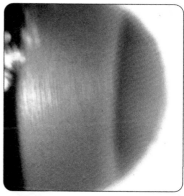

Fig 6.50

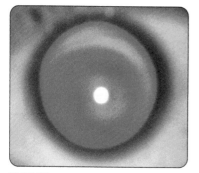

Fig 6.49

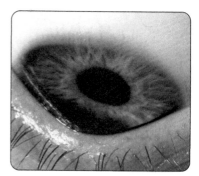

Fig 6.51

- **Acute hydrops (Fig. 6.52):** occurs when a rupture in Descemet membrane allows an influx of aqueous, causing acute discomfort and blurring; stromal scarring may develop (*Fig. 6.53*).

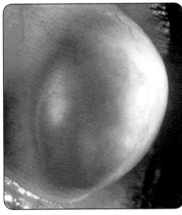

Fig 6.52

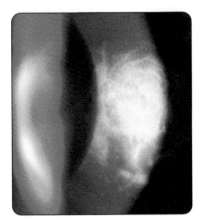

Fig 6.53

- **Investigations:** (a) keratometry shows steep readings; (b) topography detects early keratoconus and can be used to monitor progression.

Treatment

- **Optical:** spectacles or soft contact lenses in early cases, progressing to rigid lenses as the disease advances.
- **Surgery:** (a) keratoplasty in advanced disease (penetrating or deep anterior lamellar keratoplasty (DALK); (b) intracorneal ring segment (Intacs) implantation is usually of moderate benefit.
- **Corneal collagen cross-linking:** using riboflavin drops to photosensitize the eye followed by exposure to ultraviolet-A light; can be combined with Intacs insertion.
- **Of acute hydrops:** (a) cycloplegia, (b) hypertonic (5%) saline ointment, and (c) patching or a bandage contact lens.

Pellucid marginal degeneration

Definition: rare, usually bilateral, progressive peripheral corneal thinning, typically involving the inferior region.

Diagnosis

- **Presentation:** 4th or 5th decade with blurring of vision.
- **Signs:** crescentic band of slowly progressive inferior thinning (*Fig. 6.54*); acute hydrops is rare.
- **Topography:** 'butterfly' pattern with diffuse steepening inferiorly (*Fig. 6.55*).

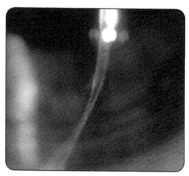

Fig 6.54

Diagnosis

- **Signs:** generalized thinning, with globular (*Fig. 6.56*) rather than conical ectasia; the cornea is more prone to rupture from relatively mild trauma, but acute hydrops is rare.
- **Differential diagnosis:** congenital glaucoma (enlarged diameter) and megalocornea (absence of thinning).

Treatment: care to protect the eyes and scleral contact lenses.

Fig 6.55

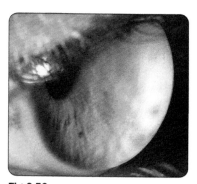

Fig 6.56

Treatment: (a) spectacles usually fail early, necessitating contact lenses; (b) surgery is more difficult than in keratoconus; options include large eccentric penetrating keratoplasty and collagen cross-linking.

Keratoglobus

Definition: extremely rare congenital condition in which the entire cornea is abnormally thin; possibly genetically related to keratoconus.

Corneal dystrophies

Epithelial dystrophies

Introduction: Cogan epithelial basement membrane dystrophy is the most common corneal dystrophy seen in clinical practice. It is usually sporadic and rarely AD. Other epithelial dystrophies (Meesmann and the clinically similar Lisch) are very rare and are not considered.

Diagnosis

- *Presentation:* in the 3rd decade with recurrent corneal erosions, often bilateral; many cases are asymptomatic.
- *Signs (Fig. 6.57):* tend to be fluid and variable and are often subtle or even absent. They may include (a) dot-like opacities, (b) epithelial microcysts, (c) subepithelial map-like patterns surrounded by a faint haze, and (d) whorled fingerprint-like lines.

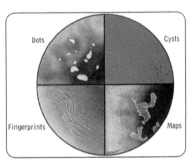

Fig 6.57

Treatment: that of recurrent corneal erosions (see above).

Bowman layer/anterior stromal dystrophies

Genetics and histology

- *Reis–Bücklers:* AD (gene TGFB1); Bowman layer and epithelial basement membrane are replaced by fibrous tissue.
- *Thiel-Behnke:* AD (two main genes implicated, including TGFB1); 'curly fibres' in Bowman layer on electron microscopy.
- *Schnyder central crystalline:* AD disorder of corneal lipid metabolism associated with raised serum cholesterol in 50%.

Diagnosis

- *Reis–Bücklers:* onset in the 1st or 2nd decade with severe recurrent corneal erosions; fine grey-white polygonal subepithelial opacities, most dense centrally (*Fig. 6.58*).
- *Thiel-Behnke:* onset at end of the 1st decade with recurrent erosions; central honeycomb pattern subepithelial opacities (*Fig. 6.59*).

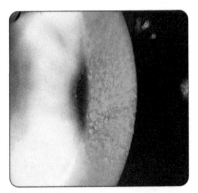

Fig 6.58

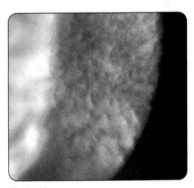

Fig 6.59

- **Schnyder central crystalline:** onset in the 2nd decade with visual impairment and glare; central subepithelial crystalline changes (*Fig. 6.60*), progressing by the 3rd decade to diffuse haze and dense corneal arcus (*Fig. 6.61*).

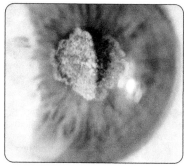

Fig 6.60

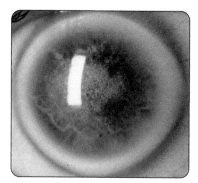

Fig 6.61

Treatment

- **Reis–Bücklers:** recurrent erosions (see above) are the main concern; excimer laser keratectomy achieves satisfactory control, as well as visual benefit, in many patients.
- **Thiel–Behnke:** surgery is required less often than in Reis–Bücklers.
- **Schnyder:** usually excimer laser keratectomy.

Stromal dystrophies

Genetics and histology

- **Lattice type I (Biber–Haab–Dimmer):** AD (gene TGFB1); stromal amyloid staining with Congo red on histology, with characteristic green birefringence when viewed with a polarizing filter.
- **Lattice type II (Meretoja syndrome):** AD; systemic and corneal amyloid.
- **Lattice type IIIA:** AD (gene TGBF1); corneal amyloid.
- **Granular type I:** AD (gene TGFB1); hyaline deposits staining with Masson trichrome.
- **Granular type II (Avellino):** AD (gene TGFB1); hyaline and amyloid deposition.
- **Macular:** rare autosomal recessive (AR) inborn error of keratan sulphate metabolism.

Diagnosis

- **Lattice type I:** onset at the end of the 1st decade with recurrent erosions, preceding stromal changes; anterior stromal refractile dots coalescing into a fine lattice (*Fig. 6.62*), sparing the periphery; vision progressively impaired by haze.
- **Lattice type II (Meretoja syndrome):** onset in the 2nd decade; erosions are rare; short, sparse, fine lattice lines more radially orientated and peripheral than type I. Systemic features

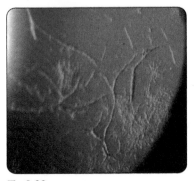

Fig 6.62

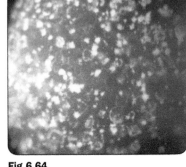

Fig 6.64

include progressive neuropathy, a characteristic 'mask-like' facial expression, and renal and cardiac problems.

- *Lattice type IIIA:* onset in old age; rope-like bands of amyloid (*Fig. 6.63*).
- *Granular type I:* onset 1st decade; vision is usually unaffected until later; small white deposits resembling sugar granules, separated by clear, but later hazy, stroma (*Fig. 6.64*).

- *Granular type II (Avellino):* onset in 2nd decade; superficial opacities resembling rings, stars, or snowflakes, most dense centrally (*Fig. 6.65*).
- *Macular:* onset in late 1st decade with visual deterioration; anterior stromal haze, initially central, with greyish-white, dense, poorly delineated lesions (*Fig. 6.66*) with eventual involvement of full-thickness stroma up to the limbus.

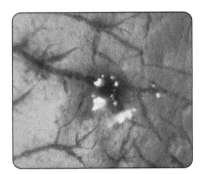

Fig 6.63

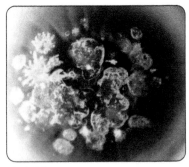

Fig 6.65

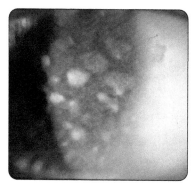

Fig 6.66

Treatment

- **Lattice type I:** penetrating or deep lamellar keratoplasty is frequently required; recurrence in the graft may occur.
- **Lattice type II (Meretoja):** keratoplasty may rarely be required in later life to improve vision.
- **Granular type I:** keratoplasty usually required by the 5th decade, with later superficial keratectomy for anterior recurrences.
- **Granular type II (Avellino):** treatment is usually not required.
- **Macular:** penetrating keratoplasty; recurrence in the graft may occur.

Endothelial dystrophies

Genetics and histology

- **Fuchs endothelial:** majority sporadic, occasionally AD; bilateral accelerated endothelial cell loss.
- **Posterior polymorphous (PPCD):** genetically heterogeneous with three distinct types; endothelial cells display characteristics similar to epithelium.

- **Congenital hereditary (CHED):** AD and AR forms; focal or generalized absence of endothelium.

Diagnosis

- **Fuchs:** (a) onset in old age initially with cornea guttata (*Fig. 6.67*, left), excrescences of Descemet membrane secreted by abnormal endothelial cells; (b) slow progression to a 'beaten metal' appearance, (c) endothelial decompensation leading to stromal then epithelial oedema with blurred vision, worse in the morning, and (d) formation of epithelial bullae (bullous keratopathy; *Fig. 6.67*, right) with discomfort on rupture; cataract surgery accelerates endothelial cell loss.

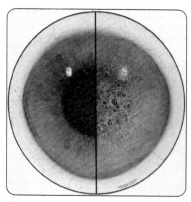

Fig 6.67

- **PPCD:** typically identified incidentally; subtle bilateral vesicular endothelial lesions of variable appearance (*Fig. 6.68*).
- **CHED:** perinatal onset; bilateral, symmetrical, diffuse corneal oedema ranging from a blue-grey,

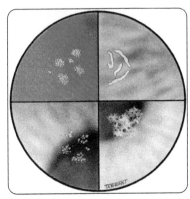

Fig 6.68

ground-glass appearance (*Fig. 6.69*) to total opacification; visual impairment is variable. Differential diagnosis includes other causes of neonatal corneal opacification: (a) congenital glaucoma, (b) birth trauma, and (c) sclerocornea.

Treatment

- *Fuchs:* topical sodium chloride 5% drops or ointment; reduction of intraocular pressure; hair dryer to speed dehydration in the morning;

bandage contact lens for comfort; keratoplasty (penetrating or Descemet stripping endothelial keratoplasty (DSEK)).
- *PPCD:* not required.
- *CHED:* early keratoplasty is technically difficult but has reasonable success; delay is likely to worsen amblyopia.

Corneal degenerations

Age-related degenerations

Diagnosis

- *Arcus senilis:* perilimbal stromal lipid deposition, initially superior and inferior, progressing circumferentially to form a band approximately 1 mm wide separated from the limbus by a clear zone (*Fig. 6.70*); extremely common in the elderly but in younger individuals may be associated with dyslipidaemia.
- *Vogt limbal girdle:* common and innocuous arc-like whitish bands of chalk-like flecks at 9 and/or 3 o'clock, more common nasally; (a) type I has a 'Swiss cheese'

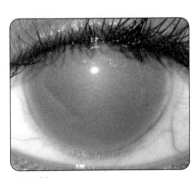

Fig 6.69

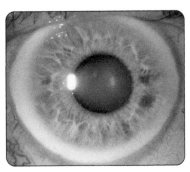

Fig 6.70

hole pattern and a clear peripheral band (*Fig. 6.71*); (b) type II does not show holes and sometimes there is no clear zone.

- *Cornea farinata:* uncommon and innocuous minute flour-like deposits in the deep stroma, most prominent centrally (*Fig. 6.72*).

- *Crocodile shagreen:* uncommon and innocuous greyish-white polygonal stromal (usually anterior) opacities, separated by relatively clear spaces (*Fig. 6.73*) resembling central cloudy dystrophy of François.

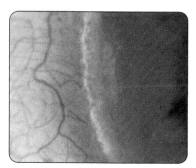

Fig 6.71

Fig 6.73

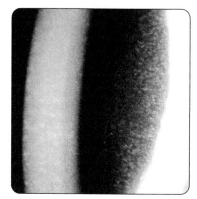

Fig 6.72

Treatment: not required, although arcus senilis in a young person should prompt investigation for a lipid abnormality.

Lipid keratopathy

Pathogenesis: secondary lipid keratopathy is associated with corneal vascularization due to injury or disease (e.g. herpes simplex and zoster); the primary form is rare and occurs spontaneously.

Diagnosis: white-yellow stromal deposits with or without vascularization, with a pattern dependent on any identifiable causative pathology (*Fig. 6.74*).

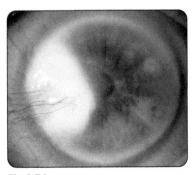

Fig 6.74

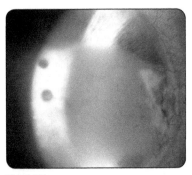

Fig 6.75

Treatment

- Control of any underlying inflammatory disease is critical.
- Photocoagulation of arterial feeder vessels may induce resorption; needle cautery is an alternative.
- Penetrating keratoplasty may be required in advanced disease, although the prognosis is often guarded.

Band keratopathy

Introduction

- *Definition:* band-like deposition of calcium salts in Bowman layer, epithelial basement membrane, and anterior stroma.
- *Ocular causes:* (a) chronic anterior uveitis, (b) phthisis bulbi, and (c) silicone oil in the anterior chamber.
- *Systemic causes:* (a) age-related (common), and metastatic calcification (very rare).

Diagnosis: (a) starts as peripheral interpalpebral calcification with a clear marginal zone; (b) gradual central spread as a plaque containing small holes (*Fig. 6.75*); (c) elevation of calcium may result in epithelial breakdown and discomfort.

Treatment

- For discomfort, or for visual compromise in a seeing eye.
- Underlying ocular or systemic disease should be addressed.
- Chelation with ethylenediaminete-traacetic acid (EDTA) 1.5–3.0%.
- Large chips of calcium can be removed with forceps and a blade.
- Other options include removal with a diamond burr, excimer laser keratectomy and lamellar keratoplasty.

Spheroidal degeneration (Labrador keratopathy)

Pathogenesis: bilateral condition typically occurring in men working outdoors; ultraviolet exposure is probably a key aetiological factor.

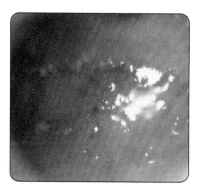

Fig 6.76

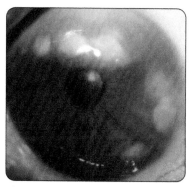

Fig 6.77

Diagnosis: (a) amber-coloured granules in the interpalpebral superficial stroma; (b) advanced lesions are nodular and the surrounding stroma often hazy (*Fig. 6.76*).

Treatment: sunglasses to reduce ultraviolet exposure, and superficial keratectomy or lamellar keratoplasty to improve vision.

Salzmann nodular degeneration

Pathogenesis: chronic corneal irritation or inflammation.

Diagnosis: blue-grey or whitish elevated nodular superficial stromal opacities in scarred cornea or at the edge of transparent cornea (*Fig. 6.77*).

Treatment: principally of the underlying cause; may require surgery as for spheroidal degeneration.

Metabolic keratopathies

Cystinosis

Pathogenesis: AR disorder characterized by widespread tissue deposition of cystine crystals; 'ocular' cystinosis is non-nephropathic.

Diagnosis

- *Presentation:* by age of 1 year with photophobia, recurrent erosions, and blepharospasm; visual impairment occurs by the end of the 1st decade.
- *Systemic features:* severe growth retardation and early renal failure; death may occur in childhood.
- *Keratopathy:* diffuse cystine crystal deposition in the conjunctiva and cornea (*Fig. 6.78*).

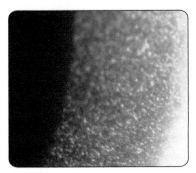

Fig 6.78

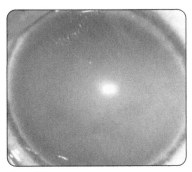

Fig 6.79

- *Other ocular features:* iris, lens, and retina may be affected later.

Treatment: systemic cysteamine may forestall renal disease; topical cysteamine to reduce corneal crystals.

Mucopolysaccharidoses

Pathogenesis: group of inherited metabolic deficiencies with accumulation of anomalous metabolite in various tissues; inheritance is mainly AR; features vary with the type.

Diagnosis
- *Systemic features:* (a) facial coarseness, (b) skeletal anomalies, (c) mental handicap, and (d) heart disease.
- *Keratopathy:* punctate corneal opacification and diffuse stromal haze (*Fig. 6.79*) occur in all mucopolysaccharidoses except Hunter and Sanfilippo, but are most severe in Hurler and Scheie syndromes.

- *Other ocular features:*
  (a) pigmentary retinopathy,
  (b) optic atrophy, and
  (c) occasionally congenital glaucoma.

Treatment: principally supportive care, although some advances have been made in specific therapies; bone marrow transplantation is helpful in some cases.

Wilson disease

Pathogenesis: deficiency of caeruloplasmin leading to widespread tissue deposition of copper.

Diagnosis
- *Presentation:* liver disease, basal ganglia dysfunction, or psychiatric disturbance.
- *Keratopathy:* zone of copper granules in peripheral Descemet membrane (Kayser–Fleischer ring; *Fig. 6.80*), best detected on gonioscopy when subtle.

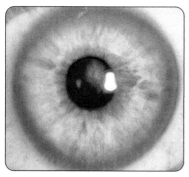

Fig 6.80

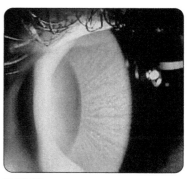

Fig 6.81

- *Other ocular feature:* anterior capsular 'sunflower' cataract is less common.

Treatment: reduction of copper absorption (e.g. zinc) or increased secretion (e.g. penicillamine); liver transplantation may be required.

Fabry disease

Pathogenesis: X-linked lysosomal storage disorder caused by deficiency of alpha-galactosidase.

Diagnosis
- *Systemic features:* (a) periodic burning pain in the extremities, (b) purple cutaneous telangiectasia (angiokeratoma corporis diffusum), (c) hypertrophic cardiomyopathy, and (d) renal disease.
- *Keratopathy:* vortex keratopathy (*Fig. 6.81*).
- *Other ocular features:* conjunctival (*Fig. 6.82*) and retinal vascular tortuosity.

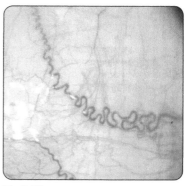

Fig 6.82

Treatment: enzyme replacement therapy and supportive measures.

Contact lenses

Therapeutic uses

- *Optical:* irregular astigmatism, and anisometropia when binocular vision cannot be achieved by spectacles.

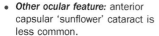

- **Promotion of epithelial healing:** persistent epithelial defects and recurrent corneal erosions.
- **Pain relief:** (a) bullous keratopathy, (b) filamentary keratitis, (c) Thygeson superficial punctate keratitis, and (d) protection from aberrant lashes.
- **Preservation of corneal integrity:** temporary capping of a descemetocele, splinting of a small corneal wound or supporting a glued larger wound.
- **Other:** maintenance of the fornices in cicatrizing conjunctivitis, and drug delivery.

Complications

- **Acute mechanical and hypoxic keratitis:** (a) superficial punctate keratitis, (b) tight lens syndrome (indentation and staining of the conjunctival epithelium in a ring around the cornea), and (c) acute hypoxia (epithelial microcysts, endothelial blebs).
- **Chronic hypoxia:** vascularization and rarely lipid deposition; superficial peripheral neovascularization of <1.5 mm is common.
- **Immune response keratitis:** mildly red eye with small, often marginal, infiltrates but no or minimal epithelial defects, probably due to a hypersensitivity response to bacterial antigen and/or lens care chemicals.
- **Acute toxic keratitis:** mild chemical trauma caused by insertion of a lens without first removing or neutralizing a cleaning agent such as hydrogen peroxide.

- **Chronic toxicity:** long-term exposure to disinfecting preservatives.
- **Suppurative keratitis:** bacterial and other microorganisms.
- **Giant papillary conjunctivitis:** (see Chapter 5).

Congenital anomalies of the cornea and globe

Microcornea

Genetics: AD.
Diagnosis

- **Signs:** unilateral or bilateral; (a) adult horizontal corneal diameter of 10 mm or less (*Fig. 6.83*), and (b) hypermetropia and shallow anterior chamber but other dimensions normal.
- **Associations:** (a) glaucoma (closed and open angle), (b) congenital cataract, (c) other anterior segment malformations, and (d) optic nerve hypoplasia.

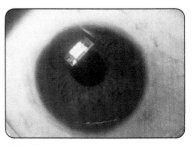

Fig 6.83

Megalocornea

Genetics: X-linked.
Diagnosis
- *Signs:* bilateral; (a) corneal diameter 13 mm or more (*Fig. 6.84*), and (b) high myopia and astigmatism but usually normal visual acuity.
- *Ocular associations:* pigment dispersion syndrome (common), and lens subluxation.
- *Systemic associations:* (a) Alport, Marfan, Ehlers–Danlos, and Down syndromes, and (b) osteogenesis imperfecta.

Diagnosis
- *Simple microphthalmos (Fig. 6.85):* no other major ocular malformations besides the short TAL.
- *Nanophthalmos:* subtype of simple microphthalmos with (a) microcornea, (b) high lens:eye volume ratio, (c) thickened abnormal sclera, and (d) increased risk of uveal effusion and angle closure glaucoma.
- *Complex microphthalmos:* with anterior and/or posterior segment dysgenesis (e.g. coloboma).

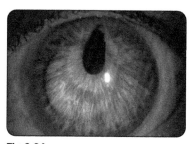

Fig 6.84

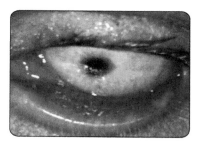

Fig 6.85

Microphthalmos

Definition: total axial length (TAL) at least two standard deviations less than normal for age; the result of stunted growth of the anterior or posterior segment or both; may be unilateral or bilateral.

- *Microphthalmos with cyst:* orbital cyst communicating with the eye.
- *Posterior microphthalmos:* normal corneal diameter.

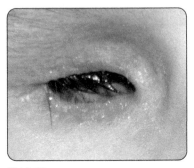

Fig 6.86

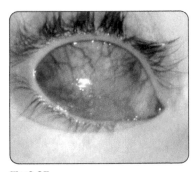

Fig 6.87

Anophthalmos

- *Simple:* complete failure of budding of the optic vesicle or early arrest in its development; associated ocular abnormalities such as the absence of extraocular muscles, a short conjunctival sac, and microblepharon (*Fig. 6.86*).
- *With cyst:* globe replaced by a cyst (*Fig. 6. 87*).

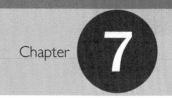

Chapter **7**

Corneal and refractive surgery

Keratoplasty

Introduction

- *Classification:* (a) partial (anterior or posterior lamellar) or (b) full-thickness (penetrating [PKP]).
- *Indications:* (a) optical, (b) tectonic, (c) therapeutic, and (d) cosmetic.
- *Donor tissue:* should be removed within 12–24 hr of death and stored under special conditions; contraindications to donation include certain infections (e.g. HIV) and some forms of ocular disease.

Penetrating keratoplasty

- *Technique:* (a) determination of graft size, (b) trephination of donor tissue, (c) excision of host tissue, and (d) fixation of donor button (*Fig. 7.1*); postoperative topical steroids and cycloplegics.
- *Early postoperative complications:* (a) persistent epithelial defect, (b) wound dehiscence, (c) uveitis, (d) elevation of intraocular pressure, (e) endophthalmitis, and (f) fixed dilated pupil (Urrets–Zavalia syndrome).
- *Late complications:* (a) astigmatism, (b) recurrence of disease in graft, (c) wound separation, (d) retrocorneal membrane formation, (e) glaucoma, and (f) cystoid macular oedema.

Corneal graft rejection

Can be endothelial, stromal, epithelial (rare), or combined.

- *Presentation:* may be asymptomatic (particularly in early stages) or with blurred vision, redness, photophobia, and pain.
- *Signs:* (a) ciliary injection, (b) anterior uveitis, (c) linear endothelial precipitates (Khodadoust line; *Fig. 7.2*), (d) elevated epithelial line (*Fig. 7.3*), (e) focal subepithelial (Krachmer) infiltrates (*Fig. 7.4*), and (f) stromal oedema.

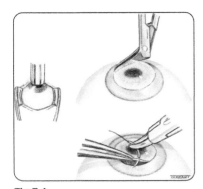

Fig 7.1

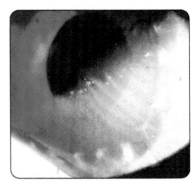

Fig 7.2

Superficial lamellar keratoplasty

- **Technique:** partial-thickness excision of the stroma.
- **Indications:** (a) opacification of the superficial one-third of the stroma, (b) marginal corneal thinning or infiltration, (c) Terrien marginal degeneration, and (d) limbal tumours.

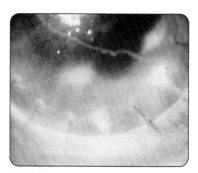

Fig 7.3

Deep anterior lamellar keratoplasty

- **Technique:** opaque corneal tissue removed almost to the level of Descemet membrane.
- **Indications:** (a) disease of the anterior 95% of corneal thickness with normal endothelium and intact Descemet membrane (e.g. no history of acute hydrops); (b) chronic inflammatory disease with a higher risk of rejection (e.g. atopic keratoconjunctivitis).
- **Advantages:** (a) no endothelial rejection, (b) less astigmatism, (c) structurally stronger globe, and (d) increased availability of graft material because endothelial quality is irrelevant.
- **Disadvantages:** technically difficult and time-consuming; interface haze may limit visual outcome.

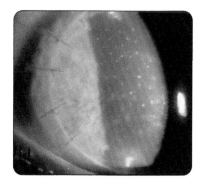

Fig 7.4

- **Treatment:** (a) topical steroid (dexamethasone 0.1% or prednisolone 1%) hourly for 24 h, tapered over months; (b) topical cycloplegics; and (c) systemic and/or subconjunctival steroids, topical ciclosporin, and systemic immunosuppressives may be used in some cases.
- **Differential diagnosis:** (a) graft failure (no inflammation), (b) infective keratitis, (c) sterile suture reaction, and (d) epithelial ingrowth.

Descemet stripping endothelial keratoplasty

- **Technique:** (a) endothelium and Descemet membrane are removed (descemetorhexis), and (b) folded donor tissue is introduced through a small limbal incision.

- *Indications:* endothelial disease (e.g. pseudophakic bullous keratopathy).
- *Advantages:* (a) little refractive change, (b) structurally stronger globe, and (c) no sutures.
- *Disadvantages:* (a) significant learning curve, (b) expensive equipment required for automated method, (c) posterior graft dislocation rate of 15%, (d) endothelial rejection can still occur, and (e) visual outcome may not be as good as with PKP.

Keratoprosthesis

- *Technique:* insertion of an artificial corneal implant such as an osteoodontokeratoprosthesis (*Fig. 7.5*) in which the patient's tooth root and alveolar bone support an optical cylinder.
- *Indications:* when conventional keratoplasty is not possible in severe but inactive corneal disease (e.g. Stevens–Johnson, chemical burns), but with intact optic nerve and retinal function.
- *Complications:* (a) glaucoma, (b) retroprosthetic membrane formation, (c) tilting, (d) extrusion, and (e) endophthalmitis.

Refractive procedures

Introduction

- *Correction of myopia:* (a) photorefractive keratectomy (PRK), (b) laser epithelial keratomileusis (LASEK),(c) laser *in situ* keratomileusis (LASIK; see *Fig. 7.11*), (d) clear lens exchange, (e) iris clip implant ('lobster claw'; *Fig. 7.6*), and (f) phakic posterior chamber implant (implantable contact lens; *Fig. 7.7*).

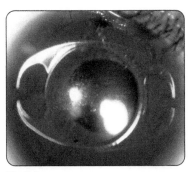

Fig 7.6

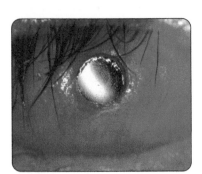

Fig 7.5

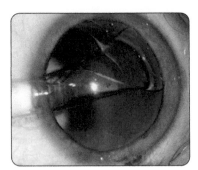

Fig 7.7

- **Correction of hypermetropia (hyperopia):** (a) PRK and LASEK (low degrees), (b) LASIK (up to 4 D, (c) conductive keratoplasty (radiofrequency energy-induced peripheral stromal shrinkage), (d) laser thermal keratoplasty, (e) intracorneal inlays (*Fig. 7.8*), (f) clear lens extraction, and (g) phakic lens implants.

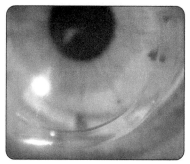

Fig 7.8

- **Correction of astigmatism:** (a) limbal relaxing incisions/arcuate keratotomy, (b) PRK and LASEK (up to 3 D), (c) LASIK (up to 5 D), (d) lens exchange using a 'toric' implant incorporating an astigmatic correction, and (e) conductive keratoplasty.
- **Correction of presbyopia:** (a) lens extraction with a multifocal or 'accommodating' implant, (b) conductive keratoplasty, (c) 'monovision' following lens or laser surgery (one eye set for emmetropia and the other for low myopia), (d) corneal multifocality (e.g. using laser), (e) scleral expansion surgery, (f) intracorneal inlays, and (g) laser to the crystalline lens to improve elasticity.

Laser refractive procedures

- **PRK:** (a) corrects myopia by ablating the central anterior corneal surface with the excimer laser so that it flattens (*Fig. 7.9*); (b) corrects hypermetropia by ablation of the periphery so that the centre steepens; complications include slowly-healing epithelial defects, corneal haze (*Fig. 7.10*), poor night vision, and regression of refractive correction.

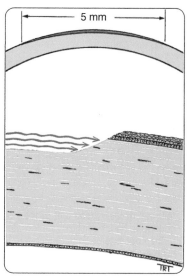

Fig 7.9

- **LASEK:** adaptation of PRK in which the epithelium is first detached and peeled back, then repositioned after laser has been applied, giving less pain, less haze, and more rapid visual recovery than PRK.
- **LASIK:** corrects higher levels of refractive error; involves creation of a superficial stromal flap (*Fig. 7.11*)

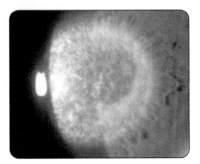

Fig 7.10

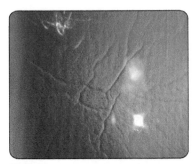

Fig 7.12

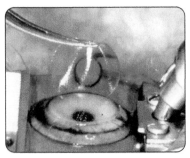

Fig 7.11

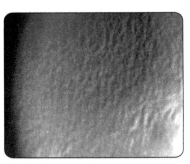

Fig 7.13

followed by laser treatment of the underlying bed; complications include (a) flap damage or amputation, (b) tear film instability, (c) flap distortion (*Fig. 7.12*), (d) subepithelial haze, (e) diffuse lamellar keratitis ('sands of Sahara'; *Fig. 7.13*), and (f) bacterial keratitis (*Fig. 7.14*).

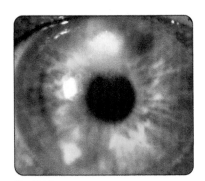

Fig 7.14

Chapter **8**

Episclera and sclera

Episcleritis

Simple episcleritis

Diagnosis
- **Presentation:** acute onset of redness and mild discomfort.
- **Signs:** hyperaemia may be sectoral (typically interpalpebral; *Fig. 8.1*) or diffuse.
- **Course:** spontaneous improvement occurs within several days, but recurrences may occur.

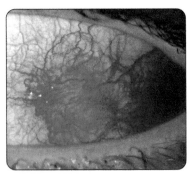

Fig 8.1

Treatment: not required if mild; otherwise lubricants or a weak steroid four times daily for 1–2 weeks.

Nodular episcleritis

Diagnosis
- **Presentation:** less acute onset than simple episcleritis with redness and discomfort worsening over 2–3 days.
- **Signs:** (a) one or more tender interpalpebral nodules (*Fig. 8.2*), and (b) absence of deeper scleral

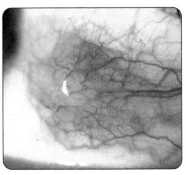

Fig 8.2

thickening; after several attacks, the vessels surrounding the inflamed area may become permanently dilated.
- **Course:** more prolonged than simple episcleritis.

Treatment: similar to that of simple episcleritis.

Immune-mediated scleritis

Anterior non-necrotizing scleritis

Definition: scleritis involves oedema and cellular infiltration of the entire thickness of the sclera; it is much less common than episcleritis and ranges from a trivial and self-limiting to a necrotizing sight-threatening condition.

Diagnosis
- **Presentation:** in 5th decade with redness, discomfort, and aching.
- **Diffuse disease:** redness; generalized (*Fig. 8.3*) or localized to one quadrant.
- **Nodular disease:** (a) single or multiple scleral nodules, of a deeper blue-red colour than

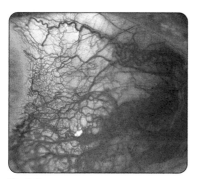

Fig 8.3

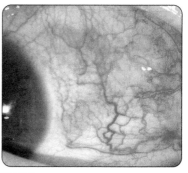

Fig 8.5

episcleral nodules, and (b) vascular congestion and dilatation with oedema and displacement of the entire beam of the slit lamp (*Fig. 8.4*).

- *Course:* as inflammation settles, the affected area often takes on a slight grey/blue appearance due to increased translucency (*Fig. 8.5*); episodes recur over several years, with the frequency decreasing after approximately 18 months.
- *Prognosis:* usually good, although more than 10% of patients with

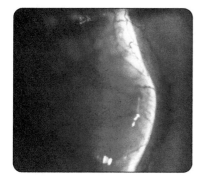

Fig 8.4

nodular scleritis develop necrotizing disease if early treatment is not instituted.

Anterior necrotizing scleritis with inflammation

Definition: aggressive form of scleritis, bilateral in 60%, which may result in severe visual morbidity unless appropriately treated.

Diagnosis

- *Presentation:* later than in non-necrotizing scleritis with the gradual onset of pain that becomes severe and radiating, often interfering with sleep and responding poorly to analgesia.
- *Vaso-occlusive type:* often associated with rheumatoid arthritis; (a) starts as isolated patches of scleral oedema with overlying nonperfused episclera and conjunctiva, and (b) may progress to scleral necrosis (*Fig. 8.6*).
- *Granulomatous type:* associated with Wegener granulomatosis and polyarteritis nodosa; (a) starts with paralimbal injection,

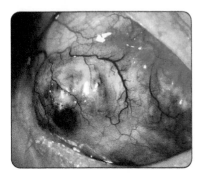

Fig 8.6

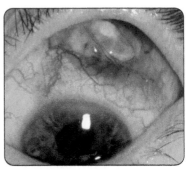

Fig 8.8

(b) subsequently extends posteriorly, and (c) within 24 h, the sclera, episclera, conjunctiva, and adjacent cornea become irregularly raised and oedematous (*Fig. 8.7*).

- *Surgically induced:* develops within weeks of ocular surgery and tends to remain localized to one segment (*Fig. 8.8* shows scleritis following sclera buckling).
- *Investigations:* (a) markers of connective tissue disease such as rheumatoid factor, antinuclear antibody, antineutrophil

cytoplasmic autoantibodies, and antiphospholipid antibodies; (b) fluorescein angiography (FA) and indocyanine green angiography (ICGA) (*Fig. 8.9*) may detect vascular nonperfusion.

- *Complications:* (a) acute and chronic keratitis, (b) uveitis, (c) glaucoma, (d) hypotony, and (e) scleral perforation (rare).

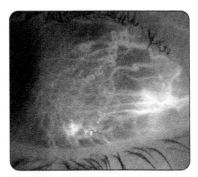

Fig 8.9

Scleromalacia perforans

Definition: specific type of necrotizing scleritis without inflammation that

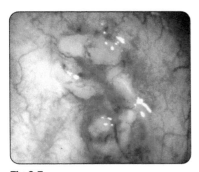

Fig 8.7

typically affects elderly women with long-standing rheumatoid arthritis; perforation of the globe is extremely rare.

Diagnosis

- **Presentation:** mild nonspecific irritation; pain is absent and vision unaffected.
- **Signs:** (a) absence of vascular congestion, (b) necrotic scleral plaques near the limbus which coalesce and enlarge, and (c) slow progression of scleral thinning and exposure of underlying uvea (*Fig. 8.10*).
- **Differential diagnosis:** scleral hyaline plaque (see below).

third of those older than age 55 years have an associated systemic disease.

- **Presentation:** pain or blurred vision; anterior scleritis may coexist.
- **Fundus signs:** (a) choroidal folds (*Fig. 8.11*), (b) uveal effusion (*Fig. 8.12*), (c) yellowish-brown subretinal mass which may be mistaken for a choroidal tumour, and (d) disc oedema.
- **Other features:** (a) myositis, (b) proptosis and periorbital oedema, (c) elevated IOP, and (d) chemosis and conjunctival injection.

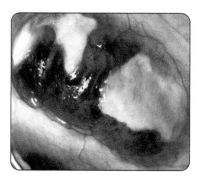

Fig 8.10

Treatment: effective in early disease but usually by presentation either no treatment is needed or it is unlikely to be effective.

Posterior scleritis

Diagnosis

- **Important facts:** (a) patients with posterior scleritis can go blind extremely rapidly, so early diagnosis is crucial, and (b) a

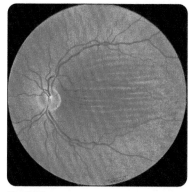

Fig 8.11

- **Imaging:** (a) ultrasonography (US) shows scleral thickening and fluid in the Tenon space gives the characteristic 'T' sign formed by the optic nerve and the fluid-containing gap (*Fig. 8.13*); (b) MR and CT (*Fig. 8.14*) may show scleral thickening.

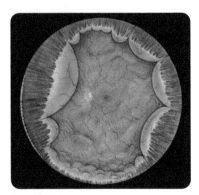

Fig 8.12

Treatment of immune-mediated scleritis

- **Topical steroids:** for symptomatic relief.
- **Periocular steroid injections:** only in selected cases.
- **Systemic NSAIDs:** only in non-necrotizing disease.
- **Systemic steroids:** (e.g. prednisolone 1.0–1.5 mg/kg/day) when NSAIDs are inappropriate or ineffective, especially in necrotizing disease; intravenous preparations are sometimes necessary.
- **Other systemic drugs:** (a) cytotoxic agents and immune modulators as an adjunct or steroid-sparing measure, and (b) specific antibodies (e.g. infliximab, rituximab) show promise.

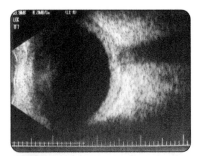

Fig 8.13

Systemic associations of scleritis

Up to half of patients with scleritis have one of the following systemic diseases:
- **Collagen vascular diseases:** (a) rheumatoid arthritis, (b) Wegener granulomatosis, (c) polyarteritis nodosa, (d) relapsing polychondritis, and (e) systemic lupus erythematosus.
- **Infections:** (a) herpes zoster (most common), (b) certain fungi, (c) syphilis, (d) leprosy, (e) Lyme disease, and (f) tuberculosis.
- **Other associations:** (a) lymphoma, (b) dysproteinaemias, (c) thyroid eye disease, (d) hyperuricaemia/gout, and (e) inflammatory bowel disease.

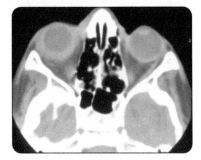

Fig 8.14

Scleral discoloration

- **Alkaptonuria:** bluish-grey or black generalized pigmentation of the sclera and the horizontal recti tendons, associated with discrete pigmented globules (*Fig. 8.15*).
- **Haemochromatosis:** rusty brown perilimbal conjunctival and scleral discoloration.
- **Blue sclera:** group of conditions featuring thinning or transparency of scleral collagen with visualization of the underlying uvea (*Fig. 8.16*) as in osteogenesis imperfecta and Ehlers–Danlos syndrome type VI.
- **Congenital ocular melanocytosis:** increased number, size, and pigmentation of melanocytes in the sclera (*Fig. 8.17*) and uvea, which may also involve the periocular skin,

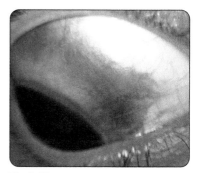

Fig 8.17

orbit, meninges, and soft palate. Classified as (a) ocular (involves only the eye), (b) dermal (only skin), and (c) oculodermal (naevus of Ota); slightly increased risk of uveal melanoma mandates observation.
- **Postinflammatory scleral changes.**
- **Scleral hyaline plaque:** innocuous oval dark greyish area located close to the insertion of the horizontal rectus muscles (*Fig. 8.18*) seen in elderly patients.

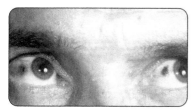

Fig 8.15

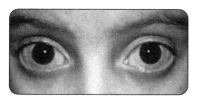

Fig 8.16

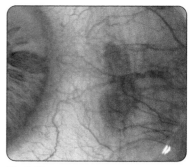

Fig 8.18

Chapter

9

Lens

Acquired cataract

Age-related cataract

- **Subcapsular** *(Fig. 9.1):* (a) anterior lies directly under the lens capsule, and (b) posterior lies just in front of the posterior capsule and appears black on retroillumination; the latter often has a more profound effect on vision than a comparable nuclear or cortical cataract, with glare and poor near vision.
- **Nuclear:** often associated with myopia due to an increase in the refractive index of the nucleus; when advanced, the nucleus appears brown (*Fig. 9.2*).
- **Cortical:** starts as clefts and vacuoles between lens fibres

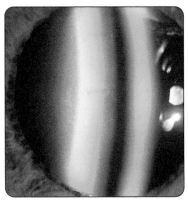

Fig 9.2

(*Fig. 9.3*) due to hydration of the cortex and evolves into wedge-shaped or radial spoke-like opacities (*Fig. 9.4*).
- **Christmas tree:** polychromatic opacities (*Fig. 9.5*).

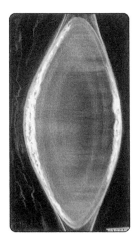

Fig 9.1

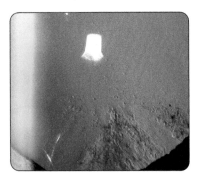

Fig 9.3

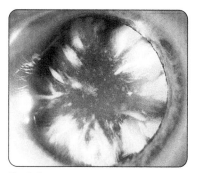

Fig 9.4

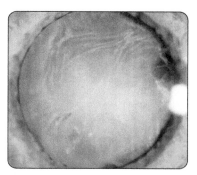

Fig 9.6

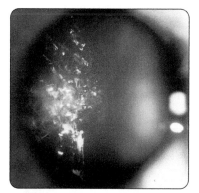

Fig 9.5

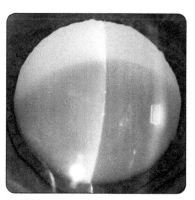

Fig 9.7

- *Cataract maturity:* (a) immature (lens is partially opaque), (b) mature (lens is completely opaque), (c) hypermature (shrunken and wrinkled capsule; *Fig. 9.6*), and (d) Morgagnian cataract (inferior sinking of nucleus in a liquefied cortex; *Fig. 9.7*).

Cataract in systemic diseases

- *Diabetes mellitus:* hyperglycaemia leads to the overaccumulation of metabolic products in the lens, initially leading to fluctuating refraction and later to cataract, particularly accelerated age-related nuclear.

- *Myotonic dystrophy:* fine cortical iridescent opacities that evolve into a visually disabling stellate posterior subcapsular cataract (*Fig. 9.8*).
- *Atopic dermatitis:* dense anterior subcapsular plaque is characteristic (*Fig. 9.9*).
- *NF2:* cataract develops in approximately 60% of patients, often prior to the age of 30 years.

Causes of secondary cataract

A secondary (complicated) cataract develops as a result of other primary ocular disease such as the following:

- *Chronic anterior uveitis:* cataract may be caused both by inflammation and by the steroids; progresses more rapidly in the presence of posterior synechiae (*Fig. 9.10*).
- *Acute congestive angle closure:* small, grey-white, anterior opacities within the pupillary area (glaukomflecken; *Fig. 9.11*).
- *High (pathological) myopia:* posterior subcapsular opacities and early onset nuclear sclerosis.
- *Hereditary fundus dystrophies:* retinitis pigmentosa, Leber congenital amaurosis, gyrate atrophy, and Stickler syndrome (see Chapter 15).

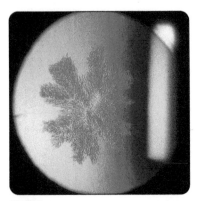

Fig 9.8

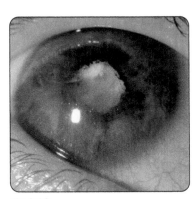

Fig 9.10

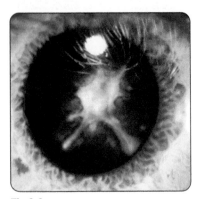

Fig 9.9

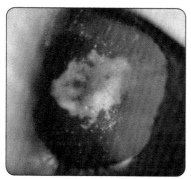

Fig 9.11

Causes of traumatic cataract

- Penetrating trauma.
- Blunt trauma may cause a characteristic flower-shaped opacity (*Fig. 9.12*).
- Electric shock.
- Infrared radiation (e.g. occupational exposure).
- Ionizing radiation (e.g. for ocular tumours).

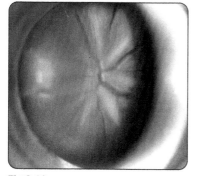

Fig 9.12

Management of age-related cataract

Preoperative considerations

- *Indications for surgery:* (a) visual improvement, (b) medical indications (e.g. phacomorphic glaucoma; see Chapter 10), and (c) to facilitate management of fundus disease (e.g. diabetic retinopathy).
- *Systemic preoperative assessment:* general medical history; investigations are not usually performed for routine local anaesthesia.
- *Ophthalmic preoperative assessment:* (a) past ophthalmic history, (b) visual acuity (VA), (c) cover testing, (d) pupillary responses, (e) slitlamp biomicroscopy, (f) ocular adnexa (e.g. chronic dacryocystitis), (f) red reflex quality, (g) fundus examination (US if poor view), and (h) refractive status (including postoperative result from an eye previously operated on).
- *Biometry:* facilitates calculation of the lens power for a planned refractive outcome by measuring corneal power (keratometry) and axial length (e.g. optical interferometry, US). Refractive outcome planning may need to take into account the refractive status of the fellow eye as well as the patient's preferences and the effect of previous ocular surgery.

Intraocular lenses

The intraocular lens (IOL) is optimized for positioning within the intact capsular bag, although complicated surgery may necessitate alternatives such as placement within the ciliary sulcus or anterior chamber.

- *Flexible IOLs:* made of silicone, acrylic, or Collamer; can be rolled or folded for introduction into the eye through a small incision.
- *Rigid IOLs:* still occasionally used.
- *Sharp/square-edged optics:* associated with a lower rate of posterior capsular opacification (PCO) compared with round-edged optics.
- *Ultraviolet filter:* routine in modern IOLs to reduce energy incident on the retina; blue light filters are also available.
- *Aspheric IOL optics:* counteract spherical aberration.
- *Heparin coating:* reduces the attraction and adhesion of inflammatory cells, which may have particular application in eyes with uveitis.
- *Multifocal, accommodative, and pseudo-accommodative IOLs:* aim to provide clear vision over a range of focal distances.
- *Toric IOLs:* integral cylindrical refractive component to compensate for pre-existing corneal astigmatism.
- *Adjustable IOLs:* alteration of refractive power following implantation.

Anaesthesia

Most cataract surgery is performed under local anaesthesia (LA), sometimes with the aid of oral or intravenous sedation. General anaesthesia is sometimes used (e.g. for children and very anxious patients).

- *Sub-Tenon periocular LA:* cannula is introduced through an incision in the conjunctiva and Tenon capsule 5 mm from the limbus inferonasally; akinesia is variable.
- *Peribulbar block:* needle is introduced through the skin or conjunctiva; provides effective anaesthesia and akinesia.
- *Topical anaesthesia:* (drops or gel) can be augmented with intracameral preservative-free lidocaine; despite the absence of akinesia, most patients can cooperate adequately.

Phacoemulsification

- *Definition:* most cataract surgery is performed using phacoemulsification ('phaco') in which the nucleus is broken down within the eye using ultrasound (Fig. 9.13).
- *Technique:* (a) a continuous curvilinear capsulorhexis (circular

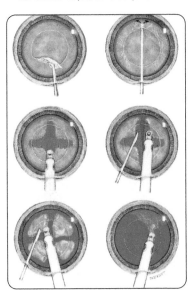

Fig 9.13

opening in the anterior lens capsule) is created to gain access to the lens, (b) emulsified nucleus is aspirated, as is the softer cortical material (irrigation/aspiration or 'I/A'), and (c) the IOL is introduced into the capsular bag, which is generally left intact (*Fig. 9.14*). A novel approach involves the use of a femtosecond laser to perform the corneal incision, the capsulorhexis and to soften the lens.

- *'Viscoelastics':* maintain intraocular cavities that would otherwise collapse, and to provide a degree of protection for delicate intraocular structures.

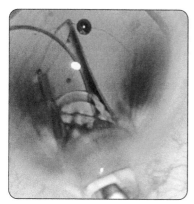

Fig 9.14

Operative complications

- *Rupture of the posterior lens capsule:* typically accompanied by the migration of vitreous gel into the anterior chamber, with an increased risk of various sequelae (e.g. chronic cystoid macular oedema, retinal detachment, uveitis, glaucoma, and endophthalmitis).

- *Dislocation of lens fragments into the vitreous cavity:* occurs after zonular dehiscence or posterior capsular rupture and may result in subsequent problems (e.g. glaucoma, chronic uveitis, retinal detachment and chronic cystoid macular oedema); large fragments may require removal by pars plana vitrectomy.
- *Dislocation of an IOL into the vitreous cavity:* very rare; removal requires pars plana vitrectomy.
- *Suprachoroidal haemorrhage:* bleeding into the suprachoroidal space from a posterior ciliary artery; if sufficiently severe may result in extrusion of intraocular contents ('expulsive' haemorrhage); if suspected intraoperatively, the operation should be terminated and the incision sutured immediately.

Acute postoperative endophthalmitis

Introduction
- *Incidence:* 0.3%.
- *Risk factors:* (a) operative complications (see above), (b) clear corneal sutureless incision, (c) temporal incision, (d) wound leak on the first day, (e) topical anaesthesia, (f) adnexal disease (e.g. chronic blepharitis, dacryocystitis), and (g) diabetes.
- *Pathogens:* 90% of isolates are gram positive (e.g. *S. epidermidis, S. aureus*), with the flora of the eyelids and conjunctiva the most frequent source.
- *Prophylaxis:* (a) preoperative 5% povidone–iodine into the conjunctival fornices, (b) treatment

of pre-existing adnexal infections, (c) preoperative antibiotics, (d) intracameral antibiotics at the end of surgery, and (e) postoperative subconjunctival antibiotic injection.

Diagnosis

- *Presentation:* within first few days of surgery with acute or subacute onset of pain, redness, eyelid swelling, and visual deterioration.
- *Signs:* (a) anterior chamber activity with fibrinous exudate and hypopyon, (b) corneal haze (*Fig. 9.15*), (c) eyelid swelling, (d) chemosis, (e) conjunctival injection and discharge, (f) relative afferent pupillary defect, and (g) vitreous inflammation with loss of the red reflex.
- *Differential diagnosis:* sterile uveitis, including secondary to retained lens material in the anterior chamber or vitreous.
- *Investigations:* vitreous and aqueous samples should be obtained under aseptic conditions and sent for urgent microscopy and culture.

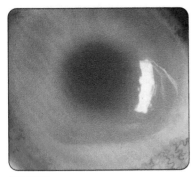

Fig 9.15

Treatment

- *Intravitreal antibiotics:* injected immediately following vitreous sampling.
- *Topical and subconjunctival antibiotics:* limited benefit but are typically given to protect the fresh wounds from re-infection.
- *Oral antibiotics:* (e.g. moxifloxacin, clarithromycin).
- *Topical steroids:* (e.g. dexamethasone 0.1% 2-hourly).
- *Oral steroids:* often commenced after 12–24 hr.
- *Topical cycloplegics:* (e.g. atropine 1% twice daily).
- *Pars plana vitrectomy:* is beneficial when VA is worse than 'hand movements'; it can also be performed to address late complications such as persistent vitreous opacities or epimacular membrane.

Delayed-onset postoperative endophthalmitis

Pathogenesis: organisms of low virulence become trapped within the capsular bag ('saccular endophthalmitis'). The pathogens can become sequestered within macrophages, protected from eradication but with continued expression of bacterial antigen; most frequent isolate is *Propionibacterium acnes*.

Diagnosis

- *Presentation:* several months following surgery with painless progressive visual deterioration and floaters.
- *Signs:* (a) low-grade anterior uveitis, sometimes with mutton-fat keratic precipitates, initially responding well to topical steroids

but recurring when treatment is stopped; (b) a white enlarging capsular plaque is characteristic (*Fig. 9.16*).

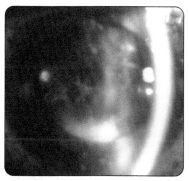

Fig 9.16

Treatment
- *Initial:* oral moxifloxacin or clarithromycin for 10–14 days.
- *Subsequent:* persistent cases may require removal of the capsular bag, residual cortex, and IOL.

Posterior capsular opacification

Pathogenesis: visually significant PCO, caused by the proliferation and migration of residual lens epithelial cells, is the most common late complication of uncomplicated cataract surgery.
Diagnosis
- *Presentation:* weeks or months following surgery with diminished VA, monocular diplopia, and glare.

- *Signs:* vacuolated opacification is the most frequently (Elschnig's pearls; *Fig. 9.17*), (b) fibrosis (*Fig. 9.18*), and (c) contraction of the anterior capsular opening (capsulophimosis; *Fig. 9.19*).

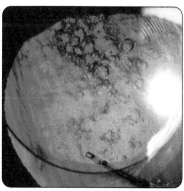

Fig 9.17

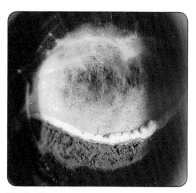

Fig 9.18

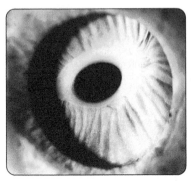

Fig 9.19

Treatment
- **Technique:** Nd:YAG laser is used to create an opening in the posterior capsule (*Fig. 9.20*).
- **Complications:** (a) 'pitting' of the IOL (typically asymptomatic), (b) cystoid macular oedema, (c) rhegmatogenous retinal detachment, (d) elevation of IOP (usually mild), and (e) posterior IOL dislocation (rare).

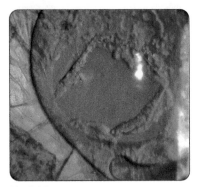

Fig 9.20

Miscellaneous postoperative complications

- **Malposition of IOL:** glare, haloes, and monocular diplopia may occur if the edge of the IOL becomes displaced into the pupil (*Fig. 9.21*); if significant, may require repositioning or replacement.

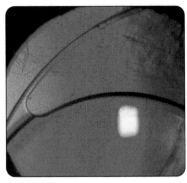

Fig 9.21

- **Cystoid macular oedema:** risk factors are (a) operative complications, (b) prior topical prostaglandin treatment, (c) diabetes, and (d) uveitis. Treatment involves (a) correction of a likely cause, if possible (e.g. anterior vitrectomy for vitreous incarceration), (b) topical NSAIDs and steroids, (c) periocular or intravitreal steroids, (d) topical or systemic carbonic anhydrase inhibitors, (e) intravitreal anti-vascular endothelial growth factor (VEGF) agents, and (f) pars plana vitrectomy in resistant cases.
- **Rhegmatogenous retinal detachment:** risk factors include (a) lattice degeneration, (b) high myopia, (c) posterior capsule rupture, and (d) early postoperative laser capsulotomy.

Congenital cataract

Introduction
- **Prevalence:** approximately 3 in 10,000 live births.
- **Laterality:** two-thirds are bilateral, with an identifiable cause in approximately half of these– usually an AD mutation; unilateral cataracts are typically sporadic with a cause identified in only 10%.
- **Morphology:** may indicate likely aetiology and visual prognosis; (a) lamellar opacities (*Fig. 9.22*) may be AD, sporadic, or occur in infants with metabolic disorders and intrauterine infections; (b) blue dot opacities (*Fig. 9.23*) are common and innocuous; (c) central 'oil droplet' opacities (*Fig. 9.24*) are characteristic of galactosaemia, and (d) posterior polar cataract may occasionally be associated with persistent hyaloid remnants (Mittendorf dot; *Fig. 9.25*) or persistent posterior fetal vasculature (hyperplastic primary vitreous).
- **Systemic metabolic associations:** (a) galactosaemia, (b) Lowe

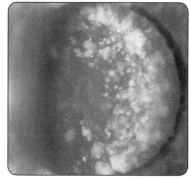

Fig 9.23

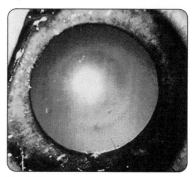

Fig 9.24

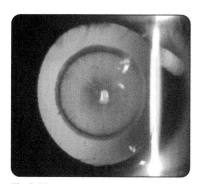

Fig 9.22

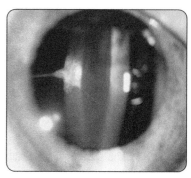

Fig 9.25

syndrome, (c) Fabry disease, (d) mannosidosis, (e) hypoparathyroidism and pseudo-hypoparathyroidism, and (f) hypo- and hyperglycaemia.

- **Associated intrauterine infections:** (a) congenital rubella, (b) toxoplasmosis, (c) cytomegalovirus, and (d) varicella.
- **Associated chromosomal abnormalities:** (a) Down syndrome (trisomy 21), (b) Edwards syndrome (trisomy 18), and (c) cri du chat syndrome (partial deletion of 5p).

Management

- **Ocular examination:** (a) estimation of the density and probable visual impact of the opacity, and (b) morphology and the presence of other ocular pathology including indicators of severe visual impairment such as nystagmus.
- **Systemic investigations:** (a) serology for intrauterine infection, (b) urinalysis (galactosaemia, Lowe syndrome), (c) glucose, and (d) electrolyte, calcium, and phosphorus analysis; other tests under the care of a paediatric specialist.
- **Treatment:** early surgery is required in dense unilateral or bilateral opacities. The cataract is removed by aspiration supplemented by posterior capsulorhexis and limited vitrectomy.
- **Postoperative complications:** (a) PCO, (b) secondary pupillary membrane formation, (c) proliferation of residual lens epithelial cells (Soemmering ring surrounding the visual axis), (d) glaucoma (20%), and (e) retinal detachment.

- **Visual rehabilitation:** (a) spectacles and contact lenses; (b) IOL implantation is safe and effective in selected cases, although refractive changes with growth must be addressed; (c) treatment of amblyopia is vital.

Ectopia lentis

Definitions: displacement of the lens from its normal position may be complete (luxation; *Fig. 9.26*) or partial (subluxation; *Fig. 9.27*), in

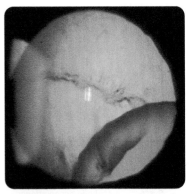

Fig 9.26

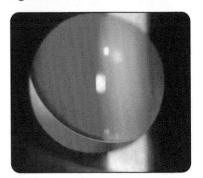

Fig 9.27

which the lens remains substantially in the pupillary area.

Aetiology

- *Acquired:* (a) trauma, (b) large eye (e.g. high myopia, buphthalmos), (c) anterior uveal tumours, and (d) hypermature cataract.
- *Hereditary without systemic associations:* (a) familial (AD, bilateral superotemporal ectopia), (b) ectopia lentis et pupillae (AR, displacement of pupil and lens in opposite directions; *Fig. 9.28*), and (c) aniridia (inferior ectopia).

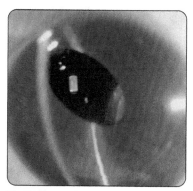

Fig 9.28

- *Hereditary with systemic associations:* (a) Marfan syndrome (AD, tall, thin stature, arachnodactyly, high-arched palate, cardiovascular lesions, bilateral superotemporal ectopia with zonule intact), (b) Weill–Marchesani syndrome (AR or AD, short stature, brachydactyly, mental handicap, inferior ectopia in 50%), (c) homocystinuria (zonules disrupted), and (d) sulphite oxidase deficiency.

Management

- *Nonsurgical:* conventional spectacle correction may be adequate in mild subluxation; aphakic spectacle or contact lens correction if appropriate.
- *Indications for surgical removal:* (a) intractable ametropia, (b) optical distortion due to astigmatism and/or lens edge effect, (c) cataract, (d) lens-induced glaucoma (see Chapter 10), (d) lens-induced uveitis (rare), and (e) endothelial touch.

Abnormalities of shape

- *Anterior lenticonus:* bilateral axial projection of the anterior surface of the lens into the anterior chamber (*Fig. 9.29*) occurs in Alport syndrome (AD or X-L), characterized by progressive sensorineural deafness and renal disease; other ocular features are fleck retinopathy and posterior polymorphous corneal dystrophy.

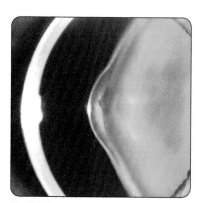

Fig 9.29

- **Posterior lenticonus:** bulging and opacification of the posterior axial zone of the lens (*Fig. 9.30*); most cases are unilateral, sporadic, and not associated with systemic abnormalities.

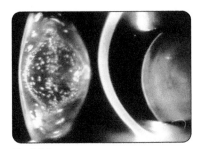

Fig 9.31

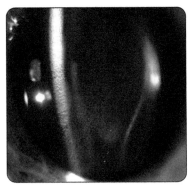

Fig 9.30

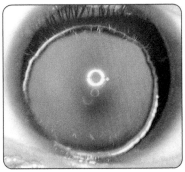

Fig 9.32

- **Lentiglobus:** very rare, usually unilateral, generalized hemispherical deformity of the lens.
- **Microspherophakia:** small spherical lens (*Fig. 9.31*); may be isolated familial or associated with (a) Peters anomaly, (b) Marfan and Weill–Marchesani syndromes, (c) hyperlysinaemia, and (d) congenital rubella.
- **Microphakia:** lens with a smaller than normal diameter (*Fig. 9.32*); may occur in Lowe syndrome.
- **Coloboma:** notching at the inferior equator (*Fig. 9.33*), with corresponding absence of zonular fibres, may be associated with iris or fundus colobomas.

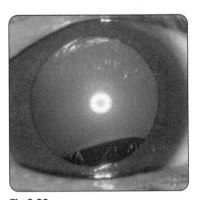

Fig 9.33

Chapter **10**

Glaucoma

Ocular hypertension

Diagnosis
- **Normal IOP:** mean IOP in the general population is 16 mm Hg; two standard deviations to either side of this gives a 'normal' IOP range of 11–21 mm Hg (*Fig. 10.1*).
- **Definition:** 4–7% of individuals older than 40 years have IOPs >21 mm Hg without detectable glaucomatous damage—'ocular hypertension' (OHT).
- **Risk factors for conversion of OHT to glaucoma:** (a) higher IOP, (b) greater age, (c) lower central corneal thickness, (d) larger C/D ratio, and (e) higher 'pattern standard deviation' on perimetry.

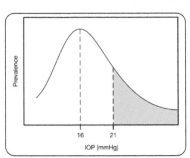

Fig 10.1

Management
- **Drug choice:** as for primary open-angle glaucoma (POAG; see below), although regimen may be less aggressive.
- **Risk of conversion to POAG:** after 5 years if untreated is 9.5%, and 4.4% if treated.
- **Other considerations:** (a) individual patient profile (e.g. age/life expectancy, patient preference, and risk factors); (b) consider treating every patient with an IOP of ≥30 mm Hg.

Primary open-angle glaucoma

Introduction
- **Definition:** POAG is a generally bilateral disease of adult onset characterized by (a) IOP >21 mm Hg at some stage, (b) glaucomatous optic neuropathy, (c) open angle, (d) characteristic visual field loss as damage progresses, and (e) absence of signs of secondary glaucoma.
- **Risk factors:** (a) elevated IOP, (b) greater age, (c) race (more common in black than white individuals), (d) family history (first-degree relatives) of POAG, (e) myopia, and (f) systemic vascular disease; elevation of IOP in response to topical steroid is more common in POAG than the general population.

Diagnosis
- **History:** usually asymptomatic until damage is advanced; (a) past ophthalmic history including refractive status, (b) family history, and (c) past medical history and current medication.
- **General examination:** (a) pupils, (b) slit lamp, (c) tonometry, (d) pachymetry for central corneal thickness (CCT), (e) gonioscopy, and (f) optic disc examination with dilated pupils.
- **Perimetry:** visual field defects include (a) small paracentral depression (70% of early defects), (b) arcuate-shaped defect,

(c) nasal step, (d) ring scotoma, and (e) end-stage changes with a small residual island of central vision.

- *Imaging:* of discs and peripapillary retinal nerve fibre layer (see below).

Optic disc changes

- Diffuse enlargement of the cup (*Fig. 10.2a*).
- Focal notching, often inferior, of the neuroretinal rim (NRR) (*Fig. 10.2b*).
- C/D ratio asymmetry may develop; comparison of overall disc diameter is critical.

- Retinal nerve fibre layer defects.
- Loss of nasal NRR.
- 'Sharpened' disc edge as adjacent NRR is lost.
- Lamina dot sign (exposed grey dot-like fenestrations in the lamina cribrosa; *Fig. 10.2c*).
- Vascular changes: (a) 'splinter' disc haemorrhages, (b) baring of circumlinear blood vessels (space between a superficial vessel and the disc margin), (c) bayoneting (double angulation of a vessel as it bends backwards due to loss of underling NRR), and (d) collateral disc vessels.

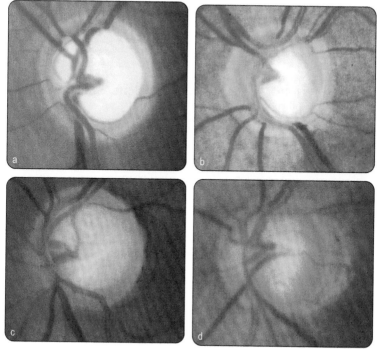

Fig 10.2

Progression of peripapillary atrophy, particularly the inner (beta) zone (*Fig. 10.2d*).

Imaging modalities: (a) stereo disc photography, (b) confocal scanning laser tomography (e.g. Heidelberg retinal tomograph), (c) scanning laser polarimetry (e.g. GDx glaucoma diagnosis), and (d) optical coherence tomography (OCT).

Management: lowering IOP is the only proven method of slowing progression. A target IOP should be set, with subsequent monitoring and target resetting if progression occurs.

- *Initial medical therapy:* with one drug in its lowest concentration, instilled as infrequently as possible consistent with the desired effect.
- *Review:* after 4–8 weeks, when response is assessed against target IOP, and if satisfactory subsequently after a further 3–6 months.
- *Causes of failure:* (a) poor compliance (25% of patients), (b) inadequate instillation technique, (c) inappropriate target pressure, and (d) IOP fluctuations including wide diurnal variation.
- *Ongoing monitoring:* optic disc assessment, perimetry (annual in most low–moderate risk cases), and annual gonioscopy (angles narrow with age).
- *Laser trabeculoplasty:* selective laser trabeculoplasty (SLT) or argon laser trabeculoplasty (ALT) can be used to replace or supplement medical treatment; indications include (a) patient preference, (b) intolerance of

medical therapy, and (c) avoidance of polypharmacy or surgery.
- *Indications for surgery:* (a) failed medical therapy, (b) intolerance of medical therapy, (c) avoidance of polypharmacy, (d) progressive deterioration despite seemingly adequate IOP control, and (e) as primary therapy in some patients.
- *Trabeculectomy:* is the most common procedure, although nonpenetrating surgery is also widely performed. If significant lens opacity is present, phacoemulsification alone may be associated with a fall in IOP; alternatively, it can be combined with a filtration procedure (e.g. phacotrabeculectomy).

Normal-pressure glaucoma

Introduction

- *Definition:* (a) glaucomatous optic neuropathy, (b) IOP consistently ≤21 mm Hg, and (c) open angle.
- *Risk factors:* (a) age (older than in POAG), (b) race (particularly prevalent in Japan), (c) family history of glaucoma, (d) CCT (thinner than in POAG), (e) systemic hypotension including nocturnal blood pressure dips, and (f) possibly abnormal vasoregulation (e.g. migraine, Raynaud phenomenon).
- *Differential diagnosis:* (a) POAG with apparently normal IOP, (b) nocturnal IOP spikes, (c) previous secondary raised IOP (trauma, uveitis, steroids, resolved pigmentary glaucoma),

(d) masking of elevated IOP by systemic treatment (e.g. beta-blocker), (e) previous acute optic nerve insult (e.g. anterior ischaemic optic neuropathy), (f) hypovolaemic or septicaemic shock, (g) progressive retinal nerve fibre defects not due to glaucoma (e.g. myopic degeneration, disc drusen), (h) congenital disc anomalies (e.g. disc pits, coloboma), and (i) chiasmal or optic nerve compression.

Diagnosis

- *Specific points in the history:* (a) migraine and Raynaud phenomenon, (b) episodes of shock, (c) headache and other neurological symptoms, and (d) systemic steroids and beta-blockers.
- *Specific points in the examination:* (a) IOP is usually in the high teens but may be lower; (b) glaucomatous cupping is similar to POAG, although acquired optic disc pits, peripapillary atrophic changes, and disc splinter haemorrhages may be more frequent than in POAG.
- *Field defects*: may be closer to fixation and more localized than in POAG.
- *Other investigations:* as for POAG, but in certain patients consider assessment of systemic vascular risk factors, 24 h ambulatory blood pressure monitoring to exclude nocturnal systemic hypotension, blood tests for other causes of nonglaucomatous optic neuropathy, and cranial MR.

Treatment

- *Indications:* visual fields are stable in 50% over 5 years without treatment, so in mild cases it may be appropriate to demonstrate progression before treating; further IOP reduction is effective in reducing progression in at least some patients.
- *Topical:* may include betaxolol thought to increases optic nerve blood flow.
- *Surgery (or laser trabeculoplasty):* if progression occurs despite reduced IOP.
- *Systemic:* (a) control of systemic vascular disease, (b) calcium channel blockers to counter vasospasm, and (c) if significant nocturnal dips in BP are detected, consider reducing antihypertensive medication (especially bedtime dosing).

Primary angle-closure glaucoma

Introduction

- *Definition:* 'angle closure' refers to occlusion of the trabecular meshwork by the peripheral iris—iridotrabecular contact (ITC), obstructing aqueous outflow. The condition is responsible for up to half of all cases of glaucoma globally and is typically associated with greater visual morbidity than POAG.
- *Mechanisms:* (a) pupillary block—failure of aqueous flow through the pupil leading to anterior bowing of the iris (*Fig. 10.3*)—is relieved by peripheral iridotomy; (b) non pupillary block relating to a thicker or more anteriorly positioned iris (*Fig. 10.4*), including plateau iris due to anteriorly positioned ciliary

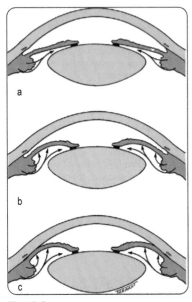

Fig 10.3

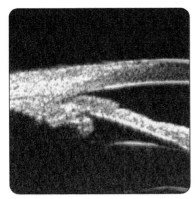

Fig 10.4

processes, is only partially relieved by iridotomy; and (c) plateau iris configuration characterized by a flat central iris plane with a normal central anterior chamber depth.

- **Risk factors:** (a) age, (b) gender (female > male), (c) race (high Far Eastern prevalence), (d) family history, (e) hypermetropia, and (f) shorter ocular and anterior chamber dimensions.

Diagnosis

- **Primary angle-closure suspect (PACS):** (a) gonioscopy shows ITC in three or more quadrants but no peripheral anterior synechiae (PAS), and (b) normal IOP, discs, and fields.
- **Primary angle closure (PAC):** (a) gonioscopy shows three or more quadrants of ITC (*Fig. 10.5*), (b) raised IOP and/or PAS, and (c) normal discs and fields.
- **Primary angle-closure glaucoma (PACG):** (a) gonioscopy shows ITC in three or more quadrants, and (b) glaucomatous optic neuropathy.
- **Chronic and subacute presentations:** typically asymptomatic although episodic mild blurring may be present; (a) IOP elevation may be intermittent,

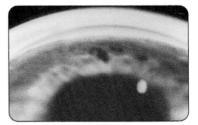

Fig 10.5

(b) disc appearance depends on severity of damage, and (c) PAS may be broad ('creeping') or discrete ('sawtooth').

- **Acute presentation:** acute onset of blurring and haloes, ocular pain and headache, sometimes malaise and gastrointestinal symptoms; (a) VA usually 6/60-HM, (b) IOP very high (50–100 mm Hg), (c) corneal epithelial oedema (*Fig. 10.6*), (d) ciliary injection, (e) shallow anterior chamber (*Fig. 10.7*), and (f) unreactive mid-dilated vertically oval pupil; fellow eye shows an occludable angle.
- **Resolved acute episode:** (a) initially, folds in Descemet membrane (*Fig. 10.8*), optic nerve head congestion, and choroidal folds; (b) later, iris atrophy with a spiral configuration, irregular pupil with posterior synechiae, glaukomflecken (*Fig. 10.9*), and optic atrophy.

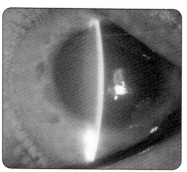

Fig 10.6

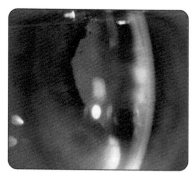

Fig 10.8

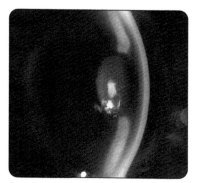

Fig 10.7

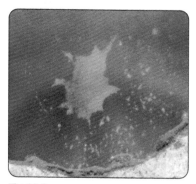

Fig 10.9

Treatment

- *PACS:* prophylactic laser iridotomy; if significant ITC persists, options include observation, laser iridoplasty, pilocarpine 1% prophylaxis, and lens extraction.
- *Chronic presentation of PAC and PACG:* as for PACS, although subsequent medical treatment (as for POAG) may be required despite an opened angle.
- *Initial treatment of acute and subacute presentation:* (a) intravenous acetazolamide 500 mg, (b) topical apraclonidine 1%, timolol 0.5%, prednisolone 1%, or dexamethasone 0.1% to the affected eye, and (c) pilocarpine 2–4% one drop to the affected eye, repeated after 30 min, with one drop of 1% as prophylaxis to the fellow eye; consider delaying pilocarpine until IOP begins to fall.
- *Subsequent treatment of acute and subacute presentation:* (a) pilocarpine 2% four times daily to the affected eye and 1% to the fellow eye, (b) ongoing treatment according to IOP with timolol 0.5% twice daily, apraclonidine 1% three times daily, and oral acetazolamide 250 mg four times daily; once cornea is clear and eye quieter, bilateral laser iridotomy is performed and medical treatment tapered.
- *Options in unresponsive acute cases:* (a) further topical pilocarpine, timolol, and apraclonidine, (b) intravenous mannitol or oral glycerol, (c) corneal indentation, (d) laser iridotomy or iridoplasty (clear oedema with glycerol 50% first), and (e) surgery (peripheral iridectomy, lens extraction, goniosynechialysis, trabeculectomy).

Differential diagnosis of acute IOP elevation: consider alternatives to angle closure, particularly if the fellow eye's angle is open.

- Lens-induced angle closure due to an intumescent or subluxated lens.
- Malignant glaucoma, especially if intraocular surgery has recently taken place.
- Other causes of secondary angle closure, with or without pupillary block (see below).
- Neovascular glaucoma sometimes presents acutely.
- Inflammatory elevation with an open angle; iridocyclitis/trabeculitis, glaucomatocyclitic crisis (Posner–Schlossman syndrome), scleritis without angle closure.
- Pigment dispersion.
- Pseudoexfoliation.
- Orbital/retro-orbital lesions (e.g. inflammation, retrobulbar haemorrhage).

Pseudoexfoliation

Pseudoexfoliation syndrome

Pathogenesis: grey-white fibrillary material is produced by abnormal basement membranes of ageing intraocular epithelial cells and deposited in structures including the trabeculum; particularly common in Scandinavia.

Diagnosis

- *Cornea:* pseudoexfoliation (PXF) material and pigment may be seen on the endothelium.
- *Iris:* PXF on the pupillary margin (*Fig. 10.10*) and 'moth-eaten' sphincter atrophy (*Fig. 10.11*).
- *Anterior lens surface:* central disc and peripheral band of PXF, with a clear zone between (*Fig. 10.12*); may be seen only with pupillary dilatation.
- *Gonioscopy:* (a) trabecular hyperpigmentation and a band

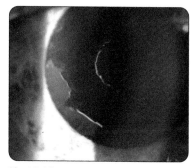

Fig 10.12

running on or anterior to the Schwalbe line (Sampaolesi line; *Fig. 10.13*); (b) dandruff-like PXF particles may be seen; there is an increased risk of angle closure, probably due to zonular laxity.

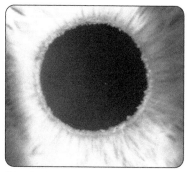

Fig 10.10

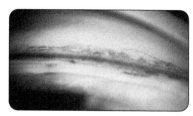

Fig 10.13

Treatment: observation at 6-monthly intervals to detect elevation of IOP.

Pseudoexfoliation glaucoma

Pathogenesis: trabecular obstruction and damage by PXF material and pigment. The cumulative risk of glaucoma in eyes with PXF is approximately 5% at 5 years and 15% at 10 years. A patient with unilateral pseudoexfoliation

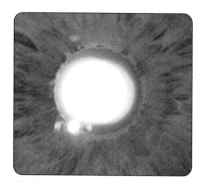

Fig 10.11

glaucoma and only PXF in the fellow eye has a 50% 5-year risk of glaucoma in the fellow eye, but only a low risk if there is no PXF.

Diagnosis

- *Presentation:* in 7th decade with chronic unilateral elevation of IOP; an acute elevation occasionally occurs due to angle closure or even with a wide-open angle.
- *Signs:* PXF and glaucomatous optic neuropathy.
- *Prognosis:* worse than in POAG because the IOP is often significantly elevated and may also exhibit great fluctuation; severe damage may therefore develop relatively rapidly.

Treatment

- *Medical:* same as for POAG but with a greater likelihood of requiring laser or surgery.
- *Laser trabeculoplasty:* effective, particularly in the medium term.
- *Surgery:* same success rate as in POAG.
- *Trabecular aspiration:* confers at least a short-term benefit, and can be performed at the same time as cataract surgery or trabeculectomy.

Pigment dispersion

Pigment dispersion syndrome

Pathogenesis: liberation of pigment granules from the iris pigment epithelium due to 'reverse pupil block,' with resultant posterior bowing of the iris and iridozonular touch. Pigment is deposited throughout the anterior segment. The condition primarily affects whites and may be inherited as AD with variable penetrance; myopia is present in the majority.

Diagnosis

- *Presentation:* typically asymptomatic, although corneal oedema with blurring and haloes may occur in response to IOP spikes; in some patients, this may be precipitated by exercise.
- *Cornea:* pigment deposition on the endothelium in a vertical spindle-shaped distribution (Krukenberg spindle; *Fig. 10.14*).

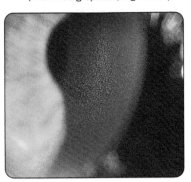

Fig 10.14

- *Anterior chamber:* usually very deep.
- *Iris:* radial slit-like transillumination defects (*Fig. 10.15*) and fine surface pigment granules.
- *Gonioscopy:* very wide angle with mid-peripheral iris concavity and homogeneous trabecular hyperpigmentation (*Fig. 10.16*); pigment may also be seen on or anterior to Schwalbe line.

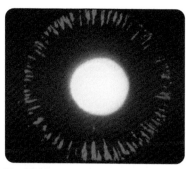

Fig 10.15

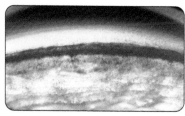

Fig 10.16

Treatment: observation at 6- to 12-monthly intervals to detect elevation of IOP.

Pigmentary glaucoma

Pathogenesis: approximately one-third of patients with pigment dispersion syndrome (PDS) develop OHT or chronic open-angle glaucoma after 15 years. Elevation of IOP appears to be caused by both pigmentary obstruction of the intertrabecular spaces and secondary damage to the trabeculum; men are affected twice as frequently as women.

Diagnosis

- **Presentation:** in 3rd and 4th decades, usually with chronic glaucoma.

- **Signs:** those of PDS, together with glaucomatous optic neuropathy; IOP may be unstable and asymmetric disease is common.
- **Differential diagnosis:** (a) POAG with a heavily pigmented trabeculum, (b) pseudoexfoliation, (c) pseudophakic pigmentary glaucoma, (d) sequelae to uveitis, and (e) subacute angle-closure glaucoma.

Treatment

- **Medical:** similar to that of POAG; miotics are theoretically of particular benefit but carry disadvantages (e.g. risk of retinal detachment) outweighing the benefits in most cases.
- **Laser trabeculoplasty:** often initially effective.
- **Trabeculectomy:** more commonly performed than in POAG, although results are variable.

Neovascular glaucoma

Introduction

- **Pathogenesis:** iris neovascularization (rubeosis iridis) occurs under the influence of growth factors produced in response to severe retinal ischaemia. Angle involvement initially impairs aqueous outflow in the presence of an open angle and later contracts resulting in angle closure.
- **Causes:** (a) ischaemic central retinal vein occlusion (most common), (b) diabetes, (c) arterial retinal vascular disease (central retinal artery occlusion, ocular ischaemic syndrome), (d) intraocular tumours, (e) long-standing retinal detachment,

and (f) chronic intraocular inflammation.
- *Classification:* (a) rubeosis iridis, (b) secondary open-angle glaucoma, and (c) secondary synechial angle-closure glaucoma.

Rubeosis iridis

Diagnosis
- Tiny dilated capillary tufts or red spots at the pupillary margin; new vessels grow radially over the surface of the iris toward the angle (*Fig. 10.17*).
- Angle neovascularization in the absence of pupillary involvement may occur, so gonioscopy without mydriasis should be performed in eyes at high risk.

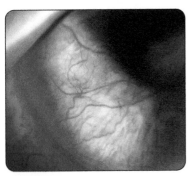

Fig 10.17

Treatment
- Early panretinal photocoagulation (PRP).
- Intravitreal anti-VEGF agents (e.g. bevacizumab) may decrease neovascularization and improve IOP control.
- Treatment of underlying cause (e.g. retinal detachment), if possible.

Secondary open-angle glaucoma

Diagnosis: neovascular tissue proliferation across the face of the angle.

Treatment
- *Medical:* (a) as for POAG (avoiding miotics and prostaglandin derivatives), (b) topical apraclonidine and/or oral acetazolamide as temporizing measures, (c) topical atropine 1% and steroids if significant inflammation is present, and (d) intravitreal anti-VEGF agents may be effective if fibrovascular angle closure has not supervened.
- *PRP:* indirect ophthalmoscopic application and/or mechanical pupillary dilatation (exceptionally) may be required.
- *Cyclodiode:* considered if medical IOP control is not possible, particularly if the eye is painful, has useful visual potential, or corneal oedema precludes PRP.

Secondary angle-closure glaucoma

Diagnosis
- As rubeosis progresses, contraction of fibrovascular tissue occludes the angle (*Fig. 10.18*).

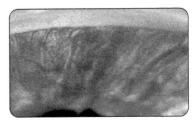

Fig 10.18

- IOP can be very high, with globe congestion and pain.
- Severe visual impairment is typical, due to the glaucoma or to the underlying cause.
- Prognosis is poor unless the neovascular process can be arrested.

Treatment

- *Medical:* as above; steroids and atropine alone may be adequate if there is no potential for vision; intravitreal anti-VEGF agents will not reverse established angle closure.
- *Retinal ablation:* (a) PRP if the fundus can be adequately visualized, or (b) trans-scleral cryotherapy or diode laser for eyes with opaque media.
- *Surgery:* (a) cyclodiode, (b) endocyclodiode, or (c) drainage surgery (enhanced trabeculectomy or shunt) to control IOP, particularly in eyes with visual potential.
- *Other:* retrobulbar alcohol injection or enucleation for intractable pain.

Inflammatory glaucoma

Angle-closure glaucoma with pupillary block

Pathogenesis: (a) formation of 360° posterior synechiae (seclusio pupillae) obstructs aqueous flow from the posterior to the anterior chamber, (b) anterior bowing of the iris (iris bombé), occurs and (c) iris becomes apposed to the trabeculum and PAS develop.

Diagnosis

- *Signs:* (a) seclusio pupillae, (b) iris bombé (*Fig. 10.19*), (c) shallow

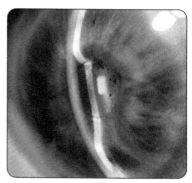

Fig 10.19

anterior chamber, and (d) signs of the underlying inflammatory condition.

- *Gonioscopy:* iridotrabecular contact; indentation may be used to assess the extent of PAS.

Angle-closure glaucoma without pupillary block

Pathogenesis: (a) inflammatory cells and debris accumulate in the angle, (b) subsequent organization and contraction of debris pulls the peripheral iris over the trabeculum, and (c) extensive PAS develop (*Fig. 10.20*) but the anterior chamber remains deep.

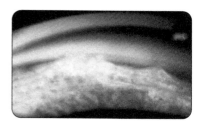

Fig 10.20

Open-angle glaucoma

Pathogenesis
- **In acute uveitis:** (a) trabecular obstruction by inflammatory cells and debris, (b) acute trabeculitis, and (c) steroid-induced IOP elevation.
- **In chronic anterior uveitis:** scarring secondary to chronic trabeculitis, although PAS are also often present.

Treatment of inflammatory glaucoma

- Medical control of IOP is more likely to be achieved if the angle is completely open.
- In steroid responders, it is important not to sacrifice control of inflammation for fear of steroid-induced IOP elevation, although long-acting preparations should be avoided.
- The IOP-lowering effect of ocular hypotensive drugs may be unpredictable (e.g. increased sensitivity to topical carbonic anhydrase inhibitors [CAI]).
- Prostaglandin analogue use is tempered by the risk of promoting inflammation and cystoid macular oedema.
- Miotics are contraindicated because they increase vascular permeability and may promote formation of posterior synechiae.
- A beta-blocker may be the drug of first choice, followed by an alpha-adrenergic agonist or a topical CAI, with a systemic CAI if needed.
- Laser iridotomy in eyes with pupillary block; occlusion of the opening may occur with active uveitis, and surgical iridectomy is sometimes necessary.
- Drainage surgery (enhanced trabeculectomy or shunt) should be preceded by aggressive control of inflammation, sometimes with systemic steroids; postoperative hypotony is a risk; steroids are tapered carefully postoperatively.
- Cyclodestructive procedures should be used with caution because overtreatment can lead to phthisis bulbi.
- Angle procedures (goniotomy and trabeculodialysis) may be successful in children.

Posner–Schlossman syndrome (glaucomatocyclitic crisis)

Pathogenesis: unilateral acute elevation of IOP associated with mild anterior uveitis and an open angle, presumed to be the result of acute trabeculitis. The cause is uncertain. Young adults are typically affected; 40% are positive for HLA-Bw54. Some will develop chronic open-angle glaucoma.

Diagnosis
- **Presentation:** subacute onset of mild discomfort, haloes, and slight blurring.
- **Signs:** (a) epithelial oedema, (b) high IOP (40–80 mm Hg), (c) a few aqueous cells, and (d) fine white central keratic precipitates.

Treatment: topical steroids and aqueous suppressants.

Lens-related glaucomas

Phacolytic glaucoma

Pathogenesis: open-angle glaucoma occurring in association with a hypermature cataract. Trabecular obstruction is caused by lens proteins leaking through the intact capsule, and macrophages.

Diagnosis

- **Presentation:** pain in an eye with very poor vision due to a hypermature cataract.
- **Signs:** (a) epithelial oedema; (b) deep anterior chamber, sometimes with white particles (*Fig. 10.21*) or pseudohypopyon (*Fig. 10.22*).

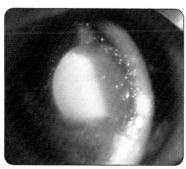

Fig 10.21

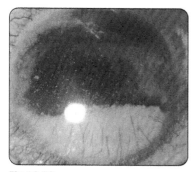

Fig 10.22

Treatment: medical control of IOP followed by cataract removal.

Phacomorphic glaucoma

Pathogenesis: acute angle-closure glaucoma precipitated by an intumescent cataract.

Diagnosis

- **Presentation:** similar to acute PACG.
- **Signs:** shallow anterior chamber, mid-dilated pupil, and cataract; fellow eye usually shows an open angle.

Treatment

- Similar to acute PACG, but miotics are omitted.
- Laser iridotomy/iridoplasty is often not possible or is ineffective.
- Cataract extraction is the definitive treatment.

Lens dislocation into the anterior chamber

Pathogenesis: blunt ocular trauma is the typical precipitant, particularly in eyes with predisposing conditions such as PXF; the dislocated lens may cause acute pupillary block.

Diagnosis: presentation is with sudden onset of visual impairment and symptoms of raised IOP.

Treatment: osmotic agents are generally included in the initial treatment. Relief of pupillary block by laser iridotomy may be sufficient in some cases. Subsequent treatment:

- **Intact zonule:** patient should lie supine with the pupil dilated to try to reposition the lens in the posterior chamber.

- **Soft lens without zonular attachments:** lensectomy through an anterior approach.
- **Hard lens without zonular attachments:** pars plana vitrectomy and lensectomy.

Traumatic glaucoma

Hyphaema

Pathogenesis: although most traumatic hyphaemas are relatively innocuous, prolonged marked elevation of IOP, principally due to trabecular obstruction, may damage the optic nerve and cause corneal blood staining. Secondary haemorrhage is often more severe than the primary bleed. The risk of complications is higher the larger the hyphaema; patients with sickle cell haemoglobinopathies are at increased risk.

Treatment

- Hospital admission and sometimes bed rest may be prudent for a large hyphaema (Fig. 10.23).

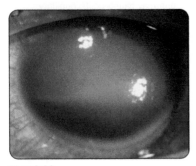

Fig 10.23

- A coagulation abnormality should be excluded and anticoagulant medication discontinued after liaison with an appropriate physician; NSAIDs should be avoided.
- IOP is treated initially with a beta-blocker and/or a topical or systemic CAI; the latter is avoided in sickle haemoglobinopathies if possible.
- Miotics and prostaglandins should be avoided; alpha-agonists are avoided in small children and patients with sickling disorders.
- Topical steroids reduce inflammation and possibly the risk of secondary haemorrhage.
- Mydriatics (e.g. atropine) may be considered to immobilize the pupil.
- Systemic or topical anti-fibrinolysis is of uncertain benefit.
- Surgical evacuation of the blood if at risk of permanent corneal staining (rare) or intractable IOP, amblyopia, or for a total hyphaema of more than 5 days' duration.
- Avoidance of activity with a risk of even minor eye trauma for several weeks; rebleed should prompt immediate review.

Angle recession glaucoma

Pathogenesis: rupture of the ciliary body between the iris root and the scleral spur due to blunt trauma; 6–9% develop glaucoma after 10 years, probably due to associated trabecular damage; the risk of glaucoma is directly related to the extent of angle recession.

Diagnosis

- Signs of previous blunt trauma may be only mild (e.g. a small sphincter rupture).
- Gonioscopy may initially show irregular widening of the ciliary body (*Fig. 10.24*), obscured by fibrosis in some long-standing cases.

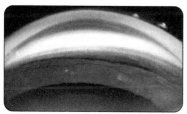

Fig 10.24

Treatment: lifelong periodic review to detect elevated IOP; medical treatment as for other types of open-angle glaucoma, although surgery is often required.

Iridocorneal endothelial syndrome

Pathogenesis: proliferation of an abnormal corneal endothelial cell layer across the angle and iris causing a spectrum of glaucoma and corneal decompensation. Iridocorneal endothelial syndrome (ICE) typically affects one eye of a middle-aged woman. The aetiology may be viral; three clinical patterns are distinguished, although overlap is common.

Diagnosis

- *Iris signs:* (a) atrophy of varying severity, (b) corectopia (malposition of the pupil; *Fig.*

10.25), and (c) pseudopolycoria (supernumerary false pupils; *Fig. 10.26*).

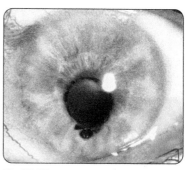

Fig 10.25

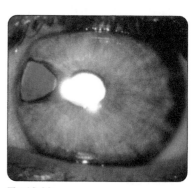

Fig 10.26

- *Glaucoma:* with broad-based PAS, extending to Schwalbe line (*Fig. 10.27*) in 50% of cases.
- *Progressive iris atrophy variant:* severe iris changes (*Fig. 10.28*).
- *Iris naevus (Cogan–Reese) syndrome:* either a diffuse naevus that covers the anterior iris or iris nodules (*Fig. 10.29*); absence of iris atrophy in 50%.

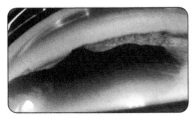

Fig 10.27

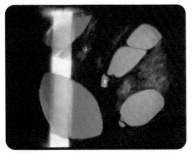

Fig 10.28

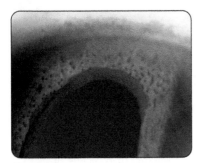

Fig 10.29

- *Chandler syndrome:* 'hammered silver' corneal endothelial abnormalities (*Fig. 10.30*), often with corneal oedema; absence of iris atrophy in 60%, and less severe glaucoma.

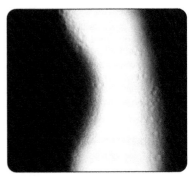

Fig 10.30

Treatment: medical treatment is often ineffective; filtering shunts or cyclodiode are eventually required.

Glaucoma associated with intraocular tumours

Pathogenesis: approximately 5% of eyes with an intraocular tumour develop a secondary elevation of IOP by one of the following mechanisms:
- *Trabecular obstruction:* direct invasion by an iris or ciliary body melanoma, or seeding from a remote tumour.
- *Trabecular blockage by macrophages* (*Fig. 10.31*) that have ingested pigment and tumour cells.

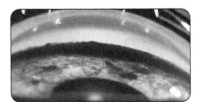

Fig 10.31

- **Secondary angle closure:** due to (a) angle neovascularization (e.g. with choroidal melanoma, retinoblastoma) or (b) anterior displacement of iris-lens diaphragm with ciliary body melanoma or a large posterior segment tumour.

Glaucoma in iridoschisis

Pathogenesis: rare condition that typically affects the elderly and is often bilateral; in most cases, the iris atrophy probably results from intermittent angle closure.

Diagnosis: (a) shallow anterior chamber and narrow angle, and (b) iris atrophy usually inferiorly (*Fig. 10.32*).

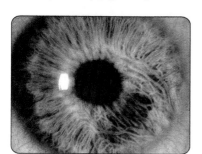

Fig 10.32

Treatment: laser iridotomy.

Primary congenital glaucoma

Pathogenesis: impaired aqueous outflow in primary congenital glaucoma is caused by maldevelopment of the anterior

chamber angle, by definition not associated with any other major ocular anomaly. Most cases are sporadic; in 40% IOP is elevated *in utero*, and by the third birthday in just over half (infantile glaucoma). Two-thirds of patients are boys, with bilateral involvement in 75%.

Diagnosis
- **Presentation:** corneal haze, lacrimation, photophobia, and blepharospasm.
- **Buphthalmos:** large eye (*Fig. 10.33*) due to elevated IOP prior to the age of 3 years; corneal diameter >11 mm before 1 year of age or >13 mm at any age is suspicious.

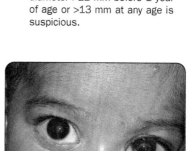

Fig 10.33

- **Haab striae:** healed curvilinear breaks in Descemet membrane (*Fig. 10.34*).
- **Optic disc cupping:** may regress in infants once the IOP is normalized; most normal infants exhibit no (or a very small) cup.
- **Evaluation under general anaesthesia:** (a) measurement of corneal diameter; (b) gonioscopy may reveal a normal-appearing or frankly abnormal angle.

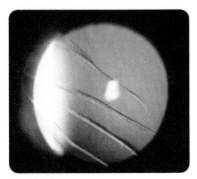

Fig 10.34

- **Differential diagnosis:** (a) lacrimation due to delayed canalization of the nasolacrimal duct, (b) other causes of corneal clouding (e.g. trauma, rubella), (c) large cornea (e.g. megalocornea), and (d) secondary infantile glaucoma (e.g. retinoblastoma, persistent posterior fetal vasculature, iridocorneal dysgenesis).

Treatment

- **Goniotomy:** horizontal incision at the midpoint of the superficial layers of the trabecular meshwork (*Fig. 10.35*); eventual success in approximately 85%.

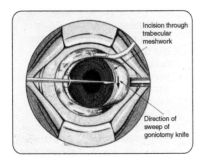

Incision through trabecular meshwork

Direction of sweep of goniotomy knife

Fig 10.35

- **Trabeculotomy:** if corneal clouding prevents visualization of the angle or when repeated goniotomy has failed: a trabeculotome is inserted into Schlemm canal via a partial thickness scleral flap and rotated into the anterior chamber (*Fig. 10.36*).

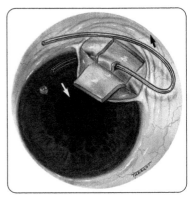

Fig 10.36

- **Trabeculectomy with adjunctive antimetabolites:** often successful.
- **Follow-up:** progressive enlargement of the corneal diameter is a key marker of uncontrolled IOP; correction of refractive errors is important.

Iridocorneal dysgenesis

Posterior embryotoxon

Definition: posterior embryotoxon is an isolated innocuous finding in 10% of the general population, consisting of a prominent and anteriorly displaced Schwalbe line and seen as a thin grey-white arcuate ridge (*Fig. 10.37*). Axenfeld–Rieger anomaly (see below)

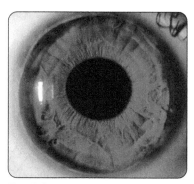

Fig 10.37

always includes posterior embryotoxon.

Axenfeld–Rieger syndrome

Definition: Axenfeld–Rieger syndrome is a spectrum of disorders featuring bilateral developmental ocular anomalies commonly including glaucoma. AD inheritance is frequent but there is no gender predilection. Several gene loci have been implicated. Individual entities are distinguished: (a) Axenfeld anomaly, (b) Rieger anomaly, and (c) Rieger syndrome.

Diagnosis

- *Axenfeld anomaly:* posterior embryotoxon with attached strands of peripheral iris tissue (*Fig. 10.38*).

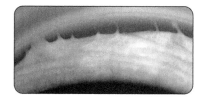

Fig 10.38

- *Rieger anomaly:* (a) posterior embryotoxon, (b) iris stromal hypoplasia (*Fig. 10.39*), (c) ectropion uveae, (d) corectopia and full-thickness iris defects (*Fig. 10.40*), and (e) gonioscopic abnormalities ranging from Axenfeld anomaly to broad leaves of iris stroma adherent to the cornea (*Fig. 10.41*); glaucoma occurs in approximately 50%, usually in childhood or early adulthood.
- *Rieger syndrome:* Rieger anomaly associated with extraocular

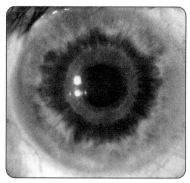

Fig 10.39

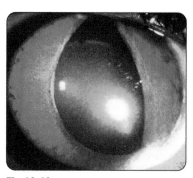

Fig 10.40

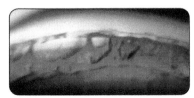

Fig 10.41

malformations such as (a) dental (hypodontia, microdontia; *Fig. 10.42*), (b) facial (maxillary hypoplasia, hypertelorism), (c) redundant paraumbilical skin, and (d) hypospadias.

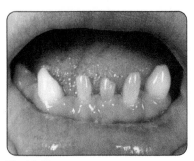

Fig 10.42

Treatment: IOP should initially be managed medically; surgery may be required.

Aniridia

Genetics: aniridia is a rare bilateral condition occurring as a result of abnormal neuroectodermal development secondary to a mutation in the PAX6 gene on chromosome 11; PAX6 is adjacent to gene WT1, mutation of which predisposes to the life-threatening Wilms tumour (nephroblastoma). AD aniridia accounts for approximately two-thirds of cases and has no systemic implications. Approximately one-third of cases are sporadic, conferring a 30% chance of developing Wilms tumour.

Diagnosis

- *Presentation:* at birth with nystagmus and photophobia; parents may have noticed absent irides or 'dilated pupils' (*Fig. 10.43*).

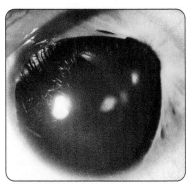

Fig 10.43

- *Gonioscopy:* hypoplastic iris, which may consist only of a rudimentary frill.
- *Cornea:* limbal stem cell deficiency may result in 'conjunctivalization' of the cornea; dry eye and epithelial defects are common; dense central scarring sometimes occurs.
- *Lens:* cataract and subluxation.
- *Fundus:* foveal and optic nerve hypoplasia, and choroidal coloboma.
- *Glaucoma:* present in 75%, which is caused by synechial angle closure (*Fig. 10.44*), and usually presents in adolescence.

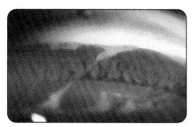

Fig 10.44

Treatment: all patients with sporadic aniridia should undergo regular abdominal ultrasonography unless absence of a predisposing WT1 mutation is confirmed.

- *Glaucoma:* can be resistant to medical treatment; (a) goniotomy may prevent a subsequent rise in IOP if performed before the development of irreversible synechial angle closure, (b) enhanced trabeculectomy or shunts may be effective in established glaucoma, but (c) cyclodiode may be necessary in many cases.
- *Opaque contact lenses:* to create an artificial pupil, may improve both vision and cosmesis.
- *Limbal stem cell transplantation.*

Glaucoma medications

Beta-blockers

- *Mechanism of action:* decrease aqueous secretion and are therefore useful in all types of glaucoma, irrespective of the state of the angle.

- *Tachyphylaxis:* occurs in approximately 10%; additional effect is limited if a topical beta blocker is used in a patient already taking a systemic beta-blocker.
- *Ocular side effects:* allergy, corneal punctate epithelial erosions, and reduced aqueous tear secretion.
- *Systemic side effects:* (a) bradycardia and hypotension (pulse must be palpated before prescribing), (b) bronchospasm, (c) sleep disorders, (d) hallucinations, (e) depression, (f) fatigue, and (g) headache. Reduction of systemic absorption may be achieved by lacrimal occlusion following instillation (digital pressure over the lacrimal sac area for approximately 3 min); closing the eyes alone for 3 min will reduce systemic absorption by approximately 50%.
- *Contraindications:* (a) asthma and obstructive airways disease, (b) bradycardia, (c) congestive cardiac failure, (d) second- or third-degree heart block, and (e) peripheral vascular disease (relative). Bedtime instillation should be avoided because a consequent nocturnal blood pressure dip may reduce optic nerve perfusion.
- *Preparations:* (a) timolol (0.25% and 0.5%) twice daily, (b) Timoptol-LA (0.25% and 0.5%) once daily, (c) Nyogel 0.1% gel once daily, (d) betaxolol 0.5% twice daily (may increase optic nerve blood flow), (e) levobunolol 0.5% once or twice daily, and (f) carteolol 1% or 2% twice daily (may induce less bradycardia than timolol).

Alpha-2 agonists

- *Mechanism of action:* reduce IOP by both decreasing aqueous secretion and enhancing uveoscleral outflow.
- *Preparations:* (a) brimonidine 0.2% twice daily is slightly less effective than timolol although may have a neuroprotective effect; main side effects are allergic conjunctivitis, xerostomia, drowsiness, and fatigue; (b) apraclonidine 1% is used mainly after laser surgery on the anterior segment to prevent an acute rise in IOP; 0.5% concentration may be used short-term, typically while a patient is awaiting glaucoma surgery; tachyphylaxis and local side effects limit long-term use.

Prostaglandin analogues

- *Mechanism of action:* principally by promoting uveoscleral outflow; bimatoprost also enhances trabecular drainage.
- *Preparations:* (a) latanoprost 0.005% once daily at bedtime provides greater IOP-lowering than timolol, although a proportion may show no response, (b) travoprost 0.004% is similar in effect to latanoprost; conjunctival hyperaemia occurs in up to 50% of patients but tends to subside with time, (c) bimatoprost (0.01% or 0.03%) is similar to latanoprost although may cause less iris pigmentation but more conjunctival hyperaemia; 0.01% may have a similar IOP-lowering effect to 0.03% but with less hyperaemia, and (d) tafluprost 0.0015% is available in preservative-free form.
- *Ocular side effects:* (a) conjunctival hyperaemia, (b) eyelash lengthening, thickening, and hyperpigmentation, (c) irreversible iris hyperpigmentation (particularly in green-brown/hazel irides), (d) hyperpigmentation of periocular skin (common but reversible), and occasionally (e) cystoid macular oedema, anterior uveitis, and herpetic keratitis.
- *Systemic side effects:* rarely mild upper respiratory tract symptoms in susceptible individuals, skin rash, and headaches/migraine; should be avoided in pregnancy.

Topical carbonic anhydrase inhibitors

- *Mechanism of action:* inhibition of aqueous secretion.
- *Preparations:* (a) dorzolamide 2% three times daily is used as monotherapy or adjunctive treatment, and it is similar in efficacy to betaxolol but inferior to timolol; main side effects are allergic blepharoconjunctivitis, and a transient bitter taste; may occasionally precipitate corneal decompensation; (b) brinzolamide 1% twice or three times daily is similar to dorzolamide, but with a lower incidence of stinging and local allergy.

Miotics

- *Mechanisms of action:* (a) in POAG, contraction of the ciliary muscle and so increase trabecular outflow; (b) in PACG, the peripheral iris is pulled away from the trabeculum and the angle opened.
- *Preparations:* (a) pilocarpine (0.5–4%) is equal in efficacy to beta blockers but for monotherapy must typically be used four times daily,

and (b) pilocarpine 4% gel instilled once daily at bedtime.

- *Ocular side effects:* miosis, brow ache, myopic shift, and exacerbation of cataract symptoms.

Combined preparations

Numerous combined 'fixed' preparations (e.g. a beta blocker and a prostaglandin analogue) offer ocular hypotensive effects close to the sum of the individual components, improve compliance, and are often more cost-effective.

Systemic carbonic acid inhibitors

- *Mechanism of action:* inhibition of aqueous secretion.
- *Indications:* principally as short-term treatment; systemic side effects limit long-term use to patients at high risk of visual loss.
- *Preparations:* (a) acetazolamide (tablets, sustained-release capsules and vials for injection), (b) dichlorphenamide tablets, and (c) methazolamide tablets (useful alternative to acetazolamide with longer duration of action).
- *Systemic side effects:* (a) paraesthesia (tingling) of the extremities, (b) malaise, (c) lowered mood, (d) gastrointestinal symptoms, (e) hypokalaemia, (f) renal stone formation, (g) Stevens–Johnson syndrome, and (h) blood dyscrasia.

Osmotic agents

- *Mechanism of action:* creation of an osmotic gradient so that water is 'drawn out' from the vitreous into the blood.
- *Indications:* when a temporary drop in IOP is required that cannot be achieved by other means (e.g. in acute angle-closure glaucoma and prior to intraocular surgery when the IOP is very high).
- *Preparations:* (a) mannitol (intravenous), (b) glycerol (oral; may be given to well-controlled diabetics), and (c) isosorbide (metabolically inert oral agent).
- *Side effects:* cardiovascular overload (use with caution in cardiac or renal disease), urinary retention, headache, backache, nausea, and confusion.

Laser therapy

Argon laser trabeculoplasty

- *Mechanism of action:* application of discrete laser burns to the trabecular meshwork enhances aqueous outflow.
- *Indications:* adult open-angle glaucomas, usually as an adjunct to medical therapy.
- *Complications:* (a) elevation of IOP, (b) anterior uveitis (usually mild), and (c) possibly an adverse effect on subsequent filtration surgery.
- *Efficacy:* in POAG, the initial success rate is 75–85%, with an average

reduction in IOP of approximately 30%; up to 50% of eyes are still controlled after 5 years, with failure occurring most frequently in the first year.

Selective laser trabeculoplasty

- SLT targets melanin pigment in the trabecular meshwork cells, leaving nonpigmented structures unscathed.
- Aiming is easier than with ALT, so may give more consistent results.
- May also be safer than ALT because there is no thermal tissue damage; repeat treatment sessions are thought to be more effective than with ALT.

Nd:YAG laser iridotomy

- *Mechanism of action:* relieves pupillary block by creating a small opening in the peripheral iris.
- *Indications:* PACS, PAC, PACG, and secondary angle-closure with pupillary block.
- *Complications:* (a) IOP elevation, (b) anterior uveitis (usually mild and transient), (c) cataract promotion, and (d) glare and diplopia, if the iridotomy is not sited under the upper eyelid.

Diode laser ablation (cyclodiode)

- *Mechanism of action:* lowers IOP by destroying part of the secretory ciliary epithelium, thereby reducing aqueous secretion.
- *Indications:* uncontrolled end-stage secondary glaucoma with minimal visual potential, mainly to control pain; lower intensity regimens can be used in eyes with good vision.
- *Complications:* (a) anterior segment inflammation, (b) IOP elevation, (c) hypotony, (d) suprachoroidal haemorrhage, and (e) corneal decompensation.

Laser iridoplasty

- *Mechanism of action:* widens the anterior chamber angle by contracting the peripheral iris away from the angle recess, often in nonpupillary block angle closure.
- *Complications:* iritis, IOP spikes, altered accommodation (common but transient).

Trabeculectomy

Definition: trabeculectomy remains the most commonly-performed surgical drainage procedure. Lowering of IOP is caused by the creation of a guarded fistula allowing aqueous outflow from the anterior chamber to the sub-Tenon space (*Fig. 10.45*); major complications are discussed below.

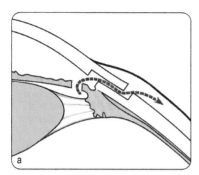

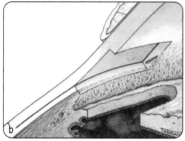

Fig 10.45

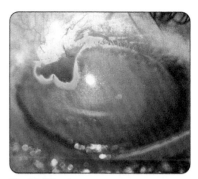

Fig 10.46

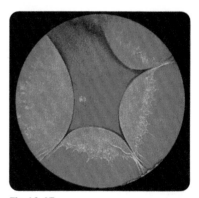

Fig 10.47

Shallow anterior chamber

- *Pupillary block:* caused by a non-patent surgical iridectomy. Signs: (a) high IOP and flat bleb, (b) negative Seidel test, and (c) iris bombé with a non-patent iridectomy. Treatment involves YAG laser to the iridectomy site.
- *Overfiltration:* caused by conjunctival bleb leakage (positive Seidel test; *Fig. 10.46*), overdrainage at the scleral flap, or a combination. Signs: (a) low IOP, bleb may be flat (conjunctival leak) or well-formed (scleral overdrainage alone); (b) choroidal detachment (*Fig. 10.47*) may be present. Treatment depends on the cause and degree of shallowing.
- *'Malignant' glaucoma:* caused by anterior rotation of the ciliary processes and iris root, often with aqueous misdirection (ciliolenticular block) in which aqueous is forced backwards into the vitreous. Signs: (a) high IOP but no bleb, and (b) negative Seidel test. Initial treatment is with mydriatics, and if necessary osmotic agents (e.g. mannitol) to

shrink the vitreous; subsequent treatment may involve YAG laser disruption of the anterior hyaloid face, cyclodiode, or pars plana vitrectomy.

Failure of filtration

- *Appearance of a normal bleb:* slightly elevated, avascular, and shows superficial microcysts (*Fig. 10.48a*).

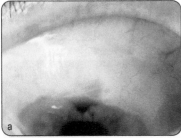

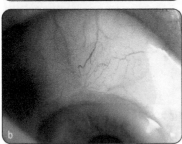

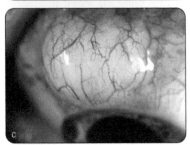

- *Poorly functioning bleb:* may be (a) flat and avascular, (b) vascularized due to episcleral fibrosis (*Fig. 10.48b*), or (c) encapsulated (Tenon cyst—dome-shaped, firm, fluid-filled; *Fig. 10.48c*).
- *Causes of failure:* (a) extrascleral (e.g. conjunctival and episcleral fibrosis), (b) scleral (e.g. overtight suturing of the scleral flap or scarring in the scleral bed), and (c) intraocular causes (e.g. blockage of the sclerostomy by vitreous, blood, uveal, or scar tissue).
- *Treatment:* (a) ocular 'massage' to encourage fistula flow, (b) suture manipulation, (c) needling of an encysted bleb, and (d) surgical revision.

Late bleb leakage

- *Cause:* disintegration of conjunctiva overlying the sclerostomy, particularly after prior mitomycin C application.
- *Complications:* infection and hypotony maculopathy (see Chapter 14).
- *Signs:* (a) low IOP, (b) avascular cystic bleb, (c) sometimes only multiple punctate staining areas ('sweating') rather than a frank leak may be seen, and (d) shallow anterior chamber and choroidal detachment in severe cases.
- *Treatment:* (a) sweating blebs may be treated by injection of autologous blood, conjunctival compression, or transconjunctival scleral flap sutures; (b) full-thickness holes usually require revisional surgery, such as conjunctival advancement or free conjunctival and/or scleral patch grafts.

Fig 10.48

Bleb-associated bacterial infection and endophthalmitis

- **Classification:** (a) limited to the bleb (blebitis), and (b) endophthalmitis.
- **Risk factors:** (a) chronic blepharitis, (b) higher dose mitomycin C, (c) long-term topical antibiotic use, (d) inferior or nasally placed bleb, and (e) bleb leak.
- **Blebitis:** (a) presents with mild discomfort and redness, (b) bleb contains whitish inflammatory material (*Fig. 10.49*), (c) anterior uveitis may be absent, and (d) red reflex is normal. Treatment is with topical and oral antibiotics.

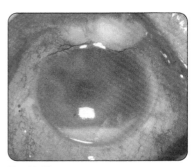

Fig 10.50

should be considered if there is no early response.

Nonpenetrating surgery

- **Definition:** in nonpenetrating surgery, the anterior chamber is not entered, reducing the incidence of postoperative hypotony.
- **Indications:** mainly POAG, although other open-angle glaucomas may also be amenable. Conventional filtration is often still the procedure of choice when the target IOP is in the low teens.
- **Deep sclerectomy:** a Descemet window is created that allows aqueous percolation from the anterior chamber to the subconjunctival space via an intrascleral chamber.
- **Viscocanalostomy:** creation of the filtering window is followed by dilatation of Schlemm canal with high-density viscoelastic, with drainage principally utilizing the canal rather than the subconjunctival space; a variation involves cannulation of the entire circumference of Schlemm canal with a microcatheter (canaloplasty).

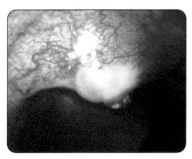

Fig 10.49

- **Endophthalmitis:** (a) presents with rapidly worsening vision, pain, and redness, (b) milky-white bleb containing pus, (c) severe anterior uveitis, often with hypopyon (*Fig. 10.50*), and (d) vitritis with impairment of the red reflex. Treatment involves topical and systemic therapy, although intravitreal antibiotics as for post-cataract surgery endophthalmitis (see Chapter 9)

- **Trabectome:** approaches the angle *ab interno* to remove a strip of trabecular meshwork; although it does not seem to lower the IOP as effectively as trabeculectomy, the safety profile is better.

Drainage shunts

Shunts using episcleral explants

- **Mechanism of action:** creation of a communication between the anterior chamber and sub-Tenon space through a tube attached to a posterior episcleral explant. Some contain pressure-sensitive valves for regulation of aqueous flow; examples include Molteno, Baerveldt, and Ahmed implants.
- **Indications:** traditionally cases in which trabeculectomy has a particularly poor prognosis (e.g. previous failed trabeculectomy, neovascular glaucoma), but the threshold for their use has recently decreased.
- **Complications:** (a) excessive drainage with hypotony, (b) tube erosion, (c) tube malposition (*Fig. 10.51*) with

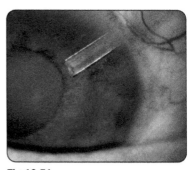

Fig 10.51

endothelial or lenticular touch, and (d) ocular motility abnormalities.

Mini shunts

- **Ex-Press mini shunt:** new device without a valve that is inserted under a scleral flap during a modified trabeculectomy; initial results are very promising.
- **iStent:** tiny titanium hooked tube inserted *ab interno* into Schlemm canal via the trabecular meshwork, often in conjunction with cataract surgery; provides a useful but frequently modest IOP reduction.

Chapter **11**

Uveitis

Terminology

- **Uveitis:** inflammation of the uveal tract.
- **Anterior uveitis:** iritis and iridocyclitis (iris and ciliary body).
- **Intermediate uveitis:** inflammation of the pars plana, the peripheral retina, and the vitreous.
- **Posterior uveitis:** inflammation posterior to the vitreous base.
- **Retinitis:** primary retinal focus of inflammation.
- **Choroiditis:** primary choroidal focus.
- **Vasculitis:** inflammation of veins, arteries, or both.
- **Panuveitis:** involvement of the entire uveal tract.
- **Endophthalmitis:** involves all intraocular tissues except the sclera.
- **Panophthalmitis:** involves the entire globe.

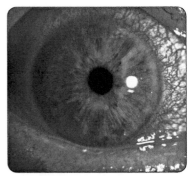

Fig 11.1

Clinical features

Acute anterior uveitis

Acute anterior uveitis (AAU) is the most common form of uveitis.

- **Presentation:** rapid onset of unilateral pain, photophobia, and redness.
- **Signs:** (a) ciliary injection, (b) miosis (Fig. 11.1), (c) endothelial dusting by inflammatory cells progresses to fine/medium keratic precipitates (KP) after a few days, (d) hypopyon in intense inflammation (Fig. 11.2), (e) anterior vitreous cells in iridocyclitis, and (f) aqueous flare (Fig. 11.3).
- **Duration:** most episodes completely resolve within 5–6 weeks.
- **Prognosis:** good with adequate treatment.

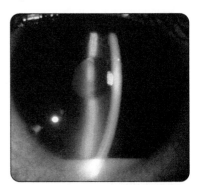

Fig 11.2

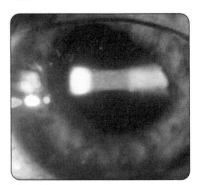

Fig 11.3

Chronic anterior uveitis

Chronic anterior uveitis (CAU) is less common than the acute type, and it is more frequently bilateral; inflammation may be granulomatous or non-granulomatous.

- **Presentation:** often insidious and may be asymptomatic until complications such as cataract or band keratopathy develop.
- **Signs:** (a) eye may be mildly injected or white, depending on the cause, (b) aqueous cells vary in number according to activity, (c) aqueous flare may be more marked than cells in eyes with prolonged activity, (d) large KP with a greasy 'mutton-fat' appearance (*Fig. 11.4*) and iris nodules in granulomatous disease (*Fig. 11.5*); (e) posterior synechiae (*Fig. 11.6*).
- **Duration:** prolonged; may last for months or even years with remissions and exacerbations.
- **Prognosis:** guarded because of complications such as cataract, glaucoma, hypotony, and phthisis bulbi (*Fig. 11.7*).

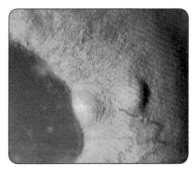

Fig 11.5

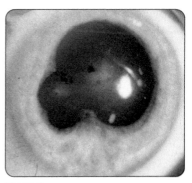

Fig 11.6

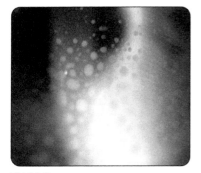

Fig 11.4

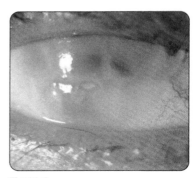

Fig 11.7

Posterior uveitis

- *Presentation:* varies according to the location of the inflammatory focus and the presence of vitritis.
- *Retinitis:* whitish retinal opacities with indistinct borders (*Fig. 11.8*) and overlying vitritis.
- *Choroiditis:* deep, round, yellow nodules (*Fig. 11.9*).
- *Vasculitis:* (periphlebitis, periarteritis) may be primary or secondary to retinitis; yellowish or grey-white patchy perivascular cuffing which may be associated with haemorrhages (*Fig. 11.10*).

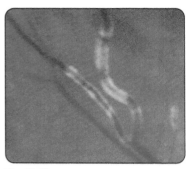

Fig 11.10

Fig 11.8

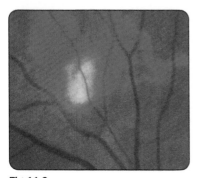

Fig 11.9

Principles of treatment

Mydriatics

- *Indications:* (a) to relieve pain caused by iridociliary spasm, and (b) prevent (or break recently formed) posterior synechiae.
- *Topical short-acting:* (a) cyclopentolate (0.5%, 1%) acts for approximately 24 hr; (b) tropicamide and phenylephrine are shorter-acting.
- *Topical long-acting:* (a) homatropine 2% (approximately 2 days); (b) and atropine 1% (up to 2 weeks).
- *Subconjunctival:* Mydricaine (adrenaline, atropine, and procaine) if no response to drops.

Topical steroids

- *Indications:* anterior uveitis.
- *Preparations:* dexamethasone, prednisolone (range of concentrations available), betamethasone, loteprednol, fluorometholone, and rimexolone.
- *Complications:* glaucoma, cataract, and corneal infection.

Periocular steroid injection

- **Advantages over topical administration:** (a) higher posterior segment concentrations may be achieved, (b) water-soluble drugs, incapable of penetrating topically, but can enter trans-sclerally, and (c) prolonged effect can be achieved with 'depot' preparations.
- **Indications:** (a) primary treatment of intermediate and certain types of posterior uveitis, (b) to supplement systemic therapy or when it is contraindicated, (c) poor compliance with topical or systemic medication, and (d) perioperatively in uveitic eyes.
- **Complications:** (a) globe penetration, (b) elevation of IOP (may be refractory with depot preparations), (c) ptosis, (d) subdermal fat atrophy, (e) ocular motility paresis, (f) optic nerve injury, (g) retinal and choroidal vascular occlusion, and (h) cutaneous hypopigmentation.
- **Technique:** via the superotemporal conjunctiva (posterior sub-Tenon; *Fig. 11.11*), or to the orbital floor via skin or conjunctiva.

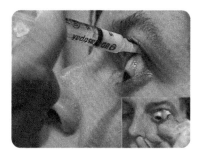

Fig 11.11

Intraocular steroids

- **Intravitreal injection:** triamcinolone acetonide can be used for some forms of posterior uveitis unresponsive to other modalities and for refractory cystoid macular oedema (CMO).
- **Complications:** (a) elevation of IOP, (b) cataract, (c) endophthalmitis (sterile or infectious), (d) haemorrhage, and (e) retinal detachment.
- **Slow-release implants:** biodegradable insert or a slow-release reservoir (fluocinolone acetonide, dexamethasone) offer the benefits of intravitreal steroid injection but over an extended period of up to 3 years; complications are similar to those of intravitreal triamcinolone injection.

Systemic steroids

- **Indications:** (a) intermediate uveitis unresponsive to periocular injection, and (b) sight-threatening posterior uveitis, particularly if bilateral.
- **Contraindications:** (a) poorly-controlled diabetes (relative contraindication), (b) peptic ulceration, (c) osteoporosis, (d) active systemic infection, and (e) psychosis on previous exposure to steroids.
- **Preparations:** oral prednisolone and intravenous methylprednisolone.
- **Common cause of failure:** inadequate dosage; a large dose should be used initially and subsequently tapered.
- **Side effects with short-term use:** (a) dyspepsia, (b) mental changes, (c) electrolyte imbalance, (d) aseptic necrosis of the head of the femur,

and (e) destabilization of diabetic control.

- **Side effects with long-term use:** (a) Cushingoid state, (b) osteoporosis, (c) limitation of growth in children, (d) reactivation of infections such as TB, (e) cataract, and (f) elevation of IOP.

Antimetabolites

- **Indications:** (a) sight-threatening uveitis, typically bilateral, non-infectious and reversible, after failure to respond to adequate steroid therapy, (b) steroid-sparing therapy in patients with intolerable side effects from systemic steroids, and (c) chronic relapsing disease requiring a daily dose of prednisolone above approximately 10 mg.
- **Preparations:** azathioprine, methotrexate, and mycophenolate mofetil.
- **Side effects:** (a) gastrointestinal disturbance, (b) bone marrow suppression, and (c) hepatotoxicity.

Other drugs

- **Ciclosporin:** drug of choice for Behçet syndrome; side effects include nephrotoxicity and hepatotoxicity.
- **Tacrolimus:** alternative to ciclosporin in intolerant or unresponsive patients.
- **Biological blockers:** interleukin receptor antagonists (daclizumab, anakinra) and tumour necrosis factor-alpha antagonists (infliximab, adalimumab).

Intermediate uveitis

Definition: intermediate uveitis (IU) is a chronic/relapsing condition that may be idiopathic or associated with systemic disease. It is typically bilateral but asymmetrical. Systemic associations include (a) multiple sclerosis (MS), (b) sarcoidosis, (c) Lyme disease, and (d) TB. The course and prognosis are very variable.

Diagnosis

- **Presentation:** in childhood or early adult life with insidious onset of blurred vision and floaters.
- **Signs:** (a) mild anterior uveitis, (b) vitreous cells with anterior predominance, (c) inferior vitreous 'snowballs' (*Fig. 11.12*), (d) peripheral phlebitis, (e) inferior 'snowbanking' (*Fig. 11.13*), and (f) neovascularization on the snowbank or the optic nerve head.

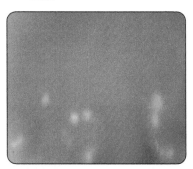

Fig 11.12

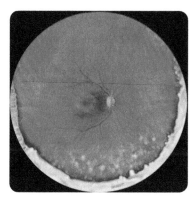

Fig 11.13

- *Complications:* (a) CMO in 30% is the major cause of visual impairment, (b) epimacular membranes, and occasionally (c) retinal detachment (tractional, rhegmatogenous, or exudative).

Treatment
- *Medical:* (a) initially topical and/or periocular steroids, (b) systemic steroids and immunosuppressive agents may be required, and (c) interferon beta for IU in MS.
- *Vitrectomy:* following failure of systemic steroids to control CMO; other indications include retinal detachment, vitreous haemorrhage, and epiretinal membranes.
- *Photocoagulation:* to peripheral retina for neovascularization at the vitreous base.

Uveitis in spondyloarthropathies

Ankylosing spondylitis

- *Definition:* an inflammatory disease leading to ossification of joints with bony ankylosis of the axial skeleton. It typically affects adult males, of whom 90% are HLA-B27 positive (6–8% of U.S. Caucasians). Radiology of the sacroiliac joints and spine reveals characteristic changes.
- *Ocular features:* AAU occurs in approximately 25% of patients with ankylosing spondylitis; conversely, 25% of males with AAU will have ankylosing spondylitis.

Reiter syndrome

- *Definition:* Reiter syndrome comprises the triad of (a) non-specific urethritis, (b) conjunctivitis, and (c) arthritis. Those affected are commonly men in the 3rd and 4th decades, of whom 85% are positive for HLA-B27.
- *Ocular features:* (a) conjunctivitis is common and usually precedes the arthritis, with spontaneous resolution occurring within 7–10 days; (b) AAU occurs in up to 12% of patients but is higher in carriers of HLA-B27.

Psoriatic arthritis

- **Definition:** arthritis developing in patients with psoriasis.
- **Ocular features:** (a) AAU occurs in approximately 7%; (b) other uncommon manifestations include conjunctivitis, marginal corneal infiltrates, and secondary Sjögren syndrome.

Uveitis in juvenile arthritis

Juvenile idiopathic arthritis

Definition: idiopathic arthritis of at least 6 weeks' duration occurring before the age of 16 years. Juvenile idiopathic arthritis (JIA) is by far the most common disease associated with childhood anterior uveitis. Girls are affected more commonly than boys. Positivity for ANA is associated with a higher risk of uveitis.

Diagnosis
- **Pauciarticular onset (60% of cases):** four or fewer joints, most commonly the knees, are involved during the first 6 months with a peak age of onset around 2 years; approximately 75% of children are ANA-positive and uveitis affects approximately 20%.
- **Polyarticular onset (20%):** five or more joints are involved; may commence throughout childhood; 40% ANA-positive and uveitis affects 5%.
- **Systemic onset (Still's disease; 20%):** presents with fever, maculopapular rash, generalized lymphadenopathy, hepatosplenomegaly, and serositis; arthritis may be absent or minimal; most are ANA-negative and uveitis does not occur.
- **Features of anterior uveitis in JIA:** (a) onset is usually asymptomatic with a white eye, (b) chronic non-granulomatous inflammation, (c) 70% bilateral, and (d) complications include band keratopathy, cataract (*Fig. 11.14*), glaucoma, and hypotony.

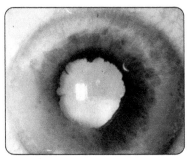

Fig 11.14

- **Differential diagnosis:** (a) idiopathic juvenile chronic iridocyclitis, (b) other types of juvenile arthritis and uveitis (e.g. juvenile spondyloarthropathies, sarcoidosis, Lyme disease, IU), and (c) masquerade syndromes (e.g. anterior segment involvement by retinoblastoma).

Treatment
- **Screening:** regular slitlamp examinations at intervals ranging from (a) 9-monthly in low-risk ANA-negative polyarticular-onset patients; (b) 2-monthly in high-risk ANA-positive pauciarticular-onset children; (c) not required in systemic-onset disease.

- *Treatment:* topical steroids are usually effective; poor responders may benefit from periocular steroids or other agents.

Uveitis in bowel disease

Ulcerative colitis

- *Definition:* idiopathic chronic inflammatory disease presenting in the 2nd and 3rd decades, affecting principally the large intestine and rectum. Extra-intestinal manifestations include mucocutaneous lesions, arthritis, and hepatic disease.
- *Ocular features:* AAU occurs in approximately 5%.

Crohn disease

- *Definition:* an idiopathic chronic granulomatous inflammatory disease of the intestinal wall, most frequently involving the ileocaecal region. Presentation is in the 2nd and 3rd decades with fever, weight loss, diarrhoea, and abdominal pain. Extra-intestinal manifestations include mucocutaneous lesions and skeletal features.
- *Ocular features:* AAU occurs in approximately 3%.

Sarcoidosis

Pathogenesis: T-lymphocyte-mediated granulomatous inflammatory disorder of unknown cause. It is most common in colder climates, although it more frequently affects patients of African descent than Caucasians. A wide range of tissues can be involved, with lung disease being common; severity varies from mild single-organ involvement to potentially fatal multisystem disease.

Diagnosis

- *Presentation:* (a) acute with fever, erythema nodosum, arthralgia, and cranial nerve palsy, or (b) insidious with symptomatic pulmonary involvement.
- *Pulmonary lesions:* vary from symptomatic hilar lymphadenopathy to severe fibrosis.
- *Skin lesions:* (a) erythema nodosum, (b) granulomas, and (c) lupus pernio.
- *Neurological disease:* (a) facial palsy, (b) seizures, (c) meningitis, (d) peripheral neuropathy, and (e) psychiatric symptoms.
- *Other:* (a) arthropathy, (b) bone cysts, (c) renal disease, (d) lymphadenopathy, and (e) liver disease.
- *Investigations:* (a) chest X-ray (abnormal in 90%), (b) biopsy (lung, lymph node, skin, conjunctiva, lacrimal gland), (c) serum angiotensin-converting enzyme and lysozyme, (d) bronchoalveolar lavage, and (e) pulmonary function tests; Mantoux test is negative in most patients.
- *Ocular features:* (a) AAU typically occurs in patients with acute-onset sarcoid, (b) CAU, typically granulomatous (*Fig. 11.15*),

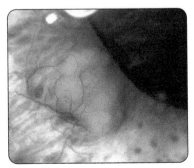

tends to affect older patients with chronic disease, (c) IU, (d) periphlebitis with 'candle wax drippings' (*Fig. 11.16*), (e) choroidal infiltrates, (f) multifocal choroiditis, (g) retinal granulomas, (h) peripheral retinal neovascularization, (i) optic nerve granulomas, and (j) disc oedema.

Fig 11.15

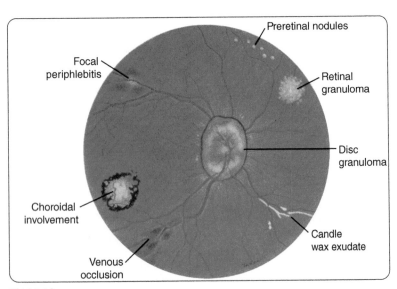

Preretinal nodules

Focal periphlebitis

Retinal granuloma

Disc granuloma

Choroidal involvement

Candle wax exudate

Venous occlusion

Fig 11.16

Treatment: anterior uveitis is treated with topical and/or periocular steroids; posterior uveitis often requires systemic steroids, and occasionally other immunosuppressive agents.

Behçet syndrome

Definition: idiopathic multisystem disease characterized by recurrent episodes of orogenital ulceration and vasculitis. It typically affects Eastern Mediterranean and Japanese individuals and is strongly associated with HLA-B51. The peak age of onset is in the 3rd decade; males are affected more frequently than females.

Diagnosis

- *Recurrent oral ulceration:* plus at least two of the following: (a) recurrent genital ulceration, (b) ocular inflammation, (c) skin lesions, and (d) positive pathergy test (pustule at needle prick site).
- *Other systemic features:* (a) vascular (aneurysms, coronary artery disease, venous thrombosis), (b) arthritis, (c) skin hypersensitivity, (d) gastrointestinal ulceration, and (e) occasionally neurological manifestations.
- *Ocular features:* common and often bilateral; (a) AAU (transient mobile hypopyon in a relatively white eye; *Fig. 11.17*), (b) persistent vitritis, (c) transient superficial white retinal infiltrates (*Fig. 11.18*), (d) diffuse retinitis, (e) retinal vasculitis (veins and arteries, often occlusive; *Fig. 11.19*), and (f) CMO, disc oedema, and optic atrophy in end-stage disease (*Fig. 11.20*).

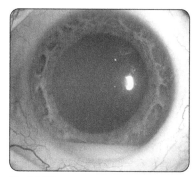

Fig 11.17

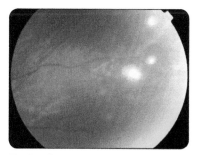

Fig 11.18

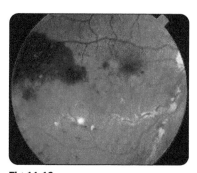

Fig 11.19

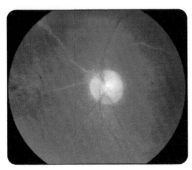

Fig 11.20

Treatment: anterior uveitis responds well to topical steroids; posterior uveitis requires systemic steroids, azathioprine, ciclosporin, subcutaneous interferon alpha, and possibly biological blockers (e.g. infliximab).

Toxoplasmosis

Pathogenesis

Toxoplasmosis is caused by the obligate intracellular protozoan *Toxoplasma gondii*.

- *Hosts:* the cat is the definitive host; intermediate hosts include mice, livestock, and humans (*Fig. 11.21*).

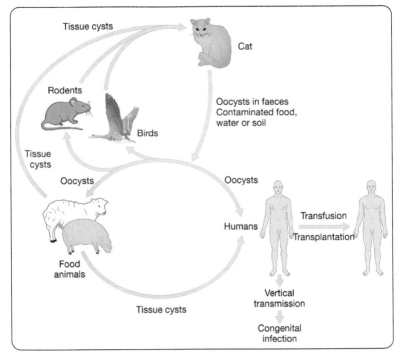

Fig 11.21

- **Sporozoites:** excreted in the faeces of the cat and spread to intermediate hosts.
- **Bradyzoites:** contained within cysts in the brain, eye, skeletal muscles, and other tissues and may lie dormant for many years.
- **Tachyzoites:** proliferating active form responsible for tissue destruction.
- **Modes of human infection:** (a) ingestion of undercooked meat from an intermediate host containing bradyzoites, (b) ingestion of sporocysts following inadvertent contamination of hands (e.g. cat litter tray), and (c) transplacental tachyzoite transfer.
- **Congenital toxoplasmosis:** follows maternal infection during pregnancy; manifestations range from stillbirth earlier in pregnancy through hydrocephalus, convulsions, paralysis, and visceral involvement to subclinical disease (may still cause intracranial calcification and chorioretinal scars).
- **Acquired toxoplasmosis:** commonly subclinical in the immunocompetent, although a lymphadenopathic syndrome, and rarely meningoencephalitis or an exanthematous form, can occur. In immunocompromised patients, infection is much more commonly life-threatening (e.g. intracerebral space-occupying lesion in AIDS).

Toxoplasma retinitis

Pathogenesis: reactivation at previously inactive cyst-containing scars. Inflammatory episodes (average age 25 years) occur when cysts rupture and release hundreds of tachyzoites into normal retina.

Diagnosis
- **Presentation:** subacute onset of floaters and blurring.
- **Signs:** (a) 'spillover' anterior uveitis may be granulomatous or resemble Fuchs syndrome, (b) solitary focal retinitis near an old pigmented scar ('satellite lesion') is typical (*Fig. 11.22*), and (c) vitritis (*Fig. 11.23*).
- **Course:** healing occurs within 6–8 weeks, with vitreous opacities taking longer to resolve; a sharply demarcated atrophic scar becomes progressively pigmented from the edges.

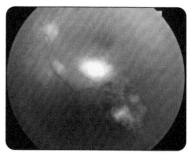

Fig 11.22

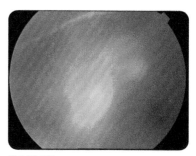

Fig 11.23

- *Causes of permanent visual loss:* (a) direct macular (*Fig. 11.24*) or optic nerve head involvement, (b) macular oedema, and (c) occlusion of a major blood vessel by the inflammatory focus.

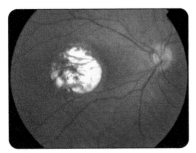

Fig 11.24

Treatment

- *Aims:* (a) limitation of the duration and severity of acute inflammation, (b) limitation of the size of scarring, and (c) reduction of recurrences.
- *Indications:* (a) sight-threatening lesion involving the macula, papillomacular bundle, optic nerve head, or a major blood vessel, (b) very severe vitritis (risk of tractional retinal detachment), and (c) immunocompromised patients (all lesions).
- *Regimen:* (a) systemic prednisolone (1 mg/kg) daily, (b) specific anti-toxoplasma agent, most frequently pyrimethamine and folinic acid, combined with (c) sulfadiazine; pyrimethamine is avoided in AIDS, and steroids are used with extreme caution in immunocompromised patients.

Toxocariasis

Pathogenesis: *Toxocara canis* is a common intestinal roundworm of dogs. Human infestation is by accidental ingestion of soil or food contaminated with ova shed in dogs' faeces, typically in young children. The ova develop into larvae that travel to various organs.

Diagnosis

- *Visceral larva migrans:* severe systemic infection (average age 2 years), which very occasionally causes death; there is leucocytosis and eosinophilia.
- *Ocular toxocariasis:* presents at an older average age in an otherwise healthy child; positive serology for *T. canis* but a normal white cell count without eosinophilia.
- *Chronic endophthalmitis:* presents at 2–9 years of age with leucocoria (*Fig. 11.25*), strabismus, or unilateral visual loss; retinoblastoma should be excluded. Prognosis is poor, with progression to tractional retinal detachment and phthisis bulbi.

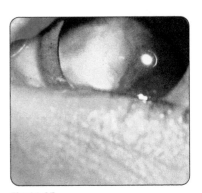

Fig 11.25

- *Posterior pole granuloma:* presents at 6–14 years of age with unilateral visual impairment; a round, yellow-white, solid granuloma one to two disc diameters in size is seen in the posterior fundus (*Fig. 11.26*); vitreoretinal traction may be present.
- *Peripheral granuloma:* may remain undetected or present with distortion of the macula or retinal detachment; a white hemispherical granuloma (*Fig. 11.27*) is evident, and may be associated with a vitreous band extending to the disc.

Treatment: with steroids, either periocular or systemic, for inflamed eyes.

Onchocerciasis

Pathogenesis: infestation with the parasitic helminth *Onchocerca volvulus*. It is the second most common cause of blindness in the world, and is endemic in parts of Africa.

Diagnosis

- *Systemic features:* (a) pruritus, (b) maculopapular rash, (c) subcutaneous onchocercomas consisting of encapsulated worms, and (d) lymphadenopathy.
- *Ocular features:* (a) anterior uveitis and pear-shaped pupillary dilatation, (b) sclerosing keratitis (see *Fig. 6.26*), (c) chorioretinitis resembling choroidal 'sclerosis' (*Fig. 11.28*); (d) live microfilariae can be seen in the anterior chamber after the patient has bent face down for a few minutes.

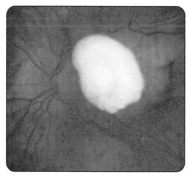

Fig 11.26

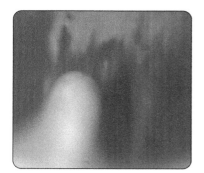

Fig 11.27

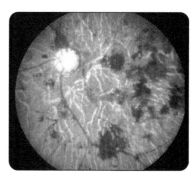

Fig 11.28

Treatment: ivermectin is given as a single dose annually; therapy targeting *Wolbachia* shows promise.

Uveitis in AIDS

AIDS

- *Pathogenesis:* human immunodeficiency virus (HIV) targets CD4+ T cells, which are vital to the initiation of the immune response to pathogens. Progressive immune deficiency is associated with a steady decline in CD4+ T cell numbers.
- *Transmission:* predominantly by heterosexual intercourse on a worldwide basis but by male homosexual contact in the Western world. Transmission may also occur by contaminated blood or needles, transplacentally, or via breast milk.
- *Course:* (a) acute seroconversion illness is followed by an asymptomatic phase; (b) symptomatic infection (AIDS) then follows and is characterized by immunosuppression with opportunistic infections and neoplasms, as well as tissue damage directly due to HIV infection.
- *Treatment:* although there is no cure for AIDS, progression of disease can be radically slowed with 'highly active antiretroviral therapy' (HAART).

Ocular involvement in AIDS

- *Eyelids:* (a) blepharitis, (b) Kaposi sarcoma, (c) severe molluscum contagiosum, (see Fig 1.45) and (d) herpes zoster ophthalmicus.
- *Orbit:* cellulitis and B cell lymphoma.
- *Anterior segment:* (a) conjunctiva (Kaposi sarcoma, squamous cell carcinoma, microangiopathy), (b) keratitis (microsporidia, herpes simplex, herpes zoster), (c) keratoconjunctivitis sicca, and (d) anterior uveitis (may be secondary to systemic drug toxicity with rifabutin or cidofovir).
- *Posterior segment:* (a) HIV microangiopathy, (b) HIV retinitis, (c) cytomegalovirus retinitis, (d) progressive retinal necrosis, (e) toxoplasmosis (frequently atypical), (f) choroidal cryptococcosis, (g) choroidal pneumocystosis, and (h) B cell intraocular lymphoma.

HIV microangiopathy

HIV microangiopathy is the most frequent retinopathy in AIDS, developing in up to 70%.

- *Pathogenesis:* immune complex deposition and HIV infection of the retinal vascular endothelium.
- *Signs:* cotton wool spots (*Fig. 11.29*), which may be associated with retinal haemorrhages and capillary

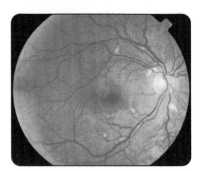

Fig 11.29

abnormalities; resolves spontaneously after several weeks.

Cytomegalovirus retinitis

Cytomegalovirus retinitis is the most common opportunistic ocular infection in AIDS, although since the advent of HAART its incidence and severity have declined.

Diagnosis

- *Indolent retinitis:* starts in the periphery and progresses slowly as granular opacification, which may be associated with a few punctate haemorrhages (*Fig. 11.30*); vasculitis is absent.

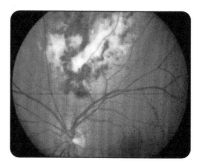

Fig 11.31

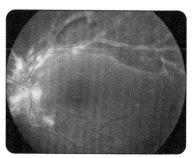

Fig 11.32

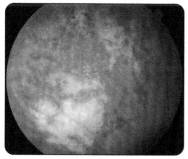

Fig 11.30

- *Fulminating retinitis:* (a) mild vitritis, (b) vasculitis with perivascular sheathing and retinal opacification, (c) well-demarcated areas of dense white opacification often associated with retinal haemorrhages (*Fig. 11.31*), (d) slow but relentless 'brushfire-like' extension along the course of the retinal vascular arcades, and (e) retinal detachment associated with large posterior breaks in uncontrolled disease (*Fig. 11.32*).

Treatment

- *Systemic:* (a) oral valganciclovir, and (b) intravenous ganciclovir, foscarnet, or cidofovir (with probenecid).
- *Ganciclovir intravitreal slow-release device (Vitrasert):* as effective as intravenous therapy with a duration of 8 months.
- *Intravitreal fomivirsen:* adverse effects include anterior uveitis, vitritis, and cataract.
- *Intravitreal cidofovir:* may occasionally cause severe uveitis.

Progressive retinal necrosis

Pathogenesis: necrotizing retinitis caused by VZV; occurs predominantly in AIDS, although also in patients with drug-induced immunosuppression.

Diagnosis

- **Presentation:** sudden onset of progressive visual loss; initially unilateral in 75%.
- **Signs:** (a) minimal anterior uveitis and vitritis, (b) yellow-white retinal infiltrates; (c) rapid confluence and full-thickness necrosis (*Fig. 11.33*).
- **Investigations:** PCR of vitreous for VZV.

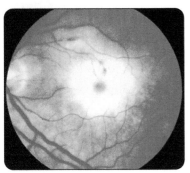

Fig 11.33

Treatment: intravenous and intravitreal ganciclovir and foscarnet, but response is often disappointing.

Acute retinal necrosis

Pathogenesis: necrotizing viral retinitis, typically affecting otherwise healthy individuals of all ages; tends to be caused by HSV in younger and by VZV in older individuals.

Diagnosis

- **Presentation:** initially unilateral; some patients develop pain with severe visual impairment over a few days, others have an insidious onset with floaters.
- **Signs:** (a) granulomatous anterior uveitis, (b) vitritis, (c) peripheral periarteritis associated with multifocal yellow-white deep retinal infiltrates, (d) circumferential progression usually sparing the posterior pole until late (*Fig. 11.34*), and (e) optic nerve involvement.

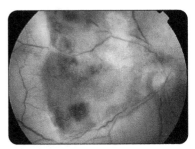

Fig 11.34

- **Course:** acute features resolve in 6–12 weeks, leaving behind transparent necrotic retina with hyperpigmented borders; without treatment, the second eye becomes involved in 30%, usually within 2 months.
- **Investigations:** PCR of vitreous for HSV and VZV.

Treatment

- **Antivirals:** (a) intravenous aciclovir for 10–14 days, then oral for 6–12 weeks (does not prevent retinal detachment), (b) oral valaciclovir and famciclovir give similar outcomes, and (c) intravitreal ganciclovir or foscarnet are also used in severe cases.

- *Systemic steroids:* may be started 24 h after initiation of antiviral therapy, particularly in severe cases (e.g. optic nerve involvement).
- *Prognosis:* 60% have final VA of less than 6/60.

Fungal uveitis

Presumed ocular histoplasmosis syndrome (POHS)

Pathogenesis: histoplasmosis is a systemic granulomatous inflammatory condition caused by *Histoplasma capsulatum,* acquired by inhalation. Although ocular histoplasmosis has never been reported in patients with active systemic infection, POHS is believed to be an immune-mediated response in individuals previously exposed to the fungus.

Diagnosis

- *Presentation:* asymptomatic in the absence of maculopathy.
- *Signs:* (a) absence of uveitis, (b) 'histo' spots consist of roundish atrophic yellow-white lesions, often associated with pigment clumps, scattered in the mid-periphery and posterior fundus, (c) peripapillary atrophy (*Fig. 11.35*), and (d) occasionally mid-peripheral linear streaks.
- *Choroidal neovascularization (CNV):* develops in approximately 5%, usually associated with an old macular histo spot in a relatively young adult.

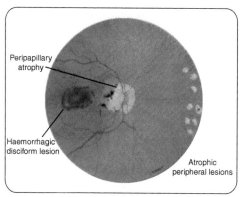

Fig 11.35

Treatment: options for CNV include (a) intravitreal anti-VEGF agents, (b) intravitreal steroids, (c) argon laser photocoagulation, (d) photodynamic therapy, and (e) surgical removal in highly selected cases.

Cryptococcosis

Pathogenesis: infection with *Cryptococcus neoformans*, which enters the body through inhalation; primarily affects patients with immune dysfunction, notably AIDS.

Diagnosis
- *Systemic features:* (a) meningitis (most important), (b) pneumonia, (c) mucocutaneous lesions, (d) pyelonephritis, (e) endocarditis, and (f) hepatitis.
- *Ocular features:* (a) papilloedema, (b) optic neuropathy, (c) ophthalmoplegia, (d) multifocal choroiditis, (e) iris infiltration, (f) keratitis, and (g) conjunctival granuloma.
- *Investigation:* central nervous system imaging, lumbar puncture, and serology.

Treatment: intravenous antifungal agents.

Endogenous fungal endophthalmitis

Pathogenesis: the major source of fungal infection within the eye is metastatic spread from a septic focus associated with a catheter, intravenous drug abuse, parenteral nutrition, and chronic lung disease such as cystic fibrosis; immunosuppression and AIDS are also major risk factors; approximately 75% of isolates show *Candida* spp.

Diagnosis
- *Presentation:* insidious onset of blurring and floaters; bilateral involvement is common.
- *Signs:* (a) creamy-white chorioretinal lesions with overlying vitritis (*Fig. 11.36*), (b) 'cotton ball' colonies (*Fig. 11.37*), (c) chronic endophthalmitis with severe vitreous infiltration (*Fig. 11.38*), and (d) proliferative

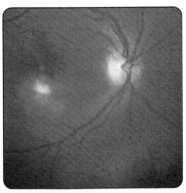

Fig 11.36

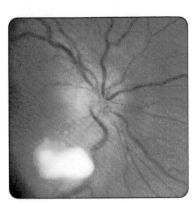

Fig 11.37

Fig 11.38

- **Cornea:** phlyctenular keratoconjunctivitis and interstitial keratitis.
- **Anterior uveitis:** usually granulomatous.
- **Choroiditis:** (a) focal or (less frequently) multifocal, (b) extensive and diffuse in AIDS, and (c) large choroidal granulomas (rare; Fig. 11.39).
- **Periphlebitis:** mild and innocuous or occlusive resulting in severe retinal ischaemia and neovascularization.

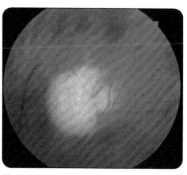

Fig 11.39

vitreoretinopathy and retinal detachment.
- **Investigations:** vitreous biopsy.

Treatment
- **Medical:** (a) oral fluconazole, and (b) oral, intravenous, or intravitreal voriconazole for cases resistant to fluconazole.
- **Pars plana vitrectomy:** with intravitreal amphotericin for severe vitreous involvement.

Bacterial uveitis

Tuberculosis

Pathogenesis: chronic granulomatous infection usually caused by *Mycobacterium tuberculosis*, acquired by inhaling infected airborne droplets. It is primarily a pulmonary disease but may spread to other sites; it is more common in immunocompromised individuals.

Diagnosis
- **Eyelids:** reddish-brown nodules (lupus vulgaris).

Treatment: (a) initially with at least three drugs (isoniazid, rifampicin, and pyrazinamide); quadruple therapy with the addition of ethambutol is necessary in some cases; (b) uveitis requires steroids.

Syphilis

Pathogenesis: caused by the spirochaete bacterium *Treponema pallidum*. In adults, the disease is usually sexually acquired when the treponemes enter through an abrasion of skin or mucous membrane; transplacental infection can occur from a mother who has become infected during or shortly before pregnancy. The natural history of untreated syphilis is variable and the condition may remain latent.

Diagnosis

- *Primary syphilis:* painless ulcer (chancre) at the site of infection, resolving in 2–6 weeks.
- *Secondary syphilis:* 6–8 weeks later is characterized by (a) generalized lymphadenopathy, (b) maculopapular rash, (c) condylomata lata, (d) snail-track ulcers (e.g. mouth), (e) meningitis, (f) nephritis, and (g) hepatitis.
- *Latent syphilis:* detected only by serology.
- *Tertiary syphilis:* (a) cardiovascular disease (e.g. aortitis), (b) neurosyphilis (e.g. tabes dorsalis), (c) Charcot joints, (d) general paresis of the insane, (e) and gummatous infiltration of bone and viscera.
- *AAU:* occurs in 4% of patients with secondary syphilis; may feature dilated iris capillaries (roseolae; *Fig. 11.40*).

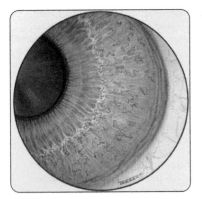

Fig 11.40

- *Posterior uveitis:* (a) chorioretinitis, often bilateral, may be multifocal or placoid with pale yellowish subretinal lesions (*Fig. 11.41*), (b) neuroretinitis, and (c) vasculitis (may be occlusive).
- *Investigations:* serology with lumbar puncture for suspected neurosyphilis.

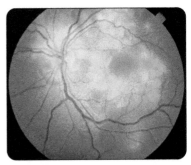

Fig 11.41

Treatment: (a) syphilis is treated with penicillin, alternatives including tetracycline or erythromycin in the penicillin-allergic; (b) uveitis requires steroids.

Lyme disease (borreliosis)

Pathogenesis: caused by the spirochaete bacterium *Borrelia burgdorferi*, transmitted through a tick bite (*Fig. 11.42*). The disease is endemic in many temperate regions and has probably been significantly underdiagnosed in the past.

Diagnosis

- *Presentation:* (a) erythema chronicum migrans, a pathognomonic annular skin lesion at the site of the tick bite,

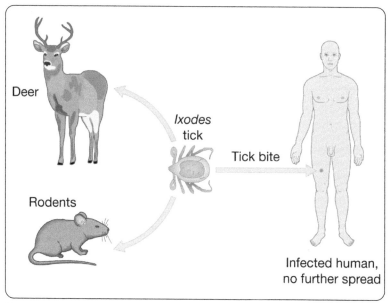

Fig 11.42

and (b) constitutional symptoms with lymphadenopathy which can last for several weeks and resolve even without treatment.

- *Early complications:* (a) neurological (cranial nerve palsies, meningitis), and (b) cardiac (conduction defects, myocarditis) may follow within 3–4 weeks.
- *Late complications:* (a) chronic arthritis, (b) polyneuropathy, and (c) encephalopathy.
- *Ocular features:* (a) uveitis (anterior, IU, peripheral multifocal choroiditis, periphlebitis, neuroretinitis), (b) follicular conjunctivitis, (c) episcleritis and scleritis, (d) keratitis, (e) orbital myositis, (f) optic neuritis, (g) ocular motor nerve palsies,

and (h) reversible Horner syndrome.
- *Investigations:* serology.

Treatment: (a) oral doxycycline (not in children) or amoxicillin for acute stage, (b) prophylaxis with doxycycline may be effective if given within 72 hr of the tick bite, and (c) intravenous ceftriaxone for ocular, cardiac, joint, or neurological disease.

Endogenous (metastatic) bacterial endophthalmitis

Pathogenesis: predisposing factors include diabetes and intravenous drug abuse. Sources of infection may be (a) indwelling catheters, (b) systemic infection (e.g. pneumonia), and (c) abdominal surgery; the most common pathogen is *Klebsiella* spp. Both eyes are involved in approximately 1 in 10 cases, and mortality from the underlying systemic disease is 5–10%.

Diagnosis

- *Systemic features:* headache, fever, and rigors.
- *Anterior segment:* discrete iris nodules or plaques, and fibrinous anterior uveitis.
- *Posterior segment:* (a) retinal infiltrates, (b) vitreous haze or abscess, and (c) retinal necrosis.
- *Investigations:* systemic infection screen, and aqueous and vitreous sampling.

Treatment

- *Systemic infection:* intravenous antibiotics according to source and infectious agent; broad-spectrum treatment if no evident source of infection (e.g. ceftazidime, vancomycin).
- *Endophthalmitis:* add oral ciprofloxacin.

Cat-scratch disease

Pathogenesis: subacute condition caused by infection with *Bartonella henselae*, transmitted by the scratch or bite of an apparently healthy cat; ocular involvement occurs in approximately 6%.

Diagnosis

- *Presentation:* red papule or pustule at the site of inoculation followed by fever, malaise, and regional lymphadenopathy.
- *Disseminated disease:* rare except in immunocompromised patients.
- *Ocular features:* (a) uveitis, (b) neuroretinitis (most common; *Fig. 11.43*), (c) Parinaud oculoglandular

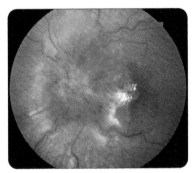

Fig 11.43

syndrome, (d) exudative maculopathy, and (e) retinal vascular occlusion.
- *Investigations:* serology for *B. henselae*.

Treatment: oral doxycycline or erythromycin, sometimes with rifampicin.

Leprosy

Pathogenesis: chronic granulomatous infection caused by *Mycobacterium leprae;* exhibits an affinity for skin, peripheral nerves, and the anterior segment of the eye. The incubation period is typically approximately 5 years.

Diagnosis

- *Lepromatous leprosy:* multisystem infection involving (a) skin, (b) peripheral nerves, (c) upper respiratory tract, (d) reticuloendothelial system, (e) eyes, (f) bones, and (g) characteristic 'leonine' facies.
- *Tuberculoid leprosy:* restricted to the skin and peripheral nerves, giving annular, anaesthetic, and

hypopigmented lesions with raised edges.

- **Lepromin test:** strongly positive in tuberculoid leprosy but negative in lepromatous disease.
- **Ocular features:** (a) CAU, (b) iris pearls, (c) miosis due to damaged dilator pupillae innervation, and (d) iris atrophy (*Fig. 11.44*).

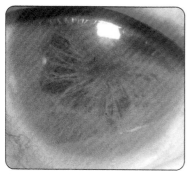

Fig 11.44

Treatment: multidrug therapy (e.g. dapsone, rifampicin, clofazimine).

White dot syndromes

Multiple evanescent white dot syndrome

Definition: usually unilateral, idiopathic self-limiting disease with a female preponderance.

Diagnosis

- **Presentation:** in 3rd and 4th decades with blurring and photopsia which may follow a viral-like illness.
- **Signs:** (a) mild vitritis, (b) numerous ill-defined small grey-white deep retinal dots at the posterior pole and mid-periphery (*Fig. 11.45a*), and (c) later granular orange macular appearance with abnormal/absent foveal reflex, and an enlarged blind spot.
- **Course:** over several weeks the dots fade and central vision recovers; foveal granularity may remain, and the enlarged blind spot persists for much longer.
- **FA:** subtle early hyperfluorescence of the dots with late staining; sometimes minimal or absent findings.
- **ICGA:** more numerous hypofluorescent spots (*Fig. 11.45b*); both FA and ICGA show

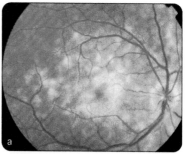

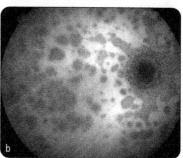

Fig 11.45

peripapillary nonperfusion, consistent with the enlarged blind spot.

- *Electroretinogram:* decrease in a-wave amplitude that returns to a normal pattern within a few weeks.

Treatment: not required.

Acute idiopathic blind spot enlargement syndrome

Definition: rare, self-limiting condition that seems to exclusively affect women.

Diagnosis

- *Presentation:* in 3rd to 6th decades with blurring and photopsia.
- *Signs:* (a) relative afferent pupillary defect, (b) enlarged blind spot, and (c) mild disc swelling or hyperaemia with peripapillary subretinal pigmentary changes.

Treatment: not required.

Acute posterior multifocal placoid pigment epitheliopathy (APMPPE)

Definition: uncommon, idiopathic, usually bilateral condition, which affects both sexes equally.

Diagnosis

- *Presentation:* in 3rd and 4th decades, following a flu-like illness in approximately one-third of patients, with subacute monocular central and paracentral scotomas; second eye is involved within days/weeks.
- *Signs:* (a) mild anterior uveitis and vitritis, and (b) multiple large yellow-white placoid lesions, which

typically begin at the posterior pole and extend to the post-equatorial fundus (*Fig. 11.46a*).

- *Course:* (a) lesions begin to fade after a few days leaving variable

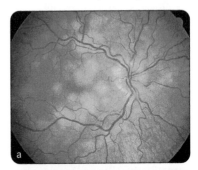

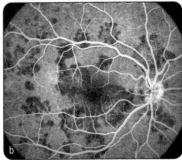

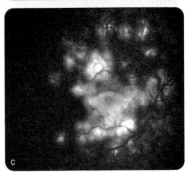

Fig 11.46

retinal pigment epithelium (RPE) disturbance; (b) VA usually recovers over months to normal or near-normal.

- *FA:* active lesions show early dense hypofluorescence (*Fig. 11.46b*) and late staining (*Fig. 11.46c*).
- *ICGA:* nonperfusion of the choriocapillaris.

Treatment: systemic steroids are sometimes given, but clear benefit has not been established.

Multifocal choroiditis and panuveitis

Definition: uncommon chronic/recurrent disease that predominantly affects myopic females; usually bilateral but asymmetrical.

Diagnosis
- *Presentation:* in 3rd and 4th decades with blurring, floaters, and photopsia.
- *Signs:* (a) anterior uveitis and vitritis, (b) multiple ovoid yellowish-grey lesions involving the posterior pole (*Fig. 11.47*) and/or periphery, with (c) evolution into

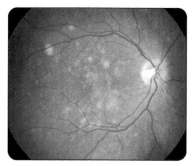

Fig 11.47

punched-out lesions with pigmented borders (*Fig. 11.48*).
- *Course:* prolonged with recurrent inflammatory episodes; complications include CNV, CMO, and occasionally subretinal fibrosis.
- *FA:* active lesions show early blockage and late staining; old lesions show RPE window defects.

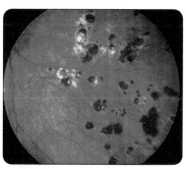

Fig 11.48

Treatment: systemic and periocular steroids are effective when administered early; other immunosuppressives are sometimes required.

Punctate inner choroidopathy

Definition: uncommon idiopathic disease typically affecting young myopic women; both eyes are frequently involved but not simultaneously.

Diagnosis
- *Presentation:* photopsia and blurring.
- *Signs:* (a) absent or minimal uveitis; (b) multiple small

yellow-white spots with fuzzy borders at the posterior pole (*Fig. 11.49a*).

- *Course:* the lesions resolve after a few weeks, leaving sharply demarcated atrophic scars; CNV develops in up to 40% of eyes, usually within 1 year.
- *FA:* active lesions show early hyperfluorescence and late staining (*Fig. 11.49b*).

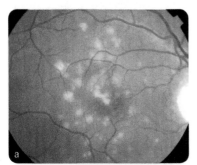

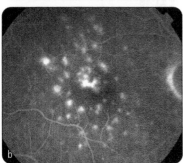

Fig 11.49

Treatment: reserved for CNV.

Serpiginous choroidopathy

Definition: uncommon chronic/recurrent disease, with a male preponderance,

which is usually bilateral although asymmetrical.

Diagnosis

- *Presentation:* in middle-age with blurring, central scotoma, or metamorphopsia.
- *Signs:* (a) mild anterior uveitis and vitritis, and (b) grey-white lesions (*Fig. 11.50*) that typically start around the optic disc and gradually spread in a serpentine manner toward the macula and periphery.
- *Course:* lesions evolve over months and years to scalloped atrophic areas (*Fig. 11.51*); CNV

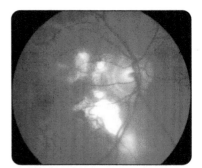

Fig 11.50

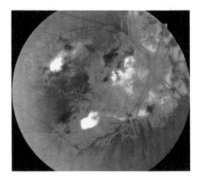

Fig 11.51

and occasionally subretinal fibrosis can occur.

- **FA:** active lesions show early hypofluorescence late hyperfluorescence, similar to APMPPE.
- **ICGA:** marked hypofluorescence.

Treatment: periocular or systemic steroids for active lesions, and long-term immunosuppression for chronic disease; prognosis is poor.

Primary stromal choroiditis

Vogt–Koyanagi–Harada syndrome (VKH)

Pathogenesis: autoimmune disease involving inflammation of melanocyte-containing tissues such as the uvea, ear, and meninges, predominantly affecting Hispanics, Japanese, and pigmented individuals. Subdivided into

- **Vogt–Koyanagi disease:** skin changes and anterior uveitis.
- **Harada disease:** neurological features and exudative retinal detachments.

Diagnosis

- **Prodromal phase:** neurological and auditory manifestations lasting a few days.
- **Acute uveitic phase:** bilateral non-granulomatous then granulomatous anterior or multifocal posterior uveitis with exudative retinal detachments (*Fig. 11.52a*) and papillitis.
- **Convalescent phase:** several weeks later with localized alopecia, poliosis, and vitiligo; focal depigmented fundus lesions

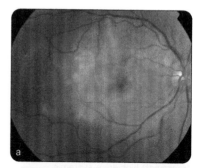

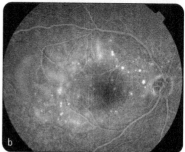

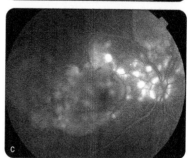

Fig 11.52

('sunset glow' fundus) and depigmented limbal lesions (Sugiura sign).

- **Chronic/recurrent phase:** smouldering anterior uveitis with exacerbations.

- **FA:** (a) acute phase shows multifocal hyperfluorescent dots at the level of the RPE, then accumulation of dye in the subretinal space (*Figs. 11.52b* and *11.52c*); (b) chronic phase shows areas of hyperfluorescent RPE window defects.
- **ICGA:** acute phase shows early regularly distributed hypofluorescent spots, with later diffuse hyperfluorescence.

Treatment: high-dose systemic steroids; ciclosporin in resistant cases.

Sympathetic ophthalmitis

Pathogenesis: bilateral granulomatous panuveitis occurring after penetrating trauma or intraocular surgery (usually multiple vitreoretinal procedures). Presentation in 65% is between 2 weeks and 3 months of the initial insult; the exciting eye is the one originally injured, and the sympathizing eye is the fellow eye.

Diagnosis
- **Presentation:** (a) irritation, (b) blurred vision, (c) photophobia, and (d) loss of accommodation in the sympathizing eye.
- **Signs:** (a) granulomatous anterior uveitis in both the exciting and sympathizing eye, (b) mid-peripheral multifocal choroidal infiltrates (*Fig. 11.53*), (c) focal sub-RPE infiltrates (Dalen–Fuchs nodules), (d) exudative retinal detachment, and (e) sunset-glow appearance similar to VKH.
- **Systemic features:** same as in VKH but less common.

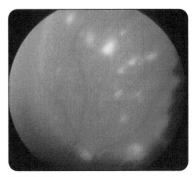

Fig 11.53

Treatment
- **Enucleation:** within first 10 days following trauma should be considered only in an eye with a hopeless visual prognosis.
- **Systemic:** steroids are usually effective; ciclosporin or azathioprine in resistant cases.

Birdshot retinochoroidopathy

Definition: uncommon idiopathic chronic/recurrent bilateral disease that predominantly affects females; 95% of patients are positive for HLA-A29.

Diagnosis
- **Presentation:** in 3rd to 6th decades with insidious impairment of central vision associated with photopsia and floaters.
- **Signs:** (a) vitritis, (b) multiple, ill-defined ovoid cream-coloured choroidal patches, in the posterior pole and mid-periphery (*Fig. 11.54a*); (c) radiate outward from

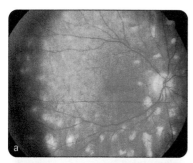

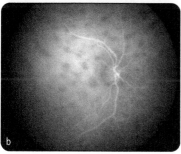

Fig 11.54

Fuchs uveitis syndrome

Definition: idiopathic, usually unilateral, chronic uveitis of insidious onset, occurring equally in young adults of both sexes.

Diagnosis

- **Presentation:** chronic floaters, gradual blurring from cataract, or on incidental detection.
- **Signs:** (a) mild anterior uveitis, (b) vitritis (may be severe), (c) KP are round or stellate and grey-white in colour, and are scattered throughout the corneal endothelium (*Fig. 11.55*), (d) absence of posterior synechiae, (e) small nodules on the pupillary border (*Fig. 11.56*) and iris stroma, and (f) diffuse iris atrophy with associated heterochromia iridis (*Fig. 11.57*).
- **Gonioscopy:** normal or shows fine radial vessels and/or small

the disc but usually spare the macula; (d) inactive lesions consist of well-delineated atrophic spots; (e) CMO is common.

- **Course:** approximately 20% of patients have a self-limited course and maintain normal VA in at least one eye.
- **FA:** disc staining, hyperfluorescence due to leakage, and CMO.
- **ICGA:** well-defined oval hypofluorescent spots (*Fig. 11.54b*).

Treatment: systemic steroids, ciclosporin, or azathioprine.

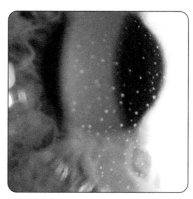

Fig 11.55

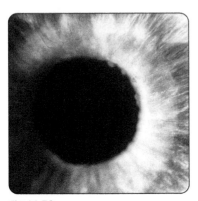

Fig 11.56

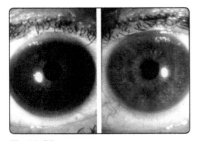

Fig 11.57

irregular peripheral anterior synechiae (*Fig. 11.58*).

- *Complications:* cataract (extremely common) and glaucoma (later manifestation).

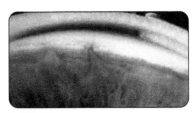

Fig 11.58

Treatment: troublesome vitreous opacities occasionally require treatment with periocular steroids and rarely vitrectomy; topical steroids are relatively ineffective for anterior uveitis.

Ocular tumours

Benign epibulbar tumours

Conjunctival naevus

Diagnosis
- **Presentation:** in 1st and 2nd decades.
- **Signs:** (a) slightly elevated pigmented bulbar lesion of variable size and pigmentation, (b) often juxtalimbal (*Fig. 12.1*); (c) cystic spaces are common.
- **Signs of potential malignancy:** (a) prominent feeder vessels, (b) sudden growth or increase in pigmentation, and (c) development after the 2nd decade, particularly in an unusual site such as palpebral or forniceal conjunctiva.

Treatment: excision, usually for cosmetic reasons; less commonly for irritation or suspicion of malignancy.

Diagnosis: (a) solitary pedunculated or sessile lesion; (b) most frequently juxtalimbal (*Fig. 12.2*), in the fornix (*Fig. 12.3*), or caruncle; (c) may occasionally be multiple and confluent.

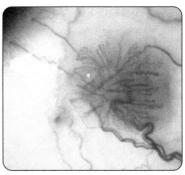

Fig 12.2

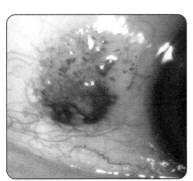

Fig 12.1

Conjunctival papilloma

Pathogenesis: often infection with human papillomavirus (especially types 6 and 11), particularly in childhood.

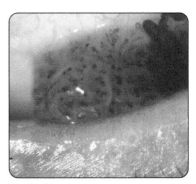

Fig 12.3

Treatment: small lesions often resolve spontaneously; large papillomas may require excision, sometimes with cryotherapy to the base and surrounding area.

Dermoid

Histology: solid mass of collagenous tissue containing dermal elements covered by stratified squamous epithelium.

Diagnosis
- *Presentation:* in early childhood.
- *Signs:* (a) smooth yellowish subconjunctival mass of soft consistency; (b) most frequently at the inferotemporal limbus; (c) protruding hair may be seen (*Fig. 12.4*).
- *Systemic associations:* Goldenhar syndrome (oculoauriculovertebral spectrum) and, less commonly, Treacher Collins syndrome.

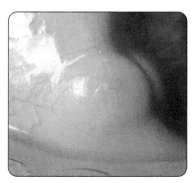

Fig 12.4

Treatment: small lesions are excised; large dermoids may require lamellar keratosclerectomy.

Pyogenic granuloma

Pathogenesis: fibrovascular proliferation in response to a conjunctival insult such as surgery, trauma, or ruptured chalazion; spontaneous lesions are rare.

Diagnosis
- *Presentation:* typically a few weeks after surgery, with a fast-growing, pink, fleshy, vascularized conjunctival mass near a wound (*Fig. 12.5*).
- *Differential diagnosis:* (a) suture granuloma, (b) vascular tumour, and (c) Tenon granuloma or cyst.

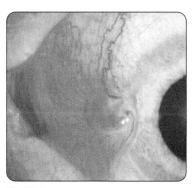

Fig 12.5

Treatment: topical steroids; excision of resistant cases.

Conjunctival (racial) epithelial melanosis

Definition: very common in dark-skinned individuals; both eyes are affected, often asymmetrically.

Diagnosis: (a) areas of flat, patchy, brownish pigmentation scattered throughout the conjunctiva, (b) more intensely at the limbus and around perforating vessels or nerves as they enter the sclera (Axenfeld loop; *Fig. 12.6*); (c) the pigment lies within the epithelium and therefore moves freely over the surface of the globe.

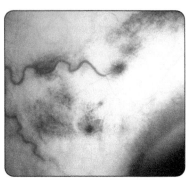

Fig 12.6

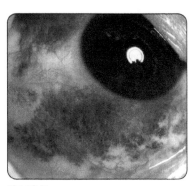

Fig 12.7

Malignant and premalignant epibulbar tumours

Primary acquired melanosis (PAM)

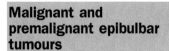

Definition: unilateral condition typically affecting white individuals older than 45 years of age. There are two histological variants which cannot be distinguished clinically.
- *PAM without atypia:* no risk of malignant transformation.
- *PAM with atypia:* regarded as melanoma *in situ* has a 50% chance of infiltrative malignancy within 5 years.

Diagnosis
- *Signs:* (a) irregular solitary or multifocal areas of flat, golden brown to dark chocolate epithelial pigmentation; (b) seen most commonly in the interpalpebral region, although any part of the conjunctiva may be affected (*Fig. 12.7*).
- *Course:* (a) PAM may expand, shrink, or remain stable for long periods, (b) may focally lighten or darken, and (c) malignant transformation should be suspected if a flat lesion becomes nodular.

Treatment: (a) small lesions may be excised; (b) large lesions should undergo incisional biopsy from various sites, with subsequent cryotherapy or topical mitomycin C for PAM with atypia.

Conjunctival melanoma

Origin: (a) from PAM with atypia (75%), (b) pre-existing naevus (20%), or (c) *de novo*.

Diagnosis
- *Presentation:* in 6th decade.
- *Signs:* (a) black, grey, or pinkish (amelanotic) vascularized nodule; may be fixed to the episclera, (b) commonly at the limbus (*Fig. 12.8*), but may develop anywhere, and (c) multifocal lesions can arise from PAM with atypia as areas of thickening and nodularity (*Fig. 12.9*).

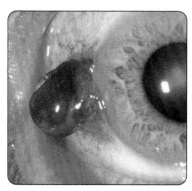

Fig 12.8

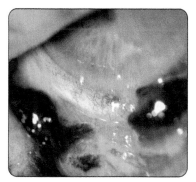

Fig 12.9

- *Poor prognostic indicators:* (a) multifocal tumour, (b) forniceal location, and (c) thickness of 2 mm or more; mortality at 10 years is 25%.
- *Differential diagnosis:* (a) large naevus, (b) ciliary body melanoma with extraocular extension, (c) melanocytoma, and (d) pigmented conjunctival carcinoma.

Treatment: excision with a wide-margin lamellar scleroconjunctivectomy and cryotherapy; radiotherapy to the base if deep extension is present histologically.

Ocular surface squamous neoplasia

Definition: spectrum of benign, premalignant and malignant unilateral slowly progressive epithelial lesions of the conjunctiva and cornea.

Risk factors: (a) excessive ultraviolet exposure, (b) human papilloma virus infection, (c) AIDS, and (d) xeroderma pigmentosum.

Diagnosis

- *Presentation:* in old age with irritation or a visible mass within the interpalpebral fissure; commonly juxtalimbal, but may involve any part of the conjunctiva or cornea.
- *Signs:* variable and limited correlation with histological type: (a) gelatinous mass with superficial vessels, (b) elevated white leucoplakic plaque (*Fig. 12.10*), (c) fleshy pink

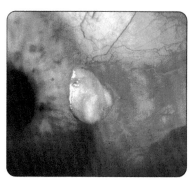

Fig 12.10

papillomatous lesion with prominent feeder and surface blood vessels (*Fig. 12.11*); (d) can masquerade as chronic conjunctivitis; corneal involvement may occur (*Fig. 12.12*).

- **Spread:** intraocular extension is uncommon and metastatic disease extremely rare.
- **Investigations:** ultrasonic biomicroscopy (UBM) to estimate the depth of invasion, and impression cytology.

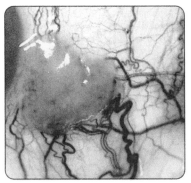

Fig 12.11

Treatment: (a) excision with 2 or 3 mm margins and assessment of clearance with frozen sections; (b) adjunctive measures aimed at reducing recurrence include cryotherapy, brachytherapy, and topical chemotherapy.

Lymphoproliferative lesions

Pathology: most conjunctival lymphoproliferative lesions consist of reactive lymphoid hyperplasia, but lymphoma may arise *de novo*, by extension from orbital disease or occasionally associated with systemic involvement. Rarely, reactive hyperplasia undergoes malignant transformation. Most conjunctival lymphomas are of B cell origin.

Diagnosis

- **Presentation:** in the 7th and 8th decades with irritation or painless swelling; may be bilateral.
- **Signs:** slow-growing salmon-pink or flesh-coloured mobile infiltrate (*Fig. 12.13*).

Treatment: radiotherapy, chemotherapy, and excision.

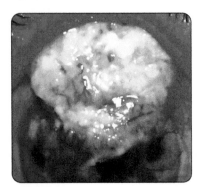

Fig 12.12

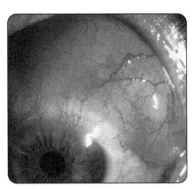

Fig 12.13

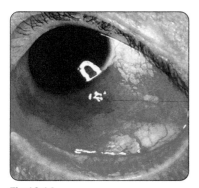

Fig 12.14

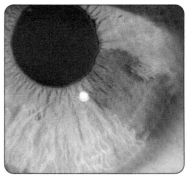

Fig 12.15

Kaposi sarcoma

Definition: slowly growing vascular tumour occurring almost exclusively in AIDS.

Diagnosis: flat bright-red lesion (*Fig. 12.14*) that may mimic a subconjunctival haemorrhage.

Treatment: radiotherapy or excision, with or without adjunctive cryotherapy.

Iris tumours

Iris naevus

Diagnosis
- *Signs:* (a) solitary pigmented, flat or slightly elevated, circumscribed lesion usually less than 3 mm in diameter, (b) typically located inferiorly (*Fig. 12.15*).
- *Signs of potential malignancy:* (a) prominent vascularity, (b) rapid growth, (c) diffuse spread, and (d) seeding.

Treatment: not required, although observation is sometimes indicated.

Iris melanoma

Pathology: approximately 8% of uveal melanomas arise in the iris. The majority are composed of spindle cells of low-grade malignancy. Predisposing factors include (a) fair skin, (b) light iris colour, (c) numerous cutaneous naevi, (d) congenital ocular and oculodermal melanocytosis (naevus of Ota), and (e) NF1.

Diagnosis
- *Presentation:* in 5th and 6th decades with enlargement of a pre-existing iris lesion.
- *Typical signs:* (a) very slowly growing pigmented or nonpigmented nodule at least 3 mm in diameter, (b) usually in the inferior half of the iris (*Fig. 12.16*), and (c) often associated with surface blood vessels.

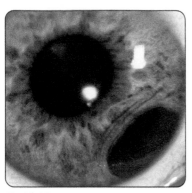

Fig 12.16

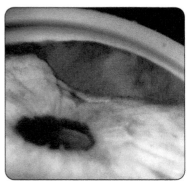

Fig 12.18

- **Associated signs:** (a) pupillary distortion, (b) ectropion uveae (*Fig. 12.17*), (c) angle invasion (*Fig. 12.18*) with glaucoma, and (d) localized cataract.

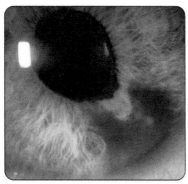

Fig 12.17

Treatment: (a) observation of suspicious lesions, (b) iridectomy for small tumours and iridocyclectomy for angle invasion, (c) brachytherapy or external proton beam irradiation, and (d) enucleation for diffusely growing tumours if radiotherapy is not possible.

Iris cysts

Primary

Diagnosis

- **Signs:** unilateral or bilateral, solitary or multiple globular brown (*Fig. 12.19*) or transparent (*Fig. 12.20*) structures located at the pupillary border, midzone, or iris root.
- **Complications:** rarely glaucoma and corneal decompensation.

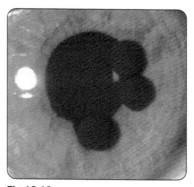

Fig 12.19

penetrating trauma or surgery; (b) extended use of long-acting miotics may be associated with formation of multiple small cysts along the pupillary border.

Diagnosis

- *Signs:* pearly and solid-appearing or serous and translucent lesions (*Fig. 12.21*).
- *Complications:* (a) corneal decompensation, (b) anterior uveitis, and (c) glaucoma.

Treatment: similar to primary cysts.

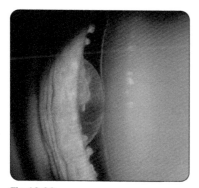

Fig 12.20

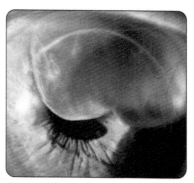

Fig 12.21

Treatment: options include (a) observation, (b) argon laser photocoagulation, (c) needle aspiration, and (d) excision.

Secondary

Pathogenesis: (a) implantation cysts originate by deposition of surface epithelial cells from the conjunctiva or cornea onto the iris following

Ciliary body melanoma

Diagnosis

- *Presentation:* in 6th decade with visual symptoms caused by pressure on the lens giving rise to astigmatism, subluxation, or cataract formation; occasionally discovered incidentally.

- **Signs:** (a) may be visible following pupillary dilatation, (b) 'sentinel' vessels in the same quadrant as the tumour (*Fig. 12. 22*), (c) erosion through the iris root may mimic an iris melanoma (*Fig. 12.23*), (d) extraocular extension may mimic a conjunctival melanoma (*Fig. 12.24*), and (e) circumferential (annular) growth.
- **Investigations:** UBM and biopsy.

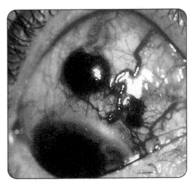

Fig 12.24

Treatment: (a) iridocyclectomy for small or medium-sized tumours, (b) brachytherapy or proton beam irradiation, and (c) enucleation for large and extensively invasive tumours.

Tumours of the choroid

Choroidal naevus

Introduction: choroidal naevi are present in 5–10% of Caucasians but are very rare in dark-skinned races. They are probably present at birth, although growth occurs mainly during prepubertal years and is extremely rare in adulthood. The risk of malignant transformation of typical small naevi is extremely low.

Diagnosis

- **Presentation:** the vast majority are asymptomatic and detected by chance.
- **Signs:** (a) usually post-equatorial, oval or circular, brown to slate-grey lesion with indistinct margins (*Fig. 12.25*); (b) surface drusen may be present.

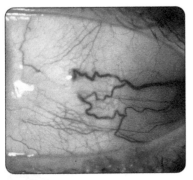

Fig 12.22

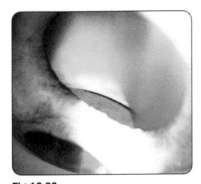

Fig 12.23

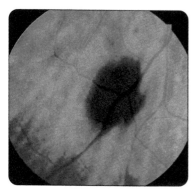

Fig 12.25

- *Features of potential malignancy:*
  (a) documented growth,
  (b) symptoms, (c) dimensions
  >5 mm diameter or >1 mm in
  thickness, (d) orange surface
  pigment, (e) absence of surface
  drusen on a thick lesion, and
  (f) associated serous retinal
  detachment.
- *Investigations:* (a) baseline
  photography, (b) FA shows
  blockage of background choroidal
  fluorescence, and (c) US shows a
  localized flat or slightly elevated
  lesion with high internal acoustic
  reflectivity.
- *Differential diagnosis:*
  (a) congenital hypertrophy of the
  RPE, (b) choroidal melanocytoma,
  and (c) small melanoma.

Treatment: baseline fundus
photography and US, with indefinite
follow-up of suspicious cases.

Choroidal melanoma

Pathology: choroidal melanoma is the
most common primary intraocular
malignancy in adults, and accounts
for 80% of all uveal melanomas.
Histologically, it may consist of
(a) spindle cells, (b) epithelioid cells,
or (c) mixed spindle and epithelioid
cells.

Diagnosis
- *Presentation:* in 7th decade with
  blurring, metamorphopsia, visual
  field loss, floaters, and photopsia;
  occasionally discovered by
  chance.
- *Signs:* (a) a solitary elevated
  dome-shaped subretinal, mass
  which may be pigmented (grey
  or brown; *Fig. 12.26*) or less
  commonly amelanotic (*Fig. 12.27*)
  often within 3 mm of the optic
  disc or fovea, (b) clumps of
  surface orange pigment (*Fig.
  12.28*); (c) has a 'collar-stud'
  appearance if the tumour breaks
  through Bruch's membrane
  (*Fig. 12.29*).

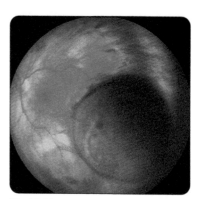

Fig 12.26

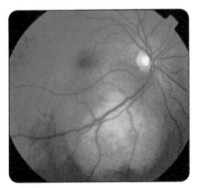

Fig 12.27

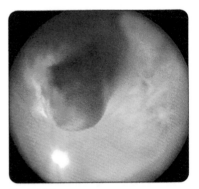

Fig 12.29

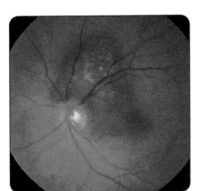

Fig 12.28

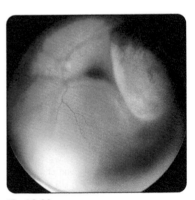

Fig 12.30

- **Associated signs:** (a) exudative retinal detachment (common; *Fig. 12.30*), (b) choroidal folds, (c) uveitis, (d) haemorrhage, (e) rubeosis iridis, (f) secondary glaucoma, and (g) cataract.
- **Tumour spread:** (a) via scleral channels to the orbit, and (b) haematogenous metastatic spread.
- **Adverse prognostic factors:** (a) large size, (b) extrascleral extension, and (c) anterior location.
- **FA:** no pathognomonic pattern, but may be useful in distinguishing simulating lesions (e.g. choroidal haemangioma).
- **US:** shows (a) internal homogeneity, (b) choroidal excavation, and (c) orbital shadowing (*Fig. 12.31*).
- **Systemic investigation:** (a) liver function tests and ultrasound, and

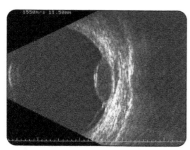

Fig 12.31

(b) chest X-ray to exclude metastatic spread to or from the choroid; only 1–2% have detectable metastasis at presentation.

- **Differential diagnosis:**
  (a) large choroidal naevus,
  (b) melanocytoma, (c) sub-RPE haemorrhage, (d) choroidal metastasis, (e) choroidal haemangioma, (f) solitary choroidal granuloma (e.g. sarcoidosis, TB), (g) posterior scleritis, (h) eccentric CNV, and (i) prominent vortex vein ampulla.

Treatment: the following factors are taken into consideration: (a) size and location of the tumour and its effects on vision, (b) state of the fellow eye, and (c) general health and age of the patient, and the patient's preferences.

- **Observation:** when it is not possible to determine clinically whether a tumour is a small melanoma or a large naevus.
- **Treatment:** (a) brachytherapy for tumours less than 20 mm in diameter and up to 10 mm thick, (b) external proton beam radiotherapy, (c) stereotactic radiotherapy, (d) transpupillary thermotherapy (TTT), (e) transscleral choroidectomy, and (f) enucleation for large tumours and in eyes with irreversible loss of useful vision.

Circumscribed choroidal haemangioma

Diagnosis

- **Presentation:** in 2nd to 4th decades with blurring, visual field defect, or metamorphopsia; in some cases, the tumour lies dormant throughout life and is discovered by chance.
- **Signs:** (a) oval orange mass with indistinct margins at the posterior pole (*Fig. 12.32*), and (b) subretinal fluid in symptomatic cases.
- **Complications:** (a) fibrous surface metaplasia, (b) cystoid retinal degeneration, (c) RPE degeneration, and (d) subretinal fibrosis.
- **FA:** spotty hyperfluorescence in the pre-arterial or early arterial

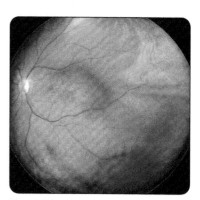

Fig 12.32

phase, and diffuse intense late hyperfluorescence.
- *US:* (a) acoustically solid lesion with a sharp anterior surface, and (b) absence of choroidal excavation and orbital shadowing (*Fig. 12.33*).
- *Differential diagnosis:* (a) amelanotic choroidal melanoma, (b) choroidal metastasis, (c) RPE detachment, and (d) posterior scleritis.

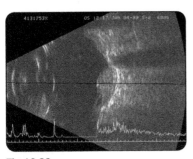

Fig 12.33

Treatment: of vision-threatening lesions may include (a) intravitreal anti-VEGF injection, (b) photodynamic therapy (PDT), (c) TTT, and (d) radiotherapy.

Diffuse choroidal haemangioma

Systemic implication: the tumour occurs almost exclusively in patients with Sturge–Weber syndrome (see Chapter 1).

Diagnosis
- *Presentation:* in 2nd decade.
- *Signs:* (a) diffuse deep red 'tomato ketchup' colour, is most marked at the posterior pole (*Fig. 12.34*);

(b) localized areas of thickening may be present.
- *Complications:* (a) cystoid retinal degeneration, (b) exudative retinal detachment, and (c) neovascular glaucoma.
- *US:* diffuse choroidal thickening.

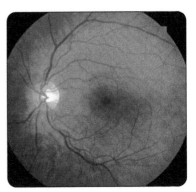

Fig 12.34

Treatment: similar to circumscribed haemangioma.

Optic disc melanocytoma

Definition: rare unilateral heavily pigmented congenital hamartoma, seen most frequently at the optic nerve head but rarely anywhere in the uvea; more common in dark-skinned individuals, and is usually asymptomatic and stable.

Diagnosis
- *Signs:* (a) dark brown or black, flat or slightly elevated lesion with feathery edges (*Fig. 12.35*); (b) a relative afferent pupillary defect may be present, even if VA is good.
- *Rare complications:* (a) malignant transformation, (b) spontaneous

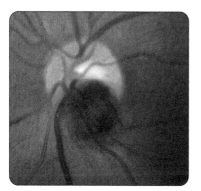

Fig 12.35

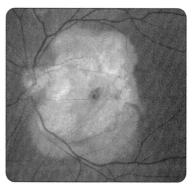

Fig 12.36

necrosis, (c) optic nerve compression, and (d) retinal vein obstruction.

Treatment: not required except for malignant transformation.

Choroidal osteoma

Definition: rare benign ossifying tumour, which grows slowly and has a strong female preponderance; bilateral in 25% of cases.

Diagnosis
- *Presentation:* in 2nd and 3rd decades with gradual visual impairment if the macula is involved; choroidal neovascularization can cause rapid visual loss.
- *Signs:* yellow-white flat or minimally elevated lesion with well-defined margins, near the disc or at the posterior pole (*Fig. 12.36*).
- *Course:* slow growth over several years; long-standing cases may develop RPE changes.

- *FA:* early diffuse mottled hyperfluorescence and late staining.
- *US:* highly reflective anterior surface and orbital shadowing.
- *Differential diagnosis:* (a) choroidal metastasis, (b) amelanotic choroidal naevus or melanoma, (c) osseous metaplasia (e.g. associated with choroidal haemangioma), and (d) sclerochoroidal calcification.

Metastatic tumours

Primary sites: 90% of uveal metastases are to the choroid, the most frequent primary sites being the breast and bronchus; less common sites include the gastrointestinal tract, kidney, and skin melanoma. Patient survival is generally poor, with a median of 8–12 months.

Diagnosis
- *Presentation:* visual impairment, though may be asymptomatic depending on location.

- **Signs:** (a) fast-growing white to orange placoid lesion with indistinct margins, most frequently located at the posterior pole (*Fig. 12.37*); (b) multifocal deposits (*Fig. 12.38*) occur in approximately 30% of patients, (c) bilateral involvement in 10–30% of cases, and (d) secondary exudative retinal detachment is common, even with small deposits.

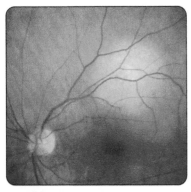

Fig 12.37

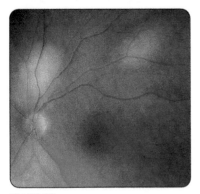

Fig 12.38

- **US:** moderately high internal acoustic reflectivity.
- **Systemic investigations:** aimed at locating the primary tumour, if unknown, together with other metastatic sites.

Treatment

- **Observation:** if the patient is asymptomatic or receiving systemic chemotherapy.
- **Treatment options:** (a) radiotherapy and (b) TTT; systemic therapy for the primary tumour may also be beneficial for choroidal lesions.

Neural retinal tumours

Retinoblastoma

Pathology: retinoblastoma is the most common primary intraocular malignancy of childhood, but is still very rare at 1:17,000 live births. It results from malignant transformation of primitive retinal cells before final differentiation. Metastatic spread is to regional nodes, lung, brain, and bone; risk factors for metastasis include advanced tumour growth, retrolaminar optic nerve invasion, massive choroidal invasion, anterior chamber involvement, and orbital spread.

Genetics: the gene predisposing to retinoblastoma, RB1, is at 13q14.

- **Heritable retinoblastoma:** accounts for 40%. The mutation is transmitted in 50% but because of incomplete penetrance only 40% of offspring will be affected. If a child has heritable retinoblastoma, the risk to siblings is only 2% if the parents are healthy but 40% if a parent is affected.

- **Nonheritable (somatic) retinoblastoma:** accounts for 60% of cases. If a patient has a solitary retinoblastoma and no positive family history, this is probably but not definitely nonheritable so that the risk in each sibling and offspring is approximately 1%.

Diagnosis

- **Presentation:** within the first year of life in bilateral cases, and approximately 2 years of age if unilateral with (a) leucocoria (60%; *Fig. 12.39*), (b) strabismus (20%; fundus examination is mandatory in all childhood strabismus), (c) secondary glaucoma, (d) tumour-induced uveitis, or (e) orbital involvement. The tumour may be revealed by routine examination of an at-risk patient.

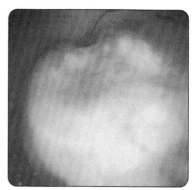

Fig 12.40

- **Exophytic tumour:** multilobular white subretinal, mass with overlying retinal detachment (*Fig. 12.41*).
- **Intraretinal tumour:** homogeneous dome-shaped whitish lesion, often with white flecks of calcification (*Fig. 12.42*).

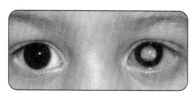

Fig 12.39

- **Differential diagnosis of leucocoria:** (a) persistent anterior fetal vasculature (persistent hyperplastic primary vitreous), (b) Coats disease, (c) retinopathy of prematurity, and (d) toxocariasis.
- **Endophytic tumour:** projects into the vitreous as a white mass (*Fig. 12.40*).

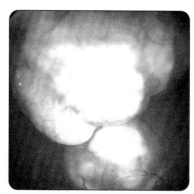

Fig 12.41

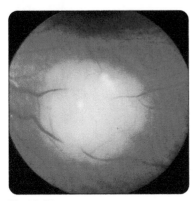

Fig 12.42

- *US:* often shows calcification; can be used to measure size.
- *MR:* superior to CT for optic nerve evaluation, detection of extraocular extension, and pinealoblastoma.
- *Other tests:* bone scans, bone marrow aspiration, and lumbar puncture to detect metastatic disease; genetic studies on patient and relatives and on tumour tissue.

Treatment
- *Screening of siblings at risk:* prenatal US, with ophthalmoscopy soon after birth, then regularly until 5 years old.
- *Small tumours:* (up to 3 mm diameter and 2 mm thick) photocoagulation, cryotherapy, or chemotherapy.
- *Medium-sized tumours:* (up to 12 mm wide and 6 mm thick) brachytherapy, chemotherapy

plus local treatment (sub-Tenon carboplatin, cryotherapy, TTT).
- *Large tumours:* chemotherapy (chemoreduction) to shrink the tumour and facilitate local treatment; enucleation (including a long piece of optic nerve) in some circumstances such as eyes with poor visual potential.
- *Extraocular extension:* adjuvant chemotherapy and external beam radiotherapy.
- *Follow-up:* regular examination and imaging, according to risk.

Astrocytoma

Systemic implications: astrocytoma is occasionally seen as a solitary lesion in normal individuals but most frequently occurs in tuberous sclerosis, and occasionally in NF1. Tuberous sclerosis (Bourneville disease) is a phacomatosis characterized by hamartomas in multiple organ systems. A classic triad of (a) epilepsy, (b) mental retardation, and (c) adenoma sebaceum is diagnostic. Approximately 60% of cases are sporadic and 40% are AD; about 50% of patients with tuberous sclerosis have fundus astrocytomas that may be multiple and bilateral.

Diagnosis
- *Presentation:* asymptomatic and detected on screening for tuberous sclerosis.
- *Signs:* (a) yellowish, round plaque or nodule (*Fig. 12.43*), (b) large

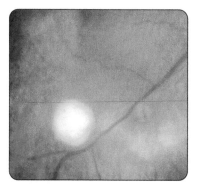

Fig 12.43

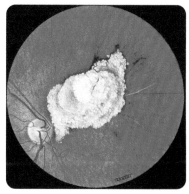

Fig 12.45

elevated mulberry-like lesion
(*Fig. 12.44*), and (c) calcification
in long-standing tumours
(*Fig. 12.45*).

- *FA:* prominent superficial vascular
  network with late leakage and
  staining.

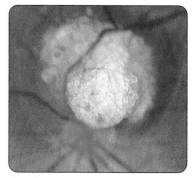

Fig 12.44

Vascular retinal tumours

Capillary haemangioma

Systemic implication: 50% of patients
with solitary tumours and virtually
all with multiple lesions have von
Hippel–Lindau syndrome (VHL), an
AD condition characterized by
(a) CNS haemangioma,
(b) phaeochromocytoma, (c) renal
carcinoma, (d) cysts in various
viscera, and (e) polycythaemia; the
prevalence of retinal tumours in VHL
is approximately 60%. The median
age at diagnosis in patients with
VHL is earlier (18 years) than in
those without (31 years).

Diagnosis

- *Presentation:* decreased vision, or
  detected by screening of those at
  risk.
- *Early tumour:* small, well-defined
  oval red lesion located between
  an arteriole and venule
  (*Fig. 12.46*).
- *Well-established tumour:* round
  orange-red mass, usually located

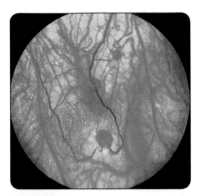

Fig 12.46

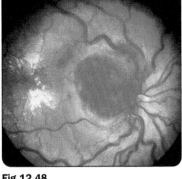

Fig 12.48

in the supero- or inferotemporal periphery with dilatation and tortuosity of the supplying artery and draining vein (*Fig. 12.47*); disc involvement may occur.

- *Complications:* (a) hard exudate formation surrounding the tumour and/or at the macula (*Fig. 12.48*), (b) exudative retinal detachment, (c) epiretinal fibrosis, (d) vitreous

haemorrhage, and (e) secondary glaucoma.
- *FA:* early hyperfluorescence and late leakage.

Treatment: (a) observation of asymptomatic juxtapapillary lesions without exudation, (b) laser photocoagulation for small lesions, (c) cryotherapy for larger peripheral lesions, (d) brachytherapy for lesions too large for cryotherapy, (e) PDT, and (f) anti-VEGF therapy.

Cavernous haemangioma

Definition: rare, unilateral, congenital hamartoma. Usually sporadic but occasionally AD; may occur in combination with lesions of the skin and CNS.

Diagnosis
- *Presentation:* usually a chance finding, rarely with vitreous haemorrhage.
- *Signs:* (a) clusters of saccular aneurysms resembling a bunch of grapes, located in the peripheral

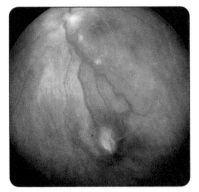

Fig 12.47

retina (*Fig. 12.49*); (b) red cells may separate from plasma, giving rise to 'fluid levels.'

- *FA:* highlights the sedimentation of erythrocytes and shows a lack of leakage.
- *Uncommon complications:* haemorrhage and epiretinal membrane formation.

Diagnosis

- *Presentation:* usually a chance finding.
- *Signs:* (a) tortuous enlarged blood vessels, the vein and artery appearing similar (*Fig. 12.50*); (b) with time become more dilated and tortuous, and may become sclerotic.

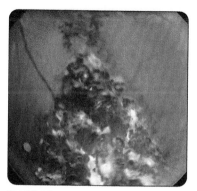

Fig 12.49

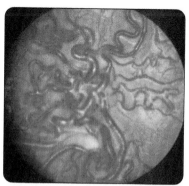

Fig 12.50

Treatment: anti-VEGF therapy may have a role.

Racemose haemangioma

Definition: racemose haemangioma (arteriovenous malformation) of the retina and optic nerve head is a rare sporadic congenital condition, usually unilateral, involving direct communication between the arteries and veins without an intervening capillary bed. Some patients have similar ipsilateral lesions involving the midbrain, basofrontal region, and posterior fossa (Wyburn–Mason syndrome).

Treatment: not required.

Primary intraocular lymphoma

Systemic implication: primary intraocular lymphoma (PIOL) represents a subset of primary CNS lymphoma, a variant of extranodal non-Hodgkin B cell lymphoma. PIOL tends to present in the 6th and 7th decades, and most patients develop CNS involvement after a mean delay of 29 months.

Diagnosis

- *Presentation:* floaters, blurred vision, red eye, or photophobia.

- **Signs:** (a) vitritis, (b) large multifocal subretinal infiltrates (*Fig. 12.51*), (c) coalescence that may occasionally form a ring encircling the equator (*Fig. 12.52*), (d) retinal vasculitis and occlusion, (e) exudative retinal detachment, and (f) optic atrophy.
- **US:** vitreous debris, elevated subretinal lesions, retinal detachment, and thickening of the optic nerves.

- **Biopsy:** of vitreous samples or subretinal nodules.

Treatment: (a) radiotherapy, (b) intravitreal methotrexate, (c) systemic chemotherapy, and (d) biological agents involving specific anti-B cell monoclonal antibodies (e.g. rituximab).

Congenital hypertrophy of the retinal pigment epithelium (CHRPE)

Classification: (a) *typical*, either solitary or grouped, and (b) *atypical*; it is important to differentiate between the two types because the latter may have important systemic implications.

Diagnosis
- **Solitary:** flat, dark grey or black, round or oval lesion with well-defined margins; depigmented lacunae are common (*Fig. 12.53*).

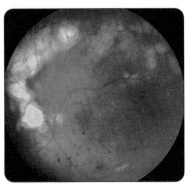

Fig 12.51

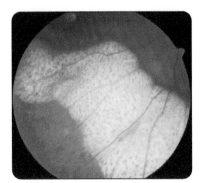

Fig 12.52

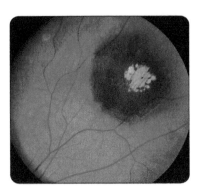

Fig 12.53

- **Grouped:** multiple lesions organized in a pattern simulating animal footprints ('bear-track' pigmentation), often confined to one sector of the fundus; smaller spots are usually located more centrally (*Fig. 12.54*).
- **Atypical:** bilateral multiple oval or spindle-shaped lesions of variable size, associated with hypopigmentation at one margin (*Fig. 12.55*).

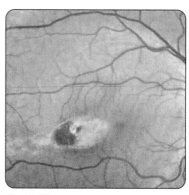

Fig 12.55

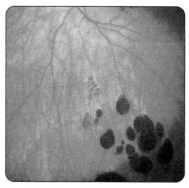

Fig 12.54

Systemic associations of atypical CHRPE

- **Familial adenomatous polyposis (FAP):** AD condition characterized by adenomatous polyps throughout the rectum and colon that develop in adolescence; if untreated, virtually all patients develop colorectal carcinoma by 50 years of age. More than 80% of patients with FAP have atypical CHRPE lesions.
- **Gardner syndrome:** FAP associated with osteomas of the skull, mandible, and long bones, and cutaneous soft tissue tumours.
- **Turcot syndrome:** AD or AR condition characterized by FAP and tumours of the CNS.

Chapter 13

Retinal vascular disease

Diabetic retinopathy

Introduction

- **Prevalence:** (a) the overall prevalence of diabetic retinopathy (DR) in diabetic patients is approximately 40%; (b) DR is more common in type 1 than in type 2 diabetes, (c) sight-threatening disease is present in up to 10%, and (d) proliferative disease affects 5–10% of the diabetic population (60% after 30 years in type 1).
- **Risk factors:** (a) duration of diabetes (50% after 10 years if diagnosed before age 30 years; 5% of type 2 diabetics have DR at presentation), (b) poor control of diabetes, (c) pregnancy, (d) hypertension, (e) nephropathy, (f) hyperlipidaemia, (g) smoking, (h) obesity, and (i) anaemia.

Classification

The classification proposed in the Early Treatment Diabetic Retinopathy Study is widely used internationally. An abbreviated version is set out in *Table 13.1*; other commonly used clinical categories are as follows:

- **Background diabetic retinopathy:** (a) microaneurysms, (b) dot and blot haemorrhages, and (c) hard exudates.
- **Diabetic maculopathy:** vision-threatening macular oedema or ischaemia.
- **Preproliferative diabetic retinopathy:** (a) cotton wool spots, (b) venous changes, (c) intraretinal microvascular anomalies (IRMA), and (d) deep retinal haemorrhages.
- **Proliferative diabetic retinopathy (PDR):** (a) neovascularization on or within one disc diameter of the disc (NVD) and/or (b) new vessels elsewhere (NVE) in the fundus.
- **Advanced diabetic eye disease:** (a) tractional retinal detachment, (b) persistent vitreous haemorrhage, and (c) neovascular glaucoma.

Table 13.1 Abbreviated early treatment diabetic retinopathy study classification of diabetic retinopathy

Category/description	Management
Nonproliferative diabetic retinopathy	
No DR	Review in 12 months.
Very mild Microaneurysms only.	Review most patients in 12 months.
Mild Any or all of: microaneurysms, retinal haemorrhages, exudates, cotton wool spots, up to the level of moderate NPDR. No IRMA or significant beading.	Review range 6–12 months, depending on severity of signs, stability, systemic factors, and patient's personal circumstances.
Moderate Severe retinal haemorrhages (more than ETDRS standard photograph 2A: approximately 20 medium–large per quadrant) in 1–3 quadrants *or* mild IRMA. • Significant venous beading can be present in no more than 1 quadrant. • Cotton wool spots commonly present.	Review in approximately 6 months. PDR occurs in up to 26%, high-risk PDR in up to 8% within 1 year.
Severe The 4-2-1 rule; one or more of: • Severe haemorrhages in all 4 quadrants. • Significant venous beading in 2 or more quadrants. • Moderate IRMA in 1 or more quadrants.	Review in 4 months. PDR in up to 50%, high-risk PDR in up to 15% within 1 year.
Very severe Two or more of the criteria for severe NPDR.	Review in 2 or 3 months. High-risk PDR in up to 45% within 1 year.
Proliferative diabetic retinopathy	
Mild/moderate NVD or NVE, but extent insufficient to meet the high-risk criteria.	Treatment considered according to severity of signs, stability, systemic factors, and patient's personal circumstances such as reliability of attendance for review. If not treated, review in up to 2 months.
High-risk • NVD greater than ETDRS standard photograph 10A (approximately one-third disc area) *or* any NVD with vitreous or preretinal haemorrhage *or* NVE also present. • Any NVD with vitreous or preretinal haemorrhage. • NVE greater than one-half disc area with vitreous or preretinal haemorrhage (or haemorrhage with presumed obscured NVD/E).	Treatment advised—see text. Should be performed immediately when possible, and certainly same day if symptomatic presentation with good retinal view.

Signs

- **Microaneurysms:** tiny red dots (*Fig. 13.1*) that tend to be the earliest signs.
- **Retinal nerve fibre layer haemorrhages:** superficial and flame-shaped (*Fig. 13.2*).
- **Intraretinal haemorrhages:** located in the compact middle layers of the retina and have a red 'dot/blot' configuration (*Fig. 13.3*).

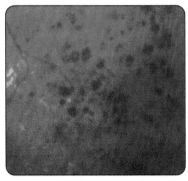

Fig 13.3

- **Deeper dark round haemorrhages:** haemorrhagic infarcts located within the middle retinal layers; risk marker for progression to retinal neovascularization.
- **Hard exudates:** waxy yellow lesions with distinct margins, often arranged in clumps and/or rings surrounding leaking microaneurysms (*Fig. 13.4*).
- **Diabetic maculopathy:** the most common cause of visual impairment in diabetics; (a) localized macular oedema is caused by focal leakage (*Fig. 13.5a*), (b) diffuse oedema is

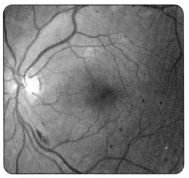

Fig 13.1

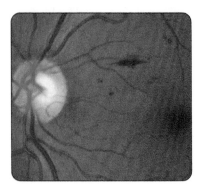

Fig 13.2

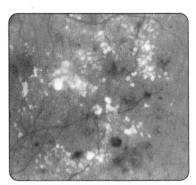

Fig 13.4

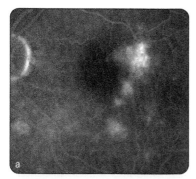

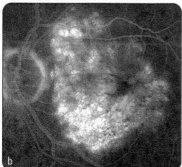

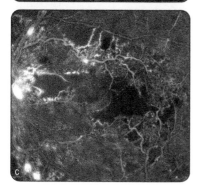

Fig 13.5

caused by leakage, often with accumulation of fluid at the fovea in cystoid configuration (CMO); FA shows diffuse late hyperfluorescence with a flower-petal pattern (*Fig. 13.5b*); (c) in ischaemic maculopathy, the macula may appear relatively normal despite reduced VA; FA shows capillary nonperfusion and an enlarged foveal avascular zone (FAZ) (*Fig. 13.5c*).

- **Cotton wool spots:** small whitish fluffy lesions consisting of focal accumulations of neuronal debris within the nerve fibre layer (*Fig. 13.6*).

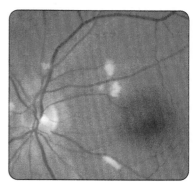

Fig 13.6

- **Venous anomalies** (*Fig. 13.7*): seen in ischaemia, consist of (a) generalized dilatation and tortuosity, (b) looping, (c) 'beading' (focal narrowing and dilatation), and (d) segmentation; the extent of the involved retinal area correlates with the risk of developing PDR.
- **IRMA:** fine irregular intraretinal arteriovenous shunts often seen adjacent to areas of capillary

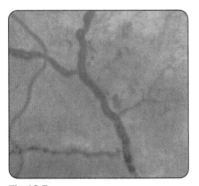

Fig 13.7

Fig 13.9

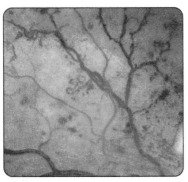

Fig 13.8

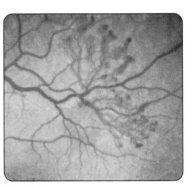

Fig 13.10

nonperfusion (*Fig. 13.8*); FA shows absence of leakage.
- *Neovascularization:* (a) NVD describes neovascularization on or within one disc diameter of the optic nerve head (*Fig. 13.9*), (b) NVE describes neovascularization further away from the disc (*Fig. 13.10*), and (c) new vessels on the iris (rubeosis iridis) carry a high risk of progression to neovascular glaucoma (see Chapter 10).

Treatment of clinically significant macular oedema (CSMO)

- *Definition:* retinal thickening within 500 μm of the centre of the macula (*Fig. 13.11a*), exudates within 500 μm of the centre of the macula, if associated with retinal thickening (*Fig. 13.11b*), or retinal thickening one disc area (1500 μm) or larger, any part of which is within one disc

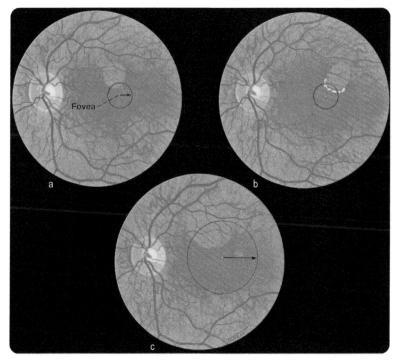

Fovea

Fig 13.11

diameter of the centre of the macula (*Fig. 13.11c*); eyes with CSMO should be considered for laser because this reduces the risk of visual loss by 50%.

- *Pretreatment FA:* delineates the area and extent of leakage, and detects ischaemic maculopathy (poor prognosis; see *Fig. 13.5c*).
- *Focal treatment:* light/moderate intensity burns (50–100 μm, 0.1 sec) applied to microaneurysms associated with CSMO; treatment as close as 300 μm from the centre of the macula may be considered in

some cases, with a lighter intensity reaction closer to the centre.

- *Grid treatment:* burns (100 μm, 0.1 sec) applied to areas of diffuse retinal thickening more than 500 μm from the centre of the macula to give a very light intensity reaction; treatment should be particularly light if significant macular ischaemia is present.
- *Results:* 70% of eyes achieve stable VA, 15% show improvement, and 15% subsequently deteriorate; it may take up to 4 months for oedema to respond.

- *Poor prognostic factors:*
  (a) significant macular ischaemia,
  (b) foveal exudates, (c) diffuse
  macular oedema, (d) CMO, (e) severe
  retinopathy at presentation,
  (f) uncontrolled systemic
  hypertension, (g) renal disease,
  (h) poorly controlled blood glucose,
  and (i) smoking.
- *Frequency-doubled micropulse
  Nd:YAG laser:* (e.g. 'pattern scan
  laser'–PASCAL); offers the potential
  for a less destructive retinal effect
  than argon, with barely visible burns
  at the level of the RPE.
- *Micropulse diode laser:* short
  duration (microseconds) burns to the
  RPE without significantly affecting the
  outer retina and choriocapillaris.
- *Intravitreal anti-VEGF agents:* show
  promise and are playing an
  increasingly prominent role.
- *Intravitreal triamcinolone:* research
  suggests that pseudophakic eyes
  with CSMO may benefit from
  intravitreal steroid injection followed
  by prompt laser.
- *Pars plana vitrectomy:* when macular
  oedema is associated with tangential
  traction from a thickened and taut
  posterior hyaloid, and possibly in
  other circumstances.
- *Lipid-lowering drugs:* may reduce the
  requirement for laser treatment.

Treatment of proliferative retinopathy

- *Risk characteristics and benefits:* The
  landmark Diabetic Retinopathy Study
  established the characteristics of
  high-risk proliferative disease and
  the effect of PRP, showing that
  (a) mild NVD with haemorrhage

carries a 26% risk of visual loss,
reduced to 4% with PRP, (b) severe
NVD without haemorrhage has a
26% risk of visual loss, reduced to
9%, (c) severe NVD with
haemorrhage carries a 37% risk of
visual loss, reduced to 20%, and
(d) severe NVE with haemorrhage
carries a 30% risk of visual loss,
reduced to 7% with treatment.
- *Complications:* visual field defects of
  sufficient severity to legally preclude
  driving; patients should also be
  made aware that there is some risk
  to central vision, and that night and
  colour vision may be affected.
- *Laser settings:* (a) spot size depends
  on the contact lens used (e.g.
  Goldmann 200–500 μm,
  panfundoscopic lens 100–300 μm),
  (b) duration 0.05–0.1 sec, and
  (c) power sufficient to produce only
  a light intensity burn (*Fig. 13.12*).
- *PRP technique:* 1500–2000 burns in
  a scatter pattern extending from the
  posterior fundus to cover the
  peripheral retina in one or more
  sessions. In eyes with severe NVD,

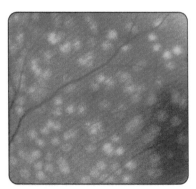

Fig 13.12

3000 or more burns may be required. Many practitioners leave two disc diameters untreated at the nasal side of the disc to preserve paracentral field. Topical anaesthesia is adequate in most patients, although a local block is sometimes necessary. Follow-up is after 4–6 weeks.

- *Intravitreal anti-VEGF therapy:* likely to have an increasing role, probably as an adjunct to PRP (e.g. to encourage resolution of persistent vitreous haemorrhage).

Advanced diabetic eye disease

Definition: serious vision-threatening complication of DR that occurs in patients in whom treatment has been inadequate or unsuccessful.

Diagnosis
- Haemorrhage–may be preretinal (retrohyaloid; *Fig. 13.13*), intragel, or both.

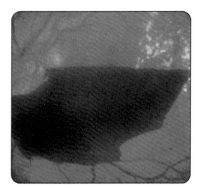

Fig 13.13

- Tractional retinal detachment is caused by progressive contraction of fibrovascular membranes at areas of vitreoretinal attachment (*Fig. 13.14*).
- Rubeosis iridis; may lead to neovascular glaucoma.

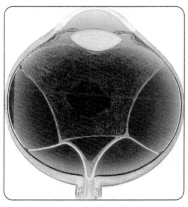

Fig 13.14

Pars plana vitrectomy (PPV)
- *Indications (Fig. 13.15):* (a) severe persistent unilateral vitreous haemorrhage precluding adequate PRP, (b) severe bilateral vitreous haemorrhage, (c) progressive tractional retinal detachment (RD) threatening or involving the macula, (d) combined tractional and rhegmatogenous RD (urgent), and (e) dense persistent premacular subhyaloid haemorrhage.
- *Visual results:* 70% achieve visual improvement, 10% worsen, and the rest are unchanged.

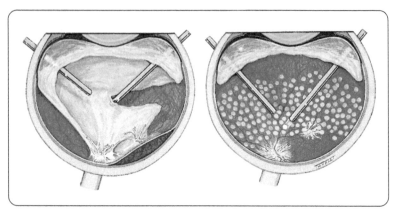

Fig 13.15

Retinal venous occlusive disease

Predisposing factors

- Age: more than 50% of patients are older than 65 years.
- Hypertension, particularly in branch retinal vein occlusion (BRVO).
- Hyperlipidaemia.
- Diabetes mellitus.
- Oral contraceptive pill: the most common association in younger females.
- Raised IOP in central retinal vein occlusion (CRVO).
- Smoking is a likely risk factor.
- Uncommon predispositions may be more important under the age of 50 years; (a) myeloproliferative disorders, (b) acquired hypercoagulable states (e.g. hyperhomocysteinaemia, lupus anticoagulant, antiphospholipid antibodies), (c) inherited hypercoagulable states (e.g. activated protein C resistance, and protein C and protein S deficiencies), (d) inflammatory disease associated with occlusive periphlebitis (e.g. Behçet syndrome, sarcoidosis), and (e) miscellaneous causes (e.g. chronic renal failure, orbital disease, dehydration).

Systemic assessment

- **All patients:** (a) blood pressure, (b) erythrocyte sedimentation rate (ESR), (c) full blood count (FBC), (d) blood glucose, (e) serum lipids, (f) plasma protein electrophoresis, (g) urea, electrolytes, and creatinine, (h) thyroid function tests (dysfunction associated), and (i) ECG (left ventricular hypertrophy associated).
- **Selected patients:** (e.g. younger than 50 years, bilateral RVO, previous thromboses, family history of thrombosis); (a) chest X-ray, (b) C-reactive protein (CRP), (c) thrombophilia screen, (d) anticardiolipin antibody (IgG and IgM), lupus anticoagulant), (e) autoantibodies, (f) serum

angiotensin-converting enzyme, (g) fasting plasma homocysteine, and (h) treponemal serology.

Branch retinal vein occlusion

Diagnosis

- *Presentation:* macular involvement may cause sudden onset of blurred vision, metamorphopsia, and a relative field defect; peripheral occlusions may be asymptomatic.
- *Acute signs:* (a) dilatation and tortuosity of the affected venous segment, (b) flame-shaped and dot/blot haemorrhages, (c) retinal oedema, and (d) sometimes cotton wool spots affecting the drained retinal sector (*Fig. 13.16a*); site of occlusion is often identifiable at an arteriovenous crossing point.
- *FA:* variable delayed venous filling, masking by blood, vessel wall staining, hypofluorescence due to capillary nonperfusion, and 'pruning' of vessels in the ischaemic areas (*Fig. 13.16b*).
- *OCT:* demonstrates and quantifies macular oedema.
- *Chronic signs:* (a) hard exudates, (b) venous sheathing and sclerosis, (c) residual haemorrhage (*Fig. 13.17*), and (d) collaterals that appear as slender tortuous venules developing locally or across the horizontal raphe between the inferior and superior vascular arcades.

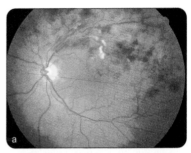
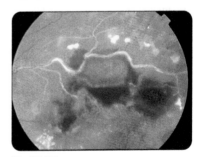

Fig 13.16

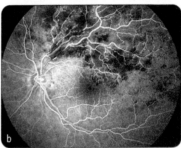

Fig 13.17

Treatment

- *Prognosis:* 50% of untreated eyes retain 6/12 or better; 25% will be <6/60.
- *Complications:* (a) chronic macular oedema—patients with visual acuity of 6/12 or worse may

benefit from laser photocoagulation, provided the macula is not significantly ischaemic; (b) retinal neovascularization (usually NVE) develops in approximately 40%, often within 6–12 months, and can lead to recurrent vitreous and preretinal haemorrhage.

- *Follow-up:* at 3 months with FA if vision is compromised, and provided retinal haemorrhages have cleared sufficiently.
- *Indications for laser:* macular oedema associated with good macular perfusion and VA 6/12 or worse after 3–6 months.
- *Relative contraindications to laser:* (a) VA less than 6/60, (b) symptoms for more than 1 year, and (c) macular ischaemia.
- *Subsequent follow-up:* 3- to 6-monthly intervals for up to 2 years to detect neovascularization.
- *Treatment of macular oedema:* (a) grid laser photocoagulation: spots of 50–100 μm, 0.1 s duration one burn width apart, to produce a gentle reaction in the area of leakage as identified on FA, up to the edge of the FAZ; (b) other options include intravitreal triamcinolone, intravitreal anti-VEGF agents, periocular steroid injection, and arteriovenous sheathotomy.
- *Neovascularization:* not normally treated unless vitreous haemorrhage occurs because early treatment does not appear to affect the visual prognosis; if appropriate, involved area is treated with scatter laser photocoagulation (200–500 μm, 0.05–0.1 s, one burn width apart, medium reaction).

Non-ischaemic central retinal vein occlusion

Diagnosis

- *Presentation:* sudden, unilateral blurred vision with moderate/ severe reduction of VA.
- *Relative afferent pupillary defect (RAPD):* absent or mild.
- *Acute signs:* (a) tortuosity and dilatation of all branches of the CRV, (b) dot/blot and flame-shaped haemorrhages throughout the fundus (*Fig. 13.18a*), (c) cotton wool spots, and (d) optic disc and macular oedema.
- *FA:* delayed arteriovenous transit time, masking by haemorrhages,

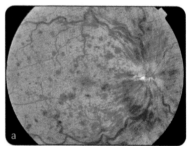

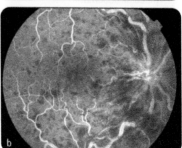

Fig 13.18

good retinal capillary perfusion (*Fig. 13.18b*), and late leakage.

- *OCT:* useful in the assessment of CMO.
- *Course:* most acute signs resolve over 6–12 months to leave disc collaterals, macular epiretinal gliosis, and macular pigmentary changes; conversion to ischaemic CRVO occurs in 34% within 3 years.
- *Prognosis:* return of VA to normal or near normal in approximately 50%; chronic macular oedema is the main cause of poor vision.

Treatment

- *Follow-up:* first review is after 3 months, with subsequent follow-up for up to 2 years.
- *Treatment of macular oedema:* (a) intravitreal steroid (triamcinolone or sustained-release implant), (b) intravitreal anti-VEGF agents, (c) experimental treatments (e.g. chorioretinal anastomosis, radial optic neurotomy, tissue plasminogen activator infusion).

Ischaemic central retinal vein occlusion

Diagnosis

- *Presentation:* sudden and severe visual loss; VA is usually CF or worse.
- *RAPD:* marked.
- *Acute signs:* (a) severe tortuosity and engorgement of all branches of the CRV, (b) extensive deep blot and flame-shaped haemorrhages involving the peripheral retina and posterior pole (*Fig. 13.19a*),

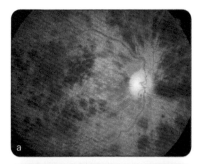
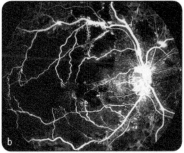

Fig 13.19

(c) severe disc oedema and hyperaemia, and (d) often prominent cotton wool spots.

- *FA:* marked delay in arteriovenous transit time, central masking by retinal haemorrhages, extensive areas of capillary nonperfusion (*Fig. 13.19b*), and vessel wall staining.
- *OCT:* useful for CMO.
- *Course:* most acute signs resolve over 9–12 months to leave disc collaterals, macular epiretinal gliosis, and macular pigmentary changes.
- *Prognosis:* extremely poor due to macular ischaemia.

- *Rubeosis iridis:* develops in approximately 50% of eyes, usually after 2–4 months, and is associated with a high risk of neovascular (100-day) glaucoma. The development of opticociliary shunts (retinochoroidal collateral veins) may protect against rubeosis iridis.

Treatment

- *Review:* (a) monthly for 6 months to detect rubeosis iridis; gonioscopy should be carried out at each visit to detect angle new vessels, and the pupillary margin should also be examined prior to mydriasis; (b) subsequent review is for up to 2 years.
- *Treatment of rubeosis:* PRP as for PDR, with 1500–3000 burns initially; intravitreal anti-VEGF agents may be used adjunctively in selected cases.
- *Treatment of macular oedema:* as for non-ischaemic CRVO, but with poorer prognosis.

Hemiretinal vein occlusion

Definition: variant of CRVO and may be ischaemic or non-ischaemic; (a) hemispheric occlusion blocks a major branch of the CRV at or near the optic disc; (b) hemicentral occlusion, which is less common, involves one trunk of a dual-trunked CRV.

Diagnosis

- *Presentation:* sudden-onset altitudinal visual field defect; VA is variable.
- *Signs:* features of BRVO, involving the superior or inferior retina (*Fig. 13.20*).

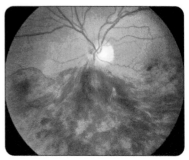

Fig 13.20

Treatment: eyes with extensive retinal ischaemia are managed in the same way as ischaemic CRVO.

Retinal arterial occlusive disease

Pathogenesis

- *Atherosclerosis-related thrombosis:* at the lamina cribrosa (80% of cases).
- *Carotid embolism:* most commonly from an atheromatous plaque at the carotid bifurcation.
- *Uncommon:* (a) giant cell arteritis (GCA), (b) cardiac embolism, (c) periarteritis (e.g. systemic lupus erythematosus, Wegener granulomatosis, Behçet syndrome), (d) thrombophilic disorders (e.g. hyperhomocysteinaemia), (e) antiphospholipid antibody syndrome, (f) inherited defects of natural anticoagulants, and (g) sickling haemoglobinopathies.

Systemic assessment

- *History:* symptoms of GCA (e.g. headache, jaw claudication, scalp tenderness, limb girdle pain, weight loss, polymyalgia rheumatica).
- *Examination:* (a) pulse (e.g. atrial fibrillation), (b) blood pressure, (c) cardiac auscultation, and (d) carotid examination (pulse, auscultation).
- *All patients:* (a) ECG, (b) ESR, (c) CRP, (d) FBC, (e) blood glucose, (f) serum lipids, urea, and electrolytes, and (g) carotid duplex scanning.
- *Selected patients:* (particularly if younger and without cardiovascular risk factors) (a) further carotid imaging, (b) cranial MR or CT, (c) echocardiography, (d) chest X-ray, (e) 24-hr ECG (Holter monitor), (f) fasting plasma homocysteine, (g) thrombophilia screen, (h) plasma protein electrophoresis, (i) thyroid function tests (associated with atrial fibrillation and dyslipidaemia), (j) autoantibodies, and (k) blood cultures.

Amaurosis fugax

- A transient ischaemic attack (TIA) is characterized by painless transient monocular loss of vision, usually lasting a few minute's.
- Often described as a 'curtain coming down over the eye'.
- Sometimes accompanied by an ipsilateral cerebral TIA, with contralateral neurological features.
- Investigation and management is as for arterial occlusion.

Branch retinal artery occlusion

Diagnosis

- *Presentation:* sudden painless altitudinal or sectoral visual field loss; VA is variable.
- *RAPD:* often present.
- *Signs:* (a) narrowing of arteries and veins, (b) segmentation of the blood column ('cattle trucking'/'boxcarting'), (c) cloudy retina corresponding to the area of ischaemia (*Fig. 13.21a*), and (d) emboli may be seen, especially at bifurcations (*Fig. 13.22*).
- *FA:* delay in arterial filling, with hypofluorescence of the involved

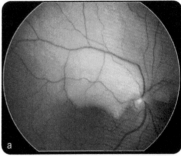

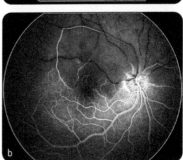

Fig 13.21

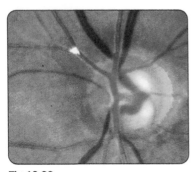

Fig 13.22

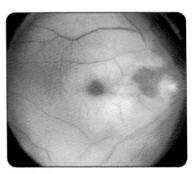

Fig 13.23

area due to masking by oedema (see *Fig. 13.21b*).

Treatment

- *Follow-up:* single follow-up assessment in 3 months may be warranted to review the fundus and provide advice on prognosis; adequate systemic management is vital (see below).
- *Prognosis:* if central vision is severely compromised, prognosis is poor unless the obstruction is relieved within a few hours (see below).

Central retinal artery occlusion

Diagnosis

- *Presentation:* (a) sudden and profound loss of vision; (b) VA is severely reduced except when a portion of the papillomacular bundle is supplied by a cilioretinal artery.
- *RAPD:* profound.
- *Signs:* (a) similar to BRAO but more extensive, and (b) an orange reflex from the intact choroid stands out at the foveola, giving a 'cherry-red spot' (*Fig. 13.23*); in

eyes with a cilioretinal artery, part of the macula will remain of normal colour.

- *Course:* (a) retinal cloudiness and cherry-red spot disappear over a few days to weeks but the arteries remain attenuated; (b) subsequent signs include optic atrophy, vessel sheathing, patchy inner retinal atrophy, and RPE changes; (c) rubeosis iridis develops in a minority of cases, and a few develop NVE or NVD.
- *FA:* delay in arterial filling and masking of background choroidal fluorescence by retinal swelling.

Treatment: follow-up at 4 weeks and again a month later to detect neovascularization; adequate systemic management is vital (see below).

Treatment of acute retinal artery occlusion

- *Aims:* theoretically, timely dissolution of thrombus or dislodgement of emboli may ameliorate visual loss. Various measures may be tried in patients with occlusions of less than

24–48 hr, although evidence of benefit is limited.

- **Ocular massage:** using a three-mirror contact lens (allows direct artery visualization) for cycles of 10 sec compression followed by 5 sec of release; self-massage through closed eyelids can be continued by the patient.
- **Anterior chamber paracentesis:** with prior povidone–iodine 5% and a short course of topical antibiotic afterwards.
- **Drug treatment:** (a) topical apraclonidine 1% and timolol 0.5%, (b) intravenous acetazolamide 500 mg, and (c) sublingual isosorbide dinitrate to induce vasodilation.
- **'Rebreathing' into a paper bag:** to elevate blood carbon dioxide and promote vasodilatation. Breathing a high oxygen (95%) and carbon dioxide (5%) mixture, 'carbogen,' may exert the dual effects of retarding ischaemia and vasodilatation.
- **Hyperosmotic agents:** mannitol or glycerol for rapid IOP lowering and increasing intravascular volume.
- **Transluminal Nd:YAG laser embolysis:** if an occluding embolus is visible; shots of 0.5–1.0 mJ or higher are applied directly to the embolus.
- **Thrombolysis:** local arterial (internal carotid and ophthalmic) or intravenous infusion.

Systemic prophylaxis following retinal arterial occlusion

The risk of stroke is relatively high in the first few days following retinal artery occlusion or amaurosis fugax, and 'fast-track' referral to a specialist stroke clinic is advisable.

- General risk factors should be addressed and smoking discontinued.
- Urgent referral is mandatory for significant cardiac arrhythmia.
- Antiplatelet therapy can be started immediately provided there are no contraindications and thrombolysis is not planned.
- Oral anticoagulation in selected patients (e.g. atrial fibrillation).
- Carotid endarterectomy may be indicated in patients with symptomatic stenosis greater than 70%.

Asymptomatic retinal embolus

A retinal embolus identified on routine examination of an asymptomatic older patient indicates a substantially increased risk of a future vascular event. Management is that of the risk factors discussed previously; a higher threshold for carotid surgery is appropriate.

Hypertensive disease

Retinopathy

Definition: spectrum of retinal vascular changes related to both transient and persistent microvascular damage from elevated blood pressure. The changes arise from a combination of acute vasoconstrictive and chronic involutional sclerotic responses.

Diagnosis

- Arteriolar narrowing; may be focal or generalized.
- Cotton wool spots and flame-shaped haemorrhages in severe hypertension (*Fig. 13.24*).

- Swelling of the optic nerve head is the hallmark of malignant (accelerated) hypertension (*Fig. 13.26*).
- Nipping at arteriovenous crossings and broadening of the vessel light reflex is characteristic of arteriolosclerosis (*Fig. 13.27*).

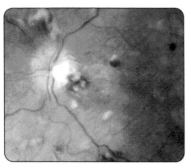

Fig 13.24

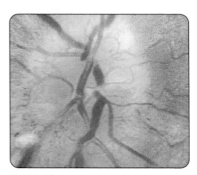

Fig 13.26

- Chronic retinal oedema may lead to deposition of hard exudates around the fovea in a star configuration (*Fig. 13.25*).

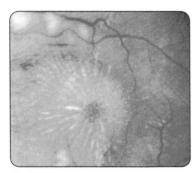

Fig 13.25

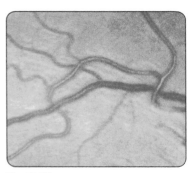

Fig 13.27

Choroidopathy

Pathogenesis: acute hypertensive crisis (accelerated/malignant hypertension) in young adults.

Diagnosis

- *Elschnig spots:* focal choroidal infarcts seen as small black spots surrounded by yellow halos.
- *Siegrist streaks:* foci of fibrinoid necrosis manifest as flecks arranged linearly along choroidal vessels.
- *Exudative retinal detachment:* sometimes bilateral, may occur in severe acute hypertension (e.g. toxaemia of pregnancy).

Sickle cell retinopathy

Pathogenesis: hypoxia and acidosis induce red blood cells containing abnormal haemoglobin to adopt an anomalous shape, resulting in microvascular occlusion.

Proliferative retinopathy

Diagnosis

- *Presentation:* asymptomatic unless vitreous haemorrhage or retinal detachment occurs.
- *Stage 1:* peripheral arteriolar occlusion and ischaemia (*Fig. 13.28*).
- *Stage 2:* peripheral arteriovenous anastomoses—dilated pre-existing capillary channels.
- *Stage 3:* sprouting of 'sea fan' new vessels from the anastomoses; 30–40% auto-infarct and appear as greyish fibrovascular lesions.
- *Stage 4:* neovascular tufts continue to proliferate, and bleed into the vitreous.

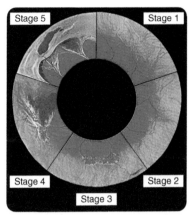

Fig 13.28

- *Stage 5:* extensive fibrovascular proliferation and retinal detachment.
- *FA:* sea fans show peripheral nonperfusion followed by leakage from new vessels (*Fig. 13.29*).

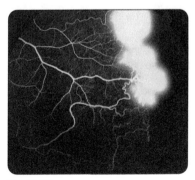

Fig 13.29

Treatment: not required in most cases; pars plana vitrectomy is occasionally required for tractional retinal detachment and/or persistent vitreous haemorrhage.

Nonproliferative retinopathy

- *Asymptomatic lesions:* (a) venous tortuosity, (b) 'silver wiring' (previously occluded peripheral arterioles), (c) 'salmon patches' (pink pre- or intraretinal haemorrhages), (d) 'black sunbursts' (patches of RPE hyperplasia) (*Fig. 13.30*), and (e) macular depression sign (oval depression of the macular reflex due to retinal atrophy).

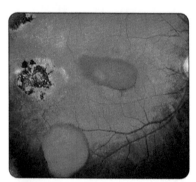

Fig 13.30

- *Symptomatic lesions:* (a) macular arteriolar occlusion, (b) RVO, (c) acute CRAO (rare), (d) choroidal vascular occlusion (usually in children), and (e) angioid streaks (rare).
- *Anterior segment features:* conjunctival corkscrew vessels and circumscribed areas of ischaemic iris atrophy, usually extending from the pupillary edge to the collarette; rubeosis is occasionally seen.

Retinopathy of prematurity

Pathogenesis: proliferative retinopathy affecting premature infants of very low birth weight, who have often been exposed to high ambient oxygen concentrations. With premature birth, normal retinal vascularization is halted and excessive VEGF production leads to the neovascular complications of retinopathy of prematurity (ROP).

Diagnosis

- *Location (Fig. 13.31):* (a) zone 1 is bounded by an imaginary circle the radius of which is twice the distance from the disc to the centre of the macula, (b) zone 2 extends concentrically from the edge of zone 1, its radius extends from the centre of the disc to the nasal ora serrata, and (c) zone 3 consists of a residual temporal crescent anterior to zone 2.
- *Extent of involvement:* determined by the number of clock hours of retina involved (30° sectors).

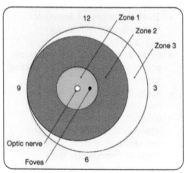

Fig 13.31

- **Staging** (*Fig. 13.32*): determined by the most severe manifestation; (a) stage 1 (demarcation line) is a thin, flat, tortuous, grey-white line running roughly parallel with the ora serrata, (b) stage 2 is a ridge arising in the region of the demarcation line, (c) stage 3 is extraretinal fibrovascular proliferation from the ridge into the vitreous, (d) stage 4 is partial retinal detachment—extrafoveal (4A) and foveal (4B), and (e) stage 5 is a total retinal detachment.
- **'Plus' disease:** (plus sign added to the stage number) signifies a tendency to progression:

  (a) failure of the pupil to dilate, (b) vascular iris engorgement, (c) vitreous haze, (d) dilated veins and tortuous arteries in at least two quadrants, and (e) increasing preretinal and vitreous haemorrhage.
- **'Threshold' disease:** five contiguous or eight cumulative clock hours of extraretinal neovascularization (stage 3) in zone 1 or 2 associated with plus disease—an indication for treatment.
- **'Rush' disease:** aggressive posterior disease.
- **Course:** spontaneous regression occurs in 80%, even in some eyes with partial retinal detachment.

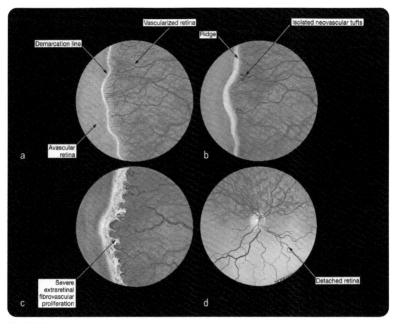

Fig 13.32

- *Screening:* infants born at or before 31 weeks' gestational age or weighing 1500 g or less should be screened for ROP, beginning 4–7 weeks postnatally with review 1–2 weekly until vascularization reaches zone 3; approximately 8% of infants screened require treatment.

Treatment

- *PRP (Fig. 13.33):* of avascular immature retina in threshold disease.
- *Intravitreal anti-VEGF agents:* increasingly being used.
- *Lens-sparing pars plana vitrectomy:* for tractional retinal detachment, especially if not involving the macula (stage 4A); visual outcome in stages 4B and 5 is often disappointing despite successful reattachment.

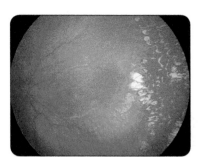

Fig 13.33

Retinal artery macroaneurysm

Definition: localized dilatation of a retinal arteriole, usually involving one eye.

Diagnosis

- *Presentation:* typically in elderly hypertensive women with (a) insidious impairment of central vision due to leakage involving the macula, (b) sudden visual loss due to haemorrhage, or (c) chance finding.
- *Signs:* (a) saccular or fusiform arteriolar dilatation, most frequently on a temporal vascular arcade, with (b) associated retinal haemorrhage in 50% (*Fig. 13.34a*).
- *FA:* immediate filling (*Fig. 13.34b*) with late leakage; incomplete filling is due to thrombosis of the lumen.

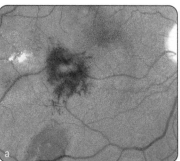

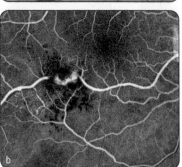

Fig 13.34

- **Course:** (a) chronic leakage with oedema and exudate (*Fig. 13.35*), (b) rupture with intra-, sub- (*Fig. 13.36*), or preretinal haemorrhage; (c) spontaneous involution may occur following thrombosis, with fibrosis (very common).
- **Prognosis:** good with vitreous or premacular haemorrhage but poor with submacular haemorrhage.

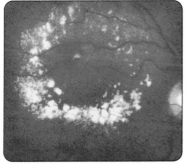

Fig 13.35

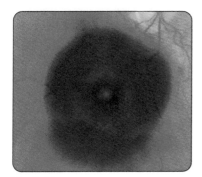

Fig 13.36

Treatment
- **Observation:** eyes with good VA.
- **Photocoagulation:** for oedema or exudates threatening or involving

the fovea; burns may be applied to the lesion itself or to the surrounding area.
- **Other:** (a) YAG laser hyaloidotomy for persistent preretinal haemorrhage overlying the macula, and (b) intravitreal injection of expandable gas with facedown positioning may shift submacular haemorrhage away from the fovea; adjunctive intravitreal tissue plasminogen activator (TPA) may be used.

Primary retinal telangiectasia

Definition: group of rare idiopathic congenital or acquired retinal vascular anomalies characterized by dilatation and tortuosity of retinal blood vessels, multiple aneurysms, vascular leakage, and deposition of hard exudates.

Idiopathic macular telangiectasia

Diagnosis
- *Type 1 (aneurysmal telangiectasia):* usually affects middle-aged males and may be related to Coats disease (see below); (a) telangiectasia, micro-aneurysms, and later larger aneurysms, with leakage leading to CMO and lipid deposition (*Fig. 13.37*); (b) peripheral retina may be involved in addition to the macula.
- *Type 2 (perifoveal telangiectasia):* affects males and females equally; (a) subtle telangiectasia (*Fig. 13.38*) progressing to cystic foveal atrophy without leakage,

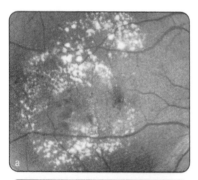

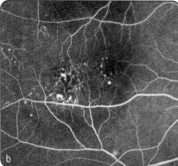

Fig 13.37

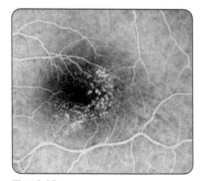

Fig 13.38

and (b) subretinal and choroidal neovascularization; worse prognosis than in type 1.

- *Occlusive telangiectasia:* extremely rare, with manifestations relating to capillary occlusion (*Fig. 13.39*) rather than telangiectasia.

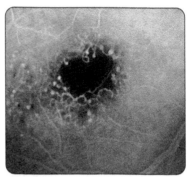

Fig 13.39

Treatment

- *Type 1:* (a) photocoagulation to areas of leakage may occasionally be beneficial; (b) intravitreal anti-VEGF agents may reduce oedema and improve vision.
- *Type 2:* intravitreal anti-VEGF agents decrease leakage on FA in the nonproliferative stage but are probably not helpful visually.

Coats disease

Diagnosis

- *Presentation:* in early childhood (typically boys, average age 5 years) with (a) unilateral visual loss, (b) strabismus, or (c) leucocoria.
- *Signs:* (a) telangiectasia, typically inferior and temporal, and anterior to the equator, (b) intra- and

subretinal exudation (*Fig. 13.40*), often in areas remote from the vascular abnormalities, particularly the macula, with (c) progression to exudative retinal detachment (*Fig. 13.41*).

- **Complications:** (a) rubeosis iridis, (b) glaucoma, (c) uveitis, (d) cataract, and (e) phthisis bulbi.
- **Prognosis:** depends on severity at presentation; the course is often milder in older children.

Treatment

- **Observation:** for mild non-vision-threatening disease.
- **Photocoagulation:** to areas of telangiectasia associated with progressive exudation.
- **Anti-VEGF therapy:** initial results are promising, although long-term safety in children remains unknown.
- **Cryotherapy:** for extensive exudative retinal detachment.
- **Pars plana vitrectomy:** for total retinal detachment.

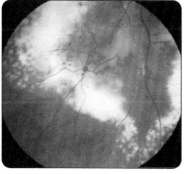

Fig 13.40

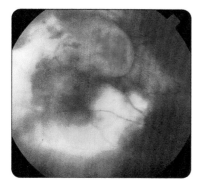

Fig 13.41

Acquired macular disorders

Age-related macular degeneration

Introduction

- **Definition:** degeneration affecting the macula; characterized by drusen and RPE changes, and sometimes CNV.
- **Classification:** non-exudative ('dry')—most common, and exudative ('wet'); the latter is associated with more rapid progression to advanced sight loss.
- **Importance:** most common cause of irreversible visual loss in industrialized countries; advanced age-related macular degeneration (AMD) in one eye confers a 50% chance of advanced AMD in the fellow eye within 5 years.
- **Risk factors:** (a) age, (b) race (higher in Caucasians), (c) family history (several genes implicated), (d) smoking (doubles risk), (e) dietary factors (e.g. high fat intake), and (f) others (cataract surgery, blue iris colour, sunlight).

Drusen

- **Pathogenesis:** extracellular deposits at the interface between the RPE and Bruch membrane, derived from immune-mediated and metabolic processes in the RPE.
- **'Hard' drusen:** well-defined and small (less than half a retinal vein width; *Fig. 14.1*); their presence in isolation carries little risk of visual loss.
- **'Soft' drusen:** less distinct and larger than hard drusen; numerous large soft drusen (*Fig. 14.2*) are associated with a high risk of visual loss, including progression to CNV.

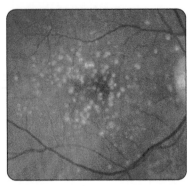

Fig 14.1

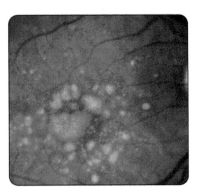

Fig 14.2

- **'Drusenoid RPE detachment':** caused by coalesce of soft drusen resulting in a localized elevation of the RPE, a 'drusenoid RPE detachment' (*Fig. 14.3*).

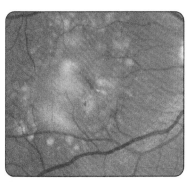

Fig 14.3

Prophylactic antioxidant supplementation in AMD

The Age-Related Eye Disease Study (AREDS) established that taking high-dose antioxidant vitamins and minerals on a regular basis can decrease the risk of AMD progression.

- *Indications:* those aged older than 55 years with one or more of the following high-risk characteristics (extensive intermediate-sized drusen, at least one druse over 125 μm, geographic atrophy, advanced AMD in one eye); treatment confers a reduction in risk of up to 25% at 5 years.
- *AREDS regimen:* vitamins C and E, beta-carotene, zinc, and copper; possible adverse effects include an increased risk of lung cancer in smokers.
- *Other measures:* (a) macular xanthophylls (lutein and zeaxanthin) and omega-3 fatty acids, (b) adequate leafy green vegetable intake; (c) cessation of smoking and avoidance of excessive sunlight should also be considered.

Non-exudative AMD

Diagnosis

- *Presentation:* gradual impairment of central vision over months or years in one or both eyes.
- *Signs:* (a) numerous intermediate–large soft drusen, (b) focal RPE changes, and (c) areas of chorioretinal atrophy (*Fig. 14.4*).
- *Course:* enlargement of atrophic areas to give 'geographical atrophy' (*Fig. 14.5*) with

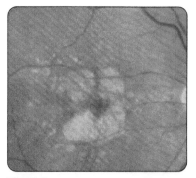

Fig 14.4

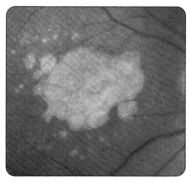

Fig 14.5

disappearance of pre-existing drusen.
- *FA:* window defect if the choriocapillaris is still intact; exposed sclera may exhibit late staining.

Treatment: prophylactic antioxidant supplementation; experimental surgical options (e.g. intraocular telescope implantation, retinal translocation, implantable photosensitive chip).

Retinal pigment epithelial detachment

Pathogenesis: separation of the RPE from Bruch's membrane caused by disruption of the physiological forces maintaining adhesion.

Diagnosis
- *Serous retinal pigment epithelial detaciment (PED):* orange dome-shaped elevation with sharply delineated edges (*Fig. 14.6a*); subretinal blood or lipid

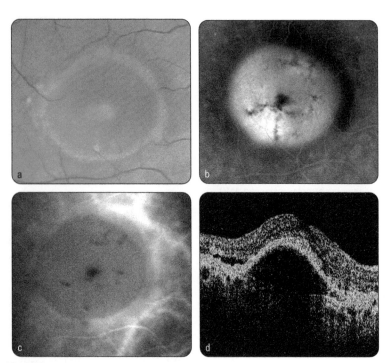

Fig 14.6

and irregularly distributed fluid are suggestive of underlying CNV.

- *Imaging of serous PED:* (a) FA shows a well-demarcated oval area of hyperfluorescence increasing in intensity but not area—'pooling'—in which a notch may indicate CNV (*Fig. 14.6b*), (b) ICGA shows an oval area of hypofluorescence and a faint ring of surrounding hyperfluorescence (*Fig. 14.6c*), and (c) OCT shows separation of the RPE from Bruch's membrane by an optically empty area (*Fig. 14.6d*).

- *Course of serous PED:* (a) gradually increasing atrophy and an eventual VA of 6/60 or less; (b) spontaneous resolution can occur, sometimes with visual improvement but often leaving geographic atrophy; and (c) rapid visual loss is typical of associated CNV (over 30%) or RPE tear formation (see below).

- *Fibrovascular PED:* (a) a form of 'occult' CNV, much more irregular in outline and elevation than serous PED; (b) FA shows markedly irregular granular or 'stippled' hyperfluorescence, with uneven filling of the PED, leakage, and late staining; (c) OCT shows an optically denser lesion than serous PED.

- *'Drusenoid' PED:* (a) shallowly elevated pale area with irregular scalloped edges; (b) FA shows diffuse hyperfluorescence, and (c) OCT shows homogeneous hyperreflectivity.

- *Haemorrhagic PED:* virtually all eyes have underlying CNV or polypoidal choroidal vasculopathy (see below); (a) presentation is

with sudden impairment of central vision, and prognosis is poor, (b) a dark red dome-shaped lesion is seen on examination, and (c) FA shows dense masking but with overlying vessels visible.

Treatment

- *Serous PED:* observation may be appropriate in eyes without CNV, especially in younger patients. Options for CNV are (a) intravitreal anti-VEGF agents, (b) PDT, and (c) intravitreal triamcinolone, often in combination.

- *Fibrovascular PED:* as for serous PED with CNV.

- *Drusenoid PED:* observation in most cases.

- *Haemorrhagic PED:* see below for management of polypoidal choroidal vasculopathy (PCV) and small CNV.

Retinal pigment epithelial tear

Pathogenesis: tearing at the junction of attached and detached RPE, either spontaneously or after interventions such as laser or intravitreal injection.

Diagnosis

- *Presentation:* sudden central visual loss.

- *Signs:* crescent-shaped pale area of RPE dehiscence, next to a darker area corresponding to the retracted and folded flap (*Fig. 14.7a*).

- *FA:* late phase shows hypofluorescence over the flap due to the thickened folded RPE, with a linear border and adjacent hyperfluorescence where the RPE is absent (*Fig. 14.7b*).

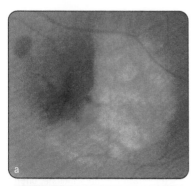

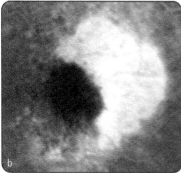

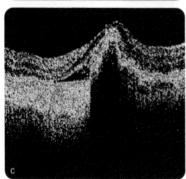

Fig 14.7

- *OCT:* hyperreflectivity adjacent to the folded RPE (*Fig. 14.7c*).
- *Prognosis:* poor in subfoveal tears.

Treatment: unproven modalities such as RPE translocation.

Exudative AMD

Pathogenesis: abnormal vessel complexes originating from the choriocapillaris (CNV) grow through Bruch's membrane; it is thought that an age-related lowering of the integrity of Bruch's membrane is a key aetiological factor.

Diagnosis

- *Presentation:* in 6th to 8th decades with blurring and/or metamorphopsia.
- *Signs:* (a) localized subretinal fluid, (b) hard exudate (*Fig. 14.8*), and (c) blood (*Fig. 14.9*) (subretinal, preretinal); (d) CNV itself is sometimes identifiable as a grey-green or pinkish-yellow subretinal lesion; later, retinal and subretinal fibrosis (*Fig. 14.10*) ensues in an evolved or treated lesion.

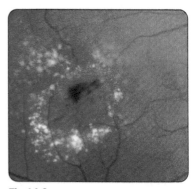

Fig 14.8

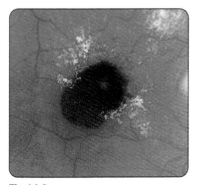

Fig 14.9

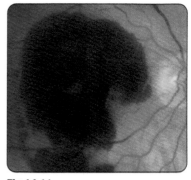

Fig 14.11

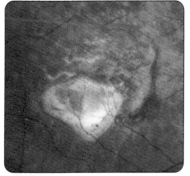

Fig 14.10

Fig 14.12

- **Prognosis of untreated CNV:** often very poor, leading to 'hand movements' vision (*Figs. 14.11–14.13*).
- **FA:** (a) 'classic' CNV is a well-defined membrane that fills

with dye in a 'lacy' pattern early, with later leakage and staining (*Fig. 14.14*): (b) 'occult' CNV is much less well-defined (*Fig. 14.15*) and often denotes a fibrovascular PED.

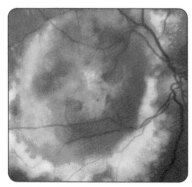

Fig 14.13

- **ICGA:** a focal hyperfluorescent 'hot spot' or 'plaque' (*Fig. 14.16*) can be a more sensitive adjunct to FA for the detection of CNV, for distinguishing other entities such as PCV, and for identification of vascular feeder complexes in some situations.
- **OCT** (*Fig. 14.17*): used to monitor response to treatment.

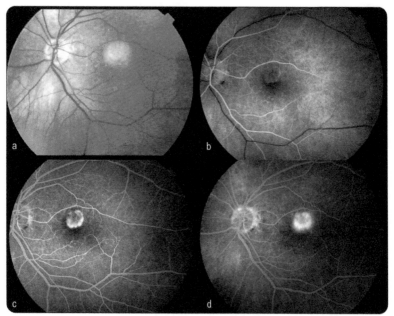

Fig 14.14

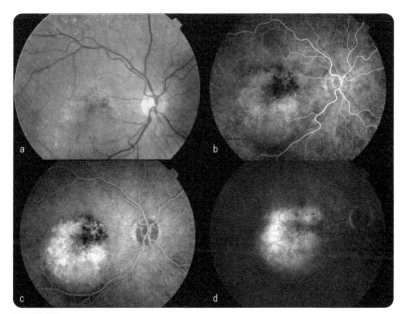

Fig 14.15

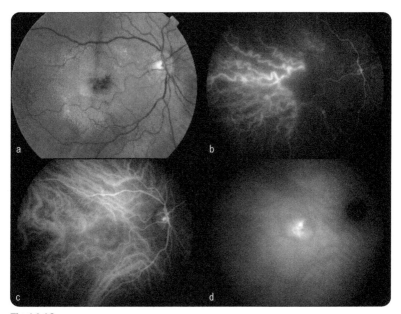

Fig 14.16

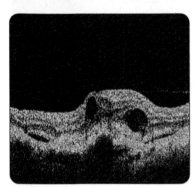

Fig 14.17

Treatment: intravitreal anti-VEGF agents have dramatically improved the visual prognosis. An eye with almost any level of vision may benefit, although better VA at the outset is associated with a superior outcome.

- *Ranibizumab (Lucentis):* monoclonal antibody fragment developed specifically for the eye.
- *Bevacizumab (Avastin):* complete antibody developed for systemic use; much cheaper, although similar in efficacy and side effect profile to ranibizumab; used 'off label' in the eye.
- *Pegaptanib (Macugen):* used less than other agents.
- *VEGF Trap-Eye:* promising newer agent with longer duration of action.
- *Complications of anti-VEGFs:* (a) retinal detachment, (b) lens damage, (c) RPE tears, (d) endophthalmitis and sterile uveitis, (e) elevated IOP, and (f) probably slightly increased incidence of stroke.

- *Treatment strategy:* long-term regular monthly injection is highly efficacious, but it is resource-intensive, inconvenient for patients, and carries a higher risk of adverse effects; overall, approximately 95% of eyes maintain vision regardless of lesion type, and 35–40% significantly improve vision, most markedly during the first 3 months.
- *Alternative treatment strategies:* (a) three initial monthly injections followed by monthly review with re-injection upon deterioration of VA or on OCT, and (b) 'treat and extend,' entailing the administration of three initial injections at monthly intervals followed by a gradual increase in the period between injections until deterioration is evident.
- *PDT:* intravenous administration of a light-activated compound (e.g. verteporfin (Visudyne)) preferentially taken up by dividing cells including neovascular tissue, and then activated focally by a low-energy laser, leading to thrombosis but sparing healthy tissue. Its use has declined following the introduction of VEGF inhibition, but it remains useful in certain circumstances.
- *Combination therapies:* (e.g. PDT plus anti-VEGFs) are under investigation and may allow a reduction in the frequency of injections.
- *Laser photocoagulation:* now rarely performed, although may still be suitable for some patients (e.g.

PCV and retinal angiomatous proliferation) (see below).

- **Investigational modalities:**
(a) sustained-release anti-VEGF systems, (b) inhibitors of other cytokines, (c) RNA strand modification of gene expression, (d) gene therapy, and (e) radiotherapy.

Retinal angiomatous proliferation

Definition: variant of exudative AMD in which the major component of the neovascular complex is initially located within the retina; often bilateral and symmetrical.

Diagnosis

- **Presentation:** similar to CNV.
- **Signs:** (a) dilated retinal vessels, typically accompanied by (b) intra-, sub-, and preretinal haemorrhage, (c) oedema, (d) hard exudate, and (e) often PED.
- **OCT:** hyperreflectivity of intraretinal neovascularization.
- **FA:** similar to occult CNV, but may show focal intraretinal hyperfluorescence.
- **ICGA:** 'hot spot' in mid or late frames, and sometimes a 'hairpin loop.'

Treatment: anti-VEGF therapy.

Polypoidal choroidal vasculopathy

Definition: idiopathic disease characterized by a dilated network of inner choroidal vessels with multiple terminal aneurysmal protuberances. It is more common in Africans and East Asians, in women, and is often bilateral but asymmetrical.

Diagnosis

- **Presentation:** in 7th decade with sudden visual impairment.
- **Signs:** (a) recurrent serosanguineous retinal and RPE detachments (*Figs. 14.18* and *14.19a*); (b) terminal swellings may be seen as reddish-orange nodules beneath the RPE.

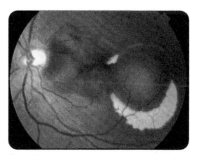

Fig 14.18

- **Course:** may be slow; up to 50% may eventually involute spontaneously.
- **ICGA:** network of large choroidal vessels with surrounding hypofluorescence, with leaking polyp-like swellings on the larger vessels (*Fig. 14.19b*).

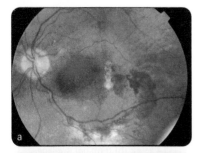

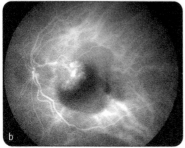

Fig 14.19

Treatment
- *Anti-VEGF therapy:* less effective than in conventional CNV.
- *PDT:* moderately effective.
- *Laser photocoagulation:* of feeder vessels or leaking lesions.

Age-related macular hole

Diagnosis
- *Presentation:* in 7th decade with a missing central patch in one eye or metamorphopsia.
- *Stage 1a ('impending' macular hole):* (a) flattening of the foveal depression with an underlying yellow spot, and (b) inner retinal layers detach from the underlying photoreceptor layer.

- *Stage 1b (occult macular hole):* (a) yellow ring (*Fig. 14.20*), and (b) centrifugal displacement of the photoreceptor layer to form a tiny schisis.
- *Stage 2 (small full-thickness hole):* (a) <400 µm central or eccentric defect (*Fig. 14.21*), and (b) dehiscence in the roof of the schitic cavity, often with persistent vitreofoveolar adhesion.

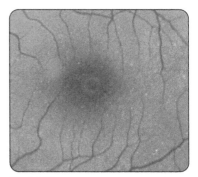

Fig 14.20

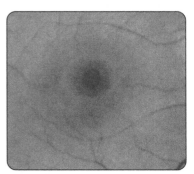

Fig 14.21

- *Stage 3 (full-size macular hole):* (a) >400 µm with a red base in which yellow-white dots may be seen, (b) surrounding grey cuff of subretinal fluid (*Fig. 14.22*), (c) overlying operculum, and (d) persistent parafoveal attachment of the vitreous cortex; VA is typically 6/60.

- *Stage 4 (full-size macular hole with complete posterior vitreous detachment; Fig. 14.23*).

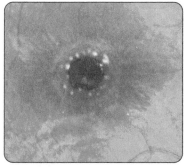

Fig 14.22

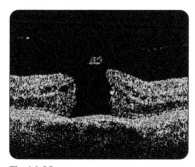

Fig 14.23

- *Watzke–Allen test:* a narrow slit beam is projected over the centre of the hole: with a macular hole, the beam appears thinned or broken; with other diagnoses it is distorted but of uniform thickness.

- *Course:* 50% of stage 1 holes resolve spontaneously and so are managed conservatively; approximately 10% of full-thickness holes also close spontaneously, with variable visual improvement.
- *OCT:* useful in diagnosis and staging (see *Fig. 14.23*).
- *FA:* full-thickness hole shows an early well-defined window defect.
- *Other causes of full-thickness macular hole:* high myopia and blunt trauma.
- *Lesions with a similar appearance:* (a) pseudohole in a macular epiretinal membrane (see *Fig. 14.33*), (b) lamellar hole in CMO, (c) foveal pseudocyst, (d) vitreomacular traction syndrome, and (e) solar maculopathy.

Treatment

- *Pars plana vitrectomy:* with peeling of the internal limiting membrane, gas tamponade and postoperative face-down posturing, for stage 2 or worse holes with VA less than 6/9; results are better in holes present for less than 6 months.
- *Results:* the hole is closed in up to 100% of cases, with visual improvement in 80–90% of eyes; VA is > 6/12 in approximately 65%, but worse in 10%.

Central serous chorioretinopathy

Pathogenesis: localized serous detachment of the sensory retina at the macula, secondary to leakage from the choriocapillaris through hyperpermeable areas in the RPE. The condition is much more common in men than in women; risk factors may include stress and steroid administration.

Diagnosis

- *Presentation:* in 4th and 5th decades with unilateral metamorphopsia and mild/moderate blurring; VA is usually 6/9–6/18, partly due to hypermetropia from retinal elevation.
- *Signs:* (a) round or oval sensory retinal elevation (*Fig. 14.24a* and *14.25a*), (b) fluid may be clear or turbid, (c) one or more depigmented RPE foci may be visible, and (d) small patches of RPE atrophy and hyperplasia

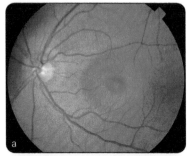
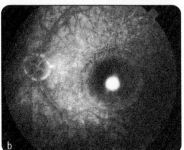

Fig 14.25

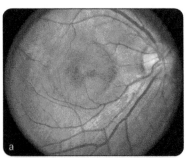
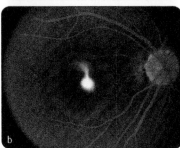

Fig 14.24

elsewhere in the posterior pole may mark the site of older lesions.

- *Course:* (a) spontaneous resolution within 3–6 months in most cases, with normal or near-normal VA in >80%, but with recurrence in up to 50%, and (b) chronic course in a minority, with gradual retinal degeneration.
- *OCT:* optically empty sensory retinal elevation (*Fig. 14.26*); RPE detachment or deficit may also be seen.
- *FA:* (a) 'smokestack' appearance with an early hyperfluorescent spot progressing to a vertical column (*Fig. 14.24b*), then diffusion throughout the detached

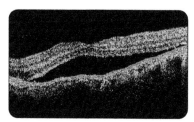

Fig 14.26

area, and (b) 'inkblot' (most common) appearance shows an early hyperfluorescent spot that gradually enlarges (*Fig. 14.25b*); an underlying PED may be demonstrated; multiple leakage points are sometimes seen.

Treatment

- *Observation:* in most cases.
- *Low-dose PDT:* now considered first-line treatment by some authorities.
- *Laser photocoagulation:* to the RPE leak speeds resolution but does not influence the visual outcome or recurrence rate; inadvisable if a leak is within the foveal avascular zone.
- *Intravitreal anti-VEGF agents:* may have utility.

Cystoid macular oedema

Pathogenesis: intraretinal leakage with the formation of cyst-like cavities in the fovea and surrounding central macula; long-standing cases may progress to lamellar hole formation with irreversible impairment of central vision. The causes are varied and include (a) ocular surgery and laser, (b) retinal vascular disease (e.g. diabetic retinopathy, retinal vein occlusion), (c) chronic uveitis (particularly intermediate), (d) drug-induced, (e) retinal dystrophies (e.g. retinitis pigmentosa), and (f) vitreomacular disease (e.g. macular epiretinal membrane).

Diagnosis

- *Presentation:* predisposing disease is generally evident, but CMO may be the presenting feature; blurring and metamorphopsia are typical; Amsler chart testing demonstrates central distortion.
- *Signs:* loss of the foveal depression and thickening of the sensory retina with multiple cystoid areas (*Fig. 14.27*).
- *FA:* early hyperfluorescent spots progressing to a characteristic petaloid pattern (*Fig. 14.28*).
- *OCT:* retinal thickening with hyporeflective spaces (*Fig. 14.29*); vitreoretinal traction and a lamellar hole will be shown if present.

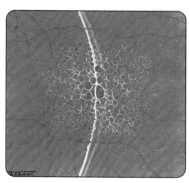

Fig 14.27

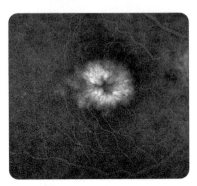

Fig 14.28

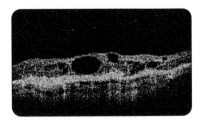

Fig 14.29

Treatment: dependent on cause.

Macular epiretinal membrane

Pathogenesis: sheet-like fibrocellular structure that develops on or above the surface of the retina. Classification: (a) idiopathic (bilateral in 10%; tends to be mild), and (b) secondary (e.g. intraocular surgery or laser, retinal detachment, trauma, inflammation).

Diagnosis

- *Presentation:* blurring and metamorphopsia but may be asymptomatic if mild; Amsler grid

in moderate–advanced cases typically shows distortion.
- *Signs:* (a) initially irregular translucent preretinal sheen ('cellophane maculopathy'; *Fig. 14.30*); (b) later the membrane thickens and contracts, typically causing mild distortion of blood vessels (*Fig. 14.31*), and (c) advanced lesions may give severe distortion of blood vessels, marked retinal wrinkling, and can obscure underlying structures

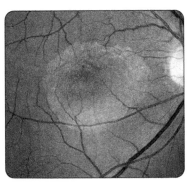

Fig 14.30

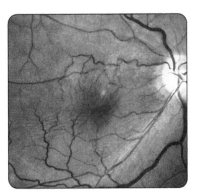

Fig 14.31

(macular pucker; *Fig. 14.32*); associated findings include macular pseudohole (*Fig. 14.33*), CMO, and small haemorrhages.

- *OCT:* highly reflective (red) surface layer associated with retinal thickening (*Fig. 14.34*); facilitates exclusion of vitreomacular traction.

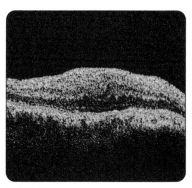

Fig 14.34

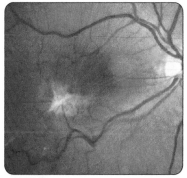

Fig 14.32

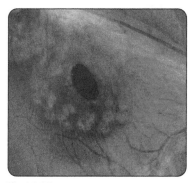

Fig 14.33

Treatment

- *Observation:* if mild and nonprogressive; spontaneous separation sometimes occurs.
- *Pars plana vitrectomy:* surgical peeling of the membrane usually improves distortion, with an improvement in VA of at least two lines in 75%; approximately 2% get worse.

Degenerative myopia

Definition: high myopia is defined as a refractive error of more than −6 dioptres and an axial length usually greater than 26 mm. Degenerative (pathological) myopia is characterized by progressive enlargement of the scleral envelope with a range of secondary ocular changes.

Diagnosis

- *Signs:* (a) fundus pallor due to diffuse attenuation of the RPE, with visible choroidal vessels, (b) focal chorioretinal atrophy and a 'tilted' disc associated with peripapillary atrophy (*Fig. 14.35*), (c) posterior staphyloma due to

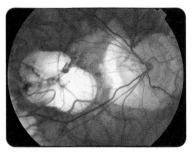

Fig 14.35

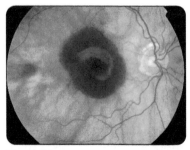

Fig 14.37

focal expansion and thinning, (d) 'lacquer cracks'; fine irregular yellow ruptures in the RPE–Bruch's membrane–choriocapillaris complex at the posterior pole (*Fig. 14.36*) that can be associated with CNV (*Fig. 14.37*) or retinal haemorrhages without CNV ('coin' haemorrhages), and (e) Fuchs spot, a circular pigmented macular lesion seen following absorption of a subretinal haemorrhage (*Fig. 14.38*).

- *Complications and associations:* (a) rhegmatogenous retinal detachment is more common

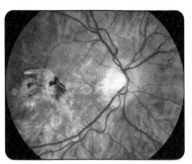

Fig 14.38

the higher the myopia and may be associated with lattice degeneration (see Chapter 16), (b) CNV, (c) macular hole, (d) cataract, and (e) increased prevalence of primary open-angle glaucoma and pigment dispersion syndrome.

Angioid streaks

Pathogenesis: band-like dehiscences in brittle, thickened, and calcified Bruch's membrane, associated with atrophy of the overlying RPE. Visual impairment occurs in more than

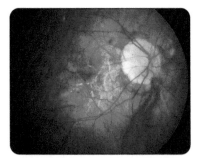

Fig 14.36

70%. Systemic associations:
(a) pseudoxanthoma elasticum
(most common), (b) Paget disease,
(c) certain haemoglobinopathies, and
(d) rarely other disorders (e.g.
familial hyperphosphataemia, lead
poisoning, Marfan syndrome,
Ehlers–Danlos syndrome).

Diagnosis

- *Signs:* (a) linear grey or dark-red
  lesions with serrated edges,
  communicating around the optic
  disc and radiating outwards (*Fig.
  14.39*), which tend to increase in
  width and extent slowly over time,
  and (b) 'peau d'orange' (orange
  skin) mottled retinal pigmentation
  (*Fig. 14.40*); optic disc drusen are
  a common association.

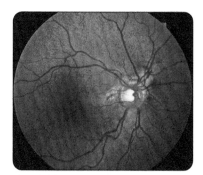

Fig 14.40

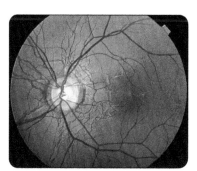

Fig 14.39

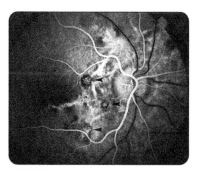

Fig 14.41

- *FA:* corresponding hyperfluorescent
  window defects due to RPE
  atrophy; may show CNV
  (*Fig. 14.41* black arrow heads).
- *Causes of visual loss:* (a) CNV
  (most common), (b) foveal
  involvement by a streak, and
  (c) choroidal rupture, which may
  occur from relatively trivial trauma
  (*Fig. 14.42*).

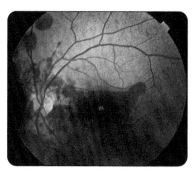

Fig 14.42

Treatment: CNV is treated with intravitreal anti-VEGF agents alone or combined with PDT; protective spectacles should be worn when appropriate, and contact sports avoided.

Choroidal folds

Pathogenesis: parallel striae involving the inner choroid, Bruch's membrane, and the RPE. Idiopathic ('congenital') folds may be present in healthy, often hypermetropic individuals in whom VA is unaffected. Causes of secondary folds: (a) chronic papilloedema, (b) orbital disease, and (c) ocular disease (e.g. choroidal tumours, posterior scleritis, hypotony); the effect on vision is variable and dependent on the cause.

Diagnosis
- *Presentation:* depends on the underlying cause.
- *Signs:* horizontally orientated parallel grooves or striae at the posterior pole (*Fig. 14.43a*); crests are less pigmented from stretching and thinning of the RPE, and troughs are darker due to RPE compression.
- *OCT:* allows differentiation between choroidal and retinal folds.
- *FA:* hyperfluorescent crests and hypofluorescent troughs (*Fig. 14.43b*).

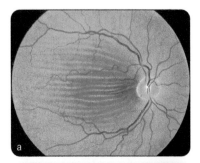
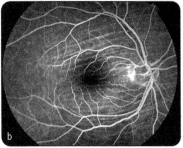

Fig 14.43

Hypotony maculopathy

Pathogenesis: very low IOP (<5 mm Hg), usually caused by excessive drainage following glaucoma filtration surgery; other causes include trauma, chronic uveitis, and retinal detachment; severe hypotony may deteriorate to phthisis bulbi.

Diagnosis
- *Signs:* (a) fine retinal folds radiating outwards from the fovea (*Fig. 14.44*), and (b) choroidal folds.
- *Other features:* depend on aetiology: (a) shallow anterior chamber, (b) uveitis,

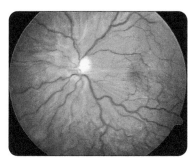

Fig 14.44

(c) trabeculectomy bleb leak,
(d) choroidal detachment, and
(e) CMO.
• **US:** to rule out a cyclitic
membrane or cyclodialysis cleft if
no cause is identified.
Treatment: aimed at restoring
normal IOP.

Vitreomacular traction syndrome

Pathogenesis: vitreous cortex remains
attached to the fovea but is
detached from the perifoveal region,
with resultant exertion of persistent
anteroposterior traction on the fovea.
Diagnosis
• *Presentation:* blurring and
metamorphopsia, photopsia,
and micropsia.
• *Signs:* macular retinal wrinkling,
epiretinal membrane, or CMO.
• *OCT:* incomplete posterior vitreous
separation with persistent
attachment of vitreous to the
fovea (*Fig. 14.45*).

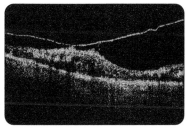

Fig 14.45

Treatment: options include observation,
intravitreal steroid and pars plana
vitrectomy to relieve macular
traction; spontaneous resolution may
occur.

Chapter **15**

Hereditary fundus dystrophies

Generalized photoreceptor dystrophies

Retinitis pigmentosa

Genetics: Typical retinitis pigmentosa (RP) is a group of retinal dystrophies initially mainly affecting the rod photoreceptor cells and subsequently cones (rod–cone dystrophy). It can be sporadic or inherited as AD, AR, or X-L; many cases are due to mutation in the rhodopsin gene. X-L has the worst prognosis with severe visual loss by the 4th decade, AR and sporadic cases have a more favourable course with retention of central vision until the 5th or 6th decade or later, and AD disease has the best outlook.

Diagnosis

- **Presentation:** decreased peripheral and night vision; age of onset is variable.
- **Signs:** (a) mid-peripheral RPE atrophy and intraretinal perivascular 'bone-spicule' pigmentary changes together with mild arteriolar narrowing (*Fig. 15.1*), (b) gradual increase in density and extent of the pigmentary change, (c) gliotic 'waxy' pallor of the optic discs (*Fig. 15.2*); (d) the macula may show atrophy, epiretinal membrane formation, or CMO.
- **Electroretinogram (ERG):** reduced scotopic rod and combined responses in early disease; later, photopic responses reduce and eventually the ERG is extinguished.
- **Electro-oculogram (EOG):** subnormal with an absence of the light rise.
- **Perimetry:** small mid-peripheral scotomas gradually coalesce, leaving a tiny central island that may eventually be extinguished.
- **Ocular associations:** (a) posterior subcapsular cataracts, (b) open-angle glaucoma, (c) myopia, (d) keratoconus, (e) Coats disease, and (f) disc drusen.
- **Atypical RP:** either closely related to typical RP or representing incomplete forms of the disease (e.g. cone–rod dystrophy, sector RP, RP sine pigmento).

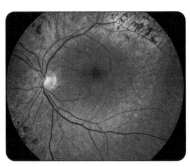

Fig 15.1

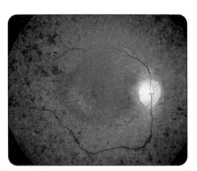

Fig 15.2

Treatment: associations such as cataract and glaucoma are treated as appropriate; CMO may respond to systemic acetazolamide.

Important systemic associations

RP, often atypical, may be associated with the following:

- *Bassen–Kornzweig syndrome (abetalipoproteinaemia):* AR lipoprotein abnormality with malabsorption of fat-soluble vitamins causing failure to thrive followed by severe spinocerebellar ataxia; blood microscopy shows 'thorny' red cells (acanthocytosis). Treatment with large vitamin doses may prevent visual loss.
- *Refsum disease:* AR enzyme deficiency resulting in phytanic acid accumulation; there are distinct infantile and adult types. Early detection and a diet low in phytanic acid can arrest progression of the potentially severe neurological and other features.
- *Kearns–Sayre syndrome:* mitochondrial inheritance; chronic progressive external ophthalmoplegia associated with systemic problems (see Chapter 19).
- *Bardet–Biedl syndrome:* genetically heterogeneous condition with systemic features including mental handicap; fundus often shows a bull's-eye maculopathy due to cone–rod dystrophy.
- *Usher syndrome:* AR, but genetically heterogeneous; accounts for approximately 5% of all cases of profound deafness in children, and approximately half of all cases of combined deafness and blindness.

Progressive cone dystrophy

Definition: a usually sporadic dystrophy predominantly affecting the cone system. In some cases, there is no evidence of rod dysfunction, whereas in others rod dysfunction subsequently develops but cone deficiency still predominates (cone–rod dystrophy).

Diagnosis

- *Presentation:* in 2nd to 4th decades with impaired central and colour vision.
- *Signs:* the macula may show (a) virtually normal appearance, (b) nonspecific pigmentary changes, or (c) bull's-eye configuration (*Table 15.1*, *Fig. 15.3*); geographic atrophy subsequently ensues (*Fig. 15.4*), with VA of 6/60 or worse.
- *ERG:* photopic responses are subnormal or unrecordable and flicker fusion frequency is reduced, but rod responses are preserved until late.
- *EOG:* normal to subnormal.

Table 15.1 **Other causes of bull's-eye macular appearance**

- Chloroquine maculopathy
- Advanced Stargardt disease
- Fenestrated sheen macular dystrophy
- Benign concentric annular macular dystrophy
- Bardet–Biedl syndrome
- Lipofuscinosis

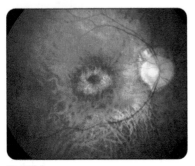

Fig 15.3

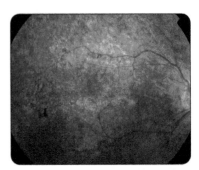

Fig 15.5

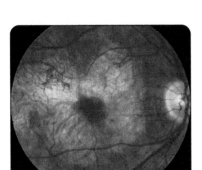

Fig 15.4

Leber congenital amaurosis

Definition: severe AR condition that is the most common genetic cause of visual impairment in children.

Diagnosis

- *Presentation:* perinatal blindness associated with nystagmus or roving eye movements.
- *Signs:* (a) absent or sluggish pupillary light reflexes; (b) mild pigmentary retinopathy may be seen initially (*Fig. 15.5*), followed by (c) coloboma-like fundus

lesions, optic atrophy, severe arteriolar narrowing, and macular pigmentation.

- *ERG:* usually nonrecordable even in early cases.
- *'Oculodigital syndrome':* constant rubbing of the eyes causing enophthalmos is characteristic (*Fig. 15.6*).

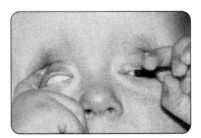

Fig 15.6

Stargardt disease and fundus flavimaculatus

Definition: Stargardt disease and fundus flavimaculatus (FFM) are variants of the same disease, characterized by diffuse accumulation of lipofuscin within the RPE. Inheritance is AR, and mutations in at least three different genes have been identified; symptoms may be disproportionate to visible fundus changes.

Diagnosis

- *Presentation:* in the 1st and 2nd decades, occasionally later, with gradual impairment of central vision; some patients may remain asymptomatic until late, especially with predominantly peripheral changes (FFM pattern).
- *Maculopathy:* (a) the macula may be normal initially and then show nonspecific mottling or an oval 'snail-slime' or 'beaten-bronze' appearance (*Fig. 15.7*), with (b) progression to geographic atrophy or bull's-eye maculopathy.
- *Flecks:* yellow-white lesions at the level of the RPE, of various size and shape such as round, oval, or pisciform (fish-shaped), at the posterior pole exclusively (*Fig. 15.8*) or extending to the mid-periphery (*Fig. 15.9*).

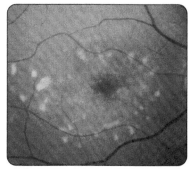

Fig 15.8

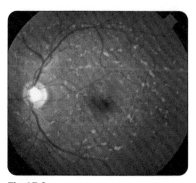

Fig 15.9

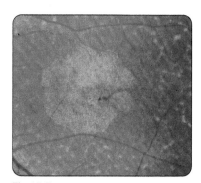

Fig 15.7

- *Course:* VA tends to stabilize at approximately 6/60; patients with only flecks have a better prognosis.
- *ERG:* photopic is normal to subnormal and scotopic normal.
- *EOG:* subnormal in advanced cases.
- *FA:* (a) maculopathy shows central hyperfluorescence; (b) generalized 'dark choroid' with prominence of the retinal vasculature is classic

(*Fig. 15.10*); (c) fresh flecks show early hypofluorescence, and old flecks show RPE window defects (*Fig. 15.11*).

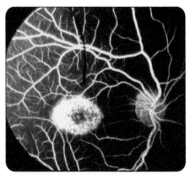

Fig 15.10

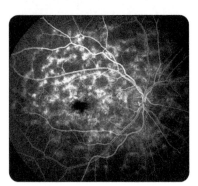

Fig 15.11

Congenital stationary night blindness

Definition: group of disorders characterized by infantile-onset nyctalopia and nonprogressive retinal dysfunction; the fundus appearance may be normal or abnormal.

Diagnosis
- *With normal fundus:* types range from complete absence of rod function with normal cone function, to mixed impairment.
- *With abnormal fundus:* (a) Oguchi disease, in which the fundus has an unusual golden-yellow colour when light-adapted, becoming normal after prolonged dark adaptation (Mizuo phenomenon), and (b) fundus albipunctatus, an innocuous AR or AD condition in which there are numerous tiny yellow-white spots sparing the fovea and extending to the periphery (*Fig. 15.12*).

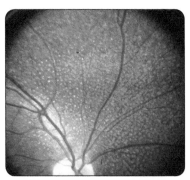

Fig 15.12

Congenital monochromatism

Definition: group of inherited conditions with abnormal colour vision as the predominant feature.
Diagnosis
- Monochromatism ranges from partial impairment of colour vision and slightly reduced VA such as blue cone monochromatism (incomplete achromatopsia) to complete absence of colour

perception and poor VA as in rod monochromatism (complete achromatopsia).

- Fundus signs are often subtle; nystagmus and photophobia are present in all but the milder forms.

Macular dystrophies

Juvenile Best macular dystrophy

Genetics: inheritance is AD (BEST1 gene). Occasionally, multifocal vitelliform lesions identical to those in Best disease may become manifest in adult life. However, in these patients the EOG is normal and the family history negative.

Diagnosis

- **Presentation:** in 5th decade with gradual onset of central blurring.
- **Signs:** (a) vitelliform appearance develops in early childhood with a round, sharply delineated ('sunny side up') macular lesion (*Fig. 15.13*), (b) slow progression to 'vitelliruptive' stage (*Fig. 15.14*)

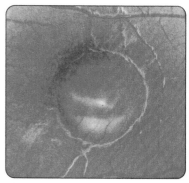

Fig 15.14

with a gradual fall in VA, and later (c) macular atrophy.

- **FA:** vitelliform lesions show corresponding hypofluorescence due to blockage.
- **OCT:** material within the RPE (*Fig. 15.15*).
- **EOG:** severely subnormal during all stages; also abnormal in carriers with normal fundi.

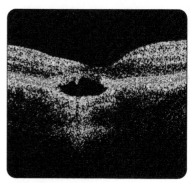

Fig 15.15

Pattern dystrophy

- **Definition:** generic term that encompasses several retinal

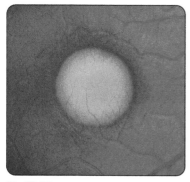

Fig 15.13

dystrophies exhibiting yellow, orange, or grey deposits at the macula in a variety of morphologies. Most are AD and have a relatively benign course; the following are two examples:

- **Adult-onset macular vitelliform dystrophy:** small foveal vitelliform lesions similar in appearance to those of Best disease (*Fig. 15.16*).
- **Butterfly-shaped macular dystrophy:** yellow pigment at the fovea in a triradiate conformation (*Fig. 15.17*).

Familial dominant drusen (malattia leventinese)

- **Definition:** early onset variant of AMD.
- **Asymptomatic stage:** (a) yellow-white radially orientated drusen develop at the macula (*Fig. 15.18*) in the 2nd decade; (b) with time they become more numerous and acquire a honeycomb configuration.
- **Symptomatic stage:** geographic atrophy and occasionally CNV during the 4th and 5th decades.

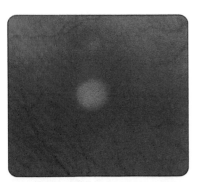

Fig 15.16

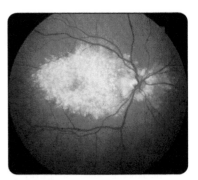

Fig 15.18

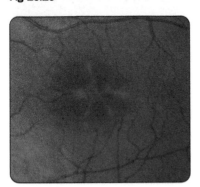

Fig 15.17

Generalized choroidal dystrophies

Choroideremia

Definition: severe and progressive diffuse degeneration of the choroid, RPE, and retinal photoreceptors. Inheritance is X-L recessive with the locus on Xq21.2 (CHM gene).

Diagnosis

- **Presentation:** in 2nd and 3rd decades with nyctalopia.

- **Signs:** (a) atrophy of the RPE and choroid, which spreads peripherally and centrally with sparing of the fovea until late (*Fig. 15.19*), (b) choroidal vessels course over bare sclera, with retinal vascular attenuation; optic atrophy; (c) severe central and peripheral visual loss occurs by the 6th decade.

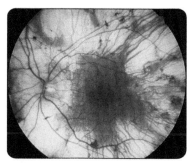

Fig 15.19

- **ERG:** markedly abnormal.
- **Signs in female carriers:** patchy mild peripheral RPE changes; VA, fields, and ERG are usually normal but nyctalopia can occur; 50% of carriers' sons will develop the condition, and 50% of daughters will be carriers.

Gyrate atrophy

Pathogenesis: AR metabolic disorder caused by a deficiency of the enzyme ornithine aminotransferase, leading to elevated ornithine levels.
Diagnosis
- **Presentation:** in 1st and 2nd decades with myopia and nyctalopia; legal blindness tends

to occur by the 4th to 6th decades.
- **Signs:** (a) sharply demarcated oval areas of chorioretinal atrophy, often with crystalline deposits at the posterior pole, (b) coalescence and extension of atrophic areas with sparing of the fovea until late (*Fig. 15.20*), and (c) extreme attenuation of retinal vasculature.

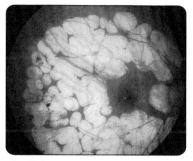

Fig 15.20

- **ERG:** subnormal in early disease and later extinguished.
Treatment: restriction of dietary arginine; pyridoxine (vitamin B_6) may normalize ornithine levels in some patients.

Vitreoretinal dystrophies

Juvenile X-linked retinoschisis

Pathogenesis: defect in Müller cell function with splitting of the retinal nerve fibre layer from the rest of the sensory retina—this differs from acquired retinoschisis, in which splitting occurs at the outer plexiform layer.

Diagnosis

- *Presentation:* (a) difficulty reading at age 5–10 years; (b) squint, nystagmus, or vitreous haemorrhage may also lead to presentation.
- *Maculopathy (universal):* 'bicycle wheel' striae radiating from the foveola, and cystoid changes (*Fig. 15.21*).

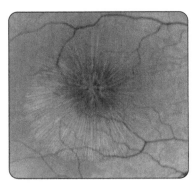

Fig 15.21

- *Peripheral retinoschisis (in 50%):* predominantly inferotemporal; does not extend but oval defects (*Fig. 15.22*) may develop and coalesce to leave retinal blood vessels floating in the vitreous ('vitreous veils').
- *Complications:* vitreous haemorrhage and rarely retinal detachment.
- *Prognosis:* poor due to progressive maculopathy.
- *OCT:* to assess maculopathy (*Fig. 15.23*).
- *ERG and EOG:* abnormal in peripheral schisis.

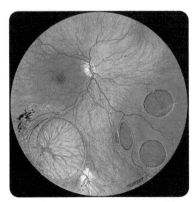

Fig 15.22

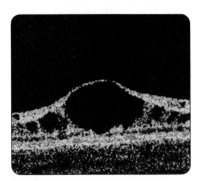

Fig 15.23

Stickler syndrome

Genetics: AD disorder of connective tissue; is the most common inherited cause of paediatric retinal detachment. It is classified into clinically and genetically distinct subtypes STL1, STL2, and STL3, the latter lacking ocular features. Wagner syndrome shows similar vitreous changes but is not associated with systemic abnormalities.

Diagnosis

- **Presentation:** early childhood with high but nonprogressive myopia.
- **Signs:** (a) optically empty vitreous (*Fig. 15.24*), (b) radial lattice-like degeneration (*Fig. 15.25*), (c) retinal detachment in approximately 50% in the 1st decade, often bilateral and with multiple or giant tears, and (d) other features (cataract, ectopia lentis, glaucoma).
- **Systemic anomalies:** (a) mid-facial hypoplasia, (b) cleft and high-arched palate, (c) joint hypermobility, and (d) deafness.

Treatment: regular screening is mandatory so that retinal breaks can be treated prophylactically.

Albinism

Tyrosinase-negative (complete) oculocutaneous albinism

Pathogenesis: inability to synthesize melanin results in lack of the pigment in all ocular structures; inheritance is usually AR.

Diagnosis

- **VA:** usually <6/60 due to foveal hypoplasia.
- **Signs:** (a) iris is diaphanous and translucent (*Fig. 15.26*), giving rise to a 'pink-eyed' appearance, (b) pale fundus with large conspicuous choroidal vessels, (c) foveal hypoplasia with absence of

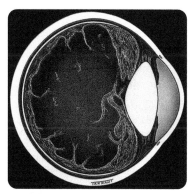

Fig 15.24

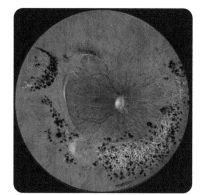

Fig 15.25

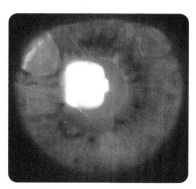

Fig 15.26

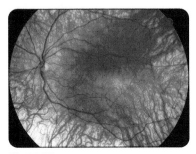

Fig 15.27

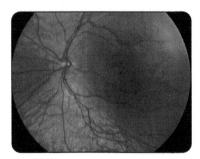

Fig 15.28

the foveal pit (*Fig. 15.27*), and
(d) nystagmus, high refractive
errors, and squint.
- *Systemic features:* (a) white hair
and very pale skin, and
(b) anomalous optic chiasm
(majority of nerve fibres from
each eye cross to the
contralateral hemisphere,
demonstrated by visual evoked
potentials).

Tyrosinase-positive (incomplete) oculocutaneous albinism

Pathogenesis: ability to synthesize
variable amounts of melanin;
inheritance is usually AR.
Diagnosis
- *VA:* usually impaired due to foveal
hypoplasia.
- *Signs:* (a) iris is blue to dark
brown, with variable translucency,
and (b) variable fundus
hypopigmentation (*Fig. 15.28*).
- *Systemic features:* (a) hair may be
white, yellow, or red—darkens with
age, (b) skin is very pale at birth
but usually darkens by 2 years;
(c) systemic conditions featuring
incomplete oculocutaneous

albinism include Chediak–Higashi,
Hermansky–Pudlak, and
Waardenburg syndromes.

Ocular albinism

- *Definition:* X-L condition in which
affected males have hypopigmented
irides and fundi, and often reduced
vision and nystagmus.
- *Female carriers:* are asymptomatic,
although often have mild signs (e.g.
partial iris translucency), macular
stippling, and mid-peripheral areas of
retinal depigmentation and
granularity (*Fig. 15.29*).

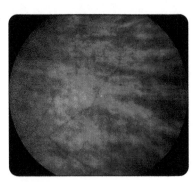

Fig 15.29

Cherry-red spot at the macula

- **Pathogenesis:** a cherry-red spot is seen when the relatively thin fovea retains transmission of the choroidal vascular hue, despite loss of transparency of the wider posterior pole retina (*Fig. 15.30*) as a result of accumulation of lipids in the ganglion cell layer. It is also a feature of central retinal artery occlusion.
- **Systemic associations:** sphingolipidoses are a group of rare inherited metabolic diseases featuring intracellular accumulation of lipid metabolites in various tissues. These include GM1 and GM2 (Tay–Sachs, Sandhoff)

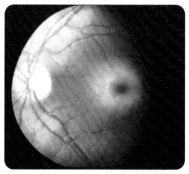

Fig 15.30

gangliosidoses, Niemann–Pick disease, and sialidosis; many have other ocular features such as corneal clouding.

Chapter **16**

Retinal detachment

Definitions

- **Retinal detachment (RD):** separation of the neurosensory retina (NSR) from the RPE, with the accumulation of subretinal fluid (SRF).
- **Rhegmatogenous RD:** occurs when a full-thickness defect in the NSR permits synchytic (liquefied) vitreous to gain access to the subretinal space.
- **Tractional RD:** involves the contraction of vitreoretinal membranes in the absence of a retinal break.
- **Exudative RD:** SRF is derived from retinal or choroidal vessels (e.g. inflammation, tumour).
- **Retinal break:** full-thickness defect in the NSR, either (a) a tear, caused by dynamic vitreoretinal traction, or (b) a hole, caused by chronic retinal atrophy.
- **U-tear:** consists of a flap with the apex pulled anteriorly by adherent vitreous, the base attached to the retina (*Figs. 16.1a–16.1c*).
- **Operculated tear:** flap has been completely torn away from the retina (*Fig. 16.1d*).
- **Dialysis:** circumferential tear along the ora serrata with vitreous gel attached to its posterior margins (*Fig. 16.1e*).
- **Giant tear:** involves 90° or more of the NSR (*Fig. 16.2*).

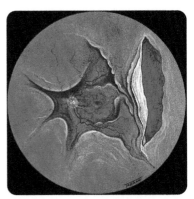

Fig 16.2

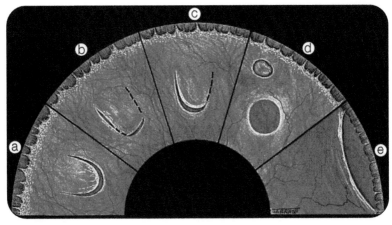

Fig 16.1

Rhegmatogenous retinal detachment

Pathogenesis: rhegmatogenous retinal detachment (RRD) affects approximately 1 in 10,000 of the population each year; both eyes are eventually involved in approximately 10%. Presentation is typically between 45 and 65 years of age but may be earlier, especially if predisposed (e.g. myopia).

- *Posterior vitreous detachment (PVD):* (a) separation of the cortical vitreous from the internal limiting membrane (ILM) of the NSR posterior to the vitreous base with the remaining solid vitreous gel collapsing inferiorly (acute PVD; *Figs. 16.3a* and *16.3b*), (b) some eyes with acute PVD develop retinal tears (*Fig. 16.3c*), and subsequent RRD; (c) occasionally avulsion of a peripheral blood vessel may

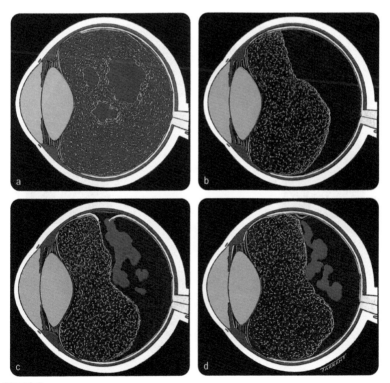

Fig 16.3

cause vitreous haemorrhage without a retinal tear (*Fig. 16.3d*).

- **RRD without PVD:** usually associated with a retinal dialysis or round holes.
- **Lattice degeneration:** present in approximately 8% of the population and in approximately 40% of eyes with RRD: (a) spindle-shaped islands of retinal thinning with a characteristic network of white lines, (b) associated RPE hyperplasia; (c) small holes within islands are common (*Figs. 16.4a–16.4d*); (d) overlying gel is liquefied, but its adhesions around the margins of lattice are exaggerated (*Fig. 16.5*); (e) tears typically occur at the posterior edge of an island.
- **Snailtrack degeneration:** (a) sharply demarcated peripheral bands of tightly packed 'snowflakes' (see *Fig. 16.4e*), (b) small holes; (c) overlying

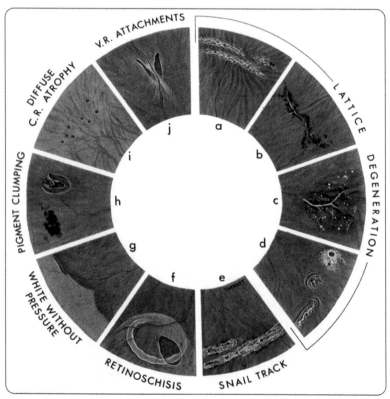

Fig 16.4

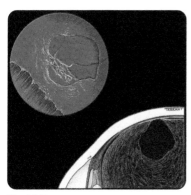

Fig 16.5

vitreous is liquefied but marked
adhesions are seldom present so
that tears are less common than
in lattice.

- **Degenerative (acquired)
  retinoschisis:** (see *Fig. 16.4f*
  and below).
- **'White with pressure':** translucent
  grey appearance of a region of
  retina induced by indenting the
  sclera that may be associated
  with abnormally strong vitreous
  attachments.
- **'White without pressure':** same
  appearance without scleral
  indentation (*Fig. 16.4g*).
- **Significance of myopia:** more than
  40% of all RRDs occur in myopic
  eyes; (a) macular holes may give
  rise to RRD in highly myopic eyes,
  (b) vitreous loss and laser
  posterior capsulotomy are more
  likely to lead to RRD than in
  non-myopic eyes, and (c)
  predisposing factors are more
  common in myopic eyes (vitreous
  degeneration, PVD, lattice and
  snailtrack degenerations).

- **Other predisposing lesions:**
  (a) pigment clumps (see *Fig.
  16.4h*), (b) diffuse chorioretinal
  atrophy (see *Fig. 16.4i*), and
  (c) abnormal paravascular
  vitreoretinal adhesions (see
  Fig. 16.4j).

Degenerative (acquired) retinoschisis

- **Pathogenesis:** (a) coalescence of
  individual lesions within areas of
  peripheral microcystoid
  degeneration, (b) the NSR splits
  into inner and outer layers with
  severing of neurons and complete
  loss of visual function in the
  affected area (absolute scotoma);
  (c) the split in 'typical'
  retinoschisis is through the outer
  plexiform layer, and in the less
  common 'reticular' form at the
  nerve fibre layer.
- **Signs:** (a) early retinoschisis
  appears as a shallowly elevated
  area of microcystoid degeneration,
  usually starting inferotemporally,
  (b) progresses to smooth
  immobile elevation of the retina
  (*Fig. 16.6*), and (c) may extend
  circumferentially, the typical form

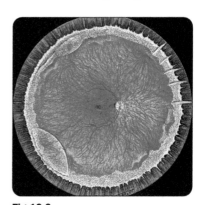

Fig 16.6

usually remaining anterior to the equator although the reticular type may spread beyond.

- **Associated features:** (a) the inner layer surface may have a snowflake-like appearance, (b) vascular sheathing and sclerosis; (c) breaks in the inner layer are small and round, whereas the less common outer layer breaks are usually larger, with rolled edges (*Fig. 16.7*).

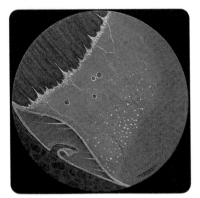

Fig 16.7

- **Prognosis:** in most cases retinoschisis is asymptomatic and innocuous, but RRD may occasionally develop in eyes with breaks in both layers; uncommon complications are progressive posterior extension and vitreous haemorrhage.

Symptoms: the classic premonitory symptoms in RRD are flashing lights (photopsia), floaters, and a shadow encroaching on the field of vision.

- **Photopsia:** caused in acute PVD by traction at sites of vitreoretinal adhesion.

- **'Floaters':** types; (a) ring-shaped (Weiss ring; *Fig. 16.8*) composed of the detached annular attachment of vitreous to the margin of the optic disc, (b) 'cobwebs' caused by condensation of vitreous collagen fibres, and (c) a shower of minute dark or red spots that may indicate vitreous haemorrhage.

- **Visual field defect:** detached retina causes a progressive relative peripheral visual field defect or 'curtain,' in many cases eventually involving central vision.

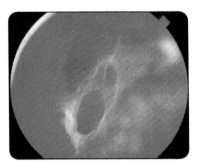

Fig 16.8

Signs

- **General:** (a) relative afferent pupillary defect, (b) intraocular pressure is lower than in the normal eye, (c) mild anterior uveitis, and (d) 'tobacco dust,' consisting of pigment cells, in the anterior vitreous (*Fig. 16.9*).

- **Retinal breaks:** appear dark orange-red; a pseudohole at the macula is frequently seen if the posterior pole is detached but rarely there may be a true macular hole.

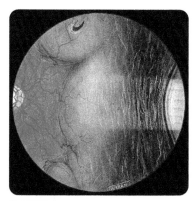

Fig 16.9

- *Fresh RD:* detached retina is convex, slightly opaque, and has a corrugated appearance (*Fig. 16.10*).
- *Long-standing RD:* (a) retinal thinning (not to be mistaken for retinoschisis), (b) secondary intraretinal cysts, and (c) subretinal demarcation lines ('high water marks') at the junction of flat and detached retina (*Fig. 16.11*).
- *Proliferative vitreoretinopathy (PVR):* refers to a process of epiretinal and subretinal membrane formation leading to retinal folds and rigidity; three grades are recognized; (a) A

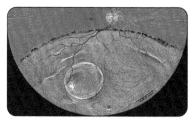

Fig 16.11

(diffuse vitreous haze and tobacco dust), (b) B (wrinkling of the inner retinal surface, tortuosity of blood vessels, retinal stiffness, decreased mobility of vitreous gel, and rolled edges of retinal breaks), and (c) C (rigid full-thickness retinal folds with heavy vitreous condensation) (*Fig. 16.12*).

- *B-scan US:* good mobility of the retina and vitreous in a fresh RRD; in long-standing cases there is reduction of mobility with retinal shortening and a characteristic triangular cross-sectional appearance.

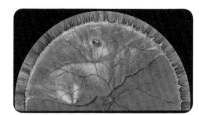

Fig 16.10

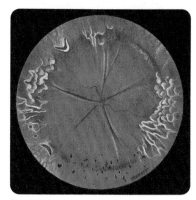

Fig 16.12

Prophylaxis: many retinal breaks require prophylactic treatment to reduce the risk of progression to RRD.

- **Risk factors:** (a) a tear is more prone to detach the retina than a hole, (b) a large break (*Fig. 16.13*) is more likely than a small one to progress to RRD, (c) symptomatic tears associated with acute PVD are more dangerous than those detected by chance, (d) superior breaks are higher risk than inferior, (e) the presence of localized SRF ('subclinical' RD; *Fig. 16.14*) is a high-risk feature in a symptomatic tear, and (f) pigmentation around a break usually indicates chronicity and lower risk (*Fig. 16.15*).

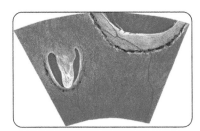

Fig 16.15

- **Other considerations:** (a) cataract surgery (particularly if associated with vitreous loss), (b) myopia, (c) family history of RRD, and (d) systemic disease associated with increased RRD risk (e.g. Marfan and Stickler syndromes).
- **Modalities:** (a) surrounding the break with laser (*Fig. 16.16*) using a slit-lamp delivery system (not for very peripheral breaks), (b) laser using an indirect ophthalmoscopic delivery system combined with scleral indentation, and (c) cryotherapy (especially in hazy media).

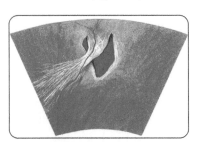

Fig 16.13

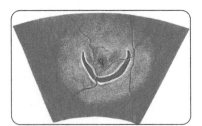

Fig 16.14

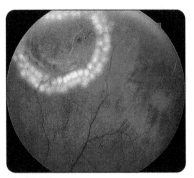

Fig 16.16

Surgery for RRD

- *Urgency:* most important consideration in an acute RRD is whether the central macula is involved ('macula on' or 'macula off'); in 'macula off' there is less urgency than in 'macula on' cases.

- *Pneumatic retinopexy:* outpatient procedure for uncomplicated RRD with a small superior break or cluster of breaks. An intravitreal gas bubble is used to reattach the retina without scleral buckling (see below), with subsequent laser or cryopexy (*Fig. 16.17*).

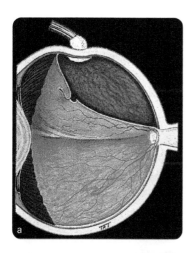
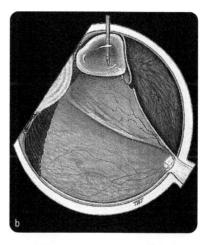
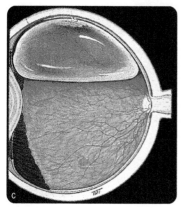
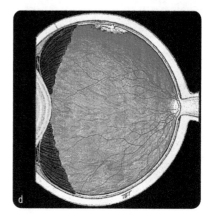

Fig 16.17

- **Scleral buckling:** silicone 'explant' sutured onto the sclera creates an inward indentation (buckle), closing a retinal break by apposing the RPE to the NSR and also reducing local vitreoretinal traction. Buckles can be (a) radial (*Fig. 16.18a*), (b) segmental circumferential (*Fig. 16.18b*), or (c) encircling circumferential (*Figs. 16.18c* and *16.18d*).

- **Indications for drainage of SRF:** (a) deep SRF preventing adequate cryotherapy, and (b) long-standing cases in which SRF is viscous and

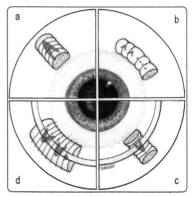

Fig 16.18

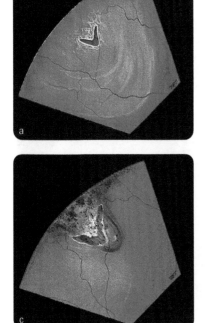

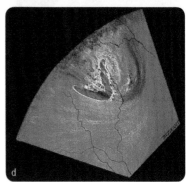

Fig 16.19

may take a long time (many months) to absorb spontaneously without drainage.

- **Causes of failure:** *Figure 16.19a* shows preoperative appearance and *Fig. 16.19b* successful reattachment. Failure may be caused by (a) inadequate explant size (*Fig. 16.19c*), (b) incorrect positioning (*Fig. 16.19d*), (c) missed breaks, (d) inadequate cryotherapy, and (e) PVR (most common cause of late failure).
- **Pars plana vitrectomy:** (see below) is generally indicated for more complex RRD.

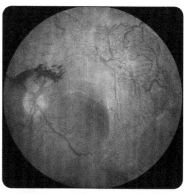

Fig 16.20

Tractional retinal detachment

Pathogenesis: progressive contraction of fibrovascular membranes over large areas of vitreoretinal adhesion; main causes are proliferative retinopathies (e.g. diabetes, retinopathy of prematurity) and penetrating posterior segment trauma (see Chapter 21).

Diagnosis
- **Presentation:** (a) photopsia and floaters are usually absent because vitreoretinal traction develops insidiously and is not associated with acute PVD; (b) any visual field defect usually progresses slowly.
- **Signs:** (a) RD has a concave configuration and breaks are absent (*Fig. 16.20*), and (b) SRF is shallow and immobile, and seldom extends to the ora serrata.
- **B-scan US:** posterior vitreous detachment and a relatively immobile retina.

Treatment: vision-threatening cases require pars plana vitrectomy (see below).

Exudative retinal detachment

Pathogenesis: there is accumulation of SRF in the absence of retinal breaks or vitreoretinal traction. The SRF is derived from leaking vessels (e.g. choroidal tumours, severe uveitis, extensive CNV).

Diagnosis
- **Presentation:** (a) photopsia is absent because traction is lacking, but (b) floaters may be present if there is associated vitritis; (c) a visual field defect may develop suddenly and progress rapidly; both eyes may be involved simultaneously, depending on the cause.
- **Signs:** (a) RD has a convex configuration but in contrast to RRD its surface is smooth (*Fig. 16.21*), (b) SRF is usually deep and highly mobile, exhibiting the

phenomenon of 'shifting fluid,' and (c) the cause of the RD may be apparent (e.g. choroidal tumour); (d) 'leopard spots' consisting of scattered subretinal pigment clumps may be seen after resolution (*Fig. 16.22*).

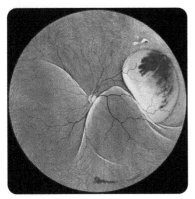

Fig 16.21

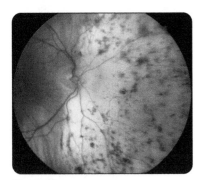

Fig 16.22

Treatment: depends on the cause.

Pars plana vitrectomy

Introduction

- *Instrumentation:* (a) vitreous cutter (*Fig. 16.23*) has an inner guillotine blade that operates extremely rapidly (up to 2500 times/minute or more), (b) intraocular fibre optic probe for illumination, (c) infusion cannula maintains intraocular pressure, and (d) accessory instruments (e.g. scissors, forceps, flute needle, endodiathermy, endolaser delivery systems).

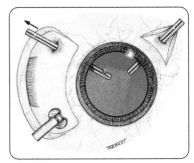

Fig 16.23

- *Tamponading agents:* achieve intraoperative retinal flattening combined with internal drainage of SRF, and produce internal tamponade of retinal breaks postoperatively: (a) air (rarely used due to short duration), (b) expanding gases such as sulphur hexafluoride (SF6) and perfluoropropane (C3F8), (c) heavy liquids (perfluorocarbons—heavier than water and so remain in a dependent position in the vitreous cavity), and (d) silicone oils (buoyant).

Indications: pars plana vitrectomy has greatly improved the prognosis for more complex RD, and the threshold for using the technique has fallen during recent years. Specific indications include the following:

- *RRD:* (a) when the retina cannot be adequately visualized (e.g. haemorrhage, posterior capsular opacification), and (b) when retinal breaks cannot be closed by scleral buckling (e.g. giant tears, large posterior breaks, PVR).
- *Tractional RD:* diabetic retinopathy (e.g. when the macula is involved or threatened) and secondary to penetrating trauma.

Postoperative complications

- *Raised intraocular pressure:* may be caused by (a) overexpansion of intraocular gas, (b) pupillary block by silicone oil (prevented by performing an inferior [Ando] iridotomy), (c) late silicone glaucoma caused by trabecular blockage with emulsified droplets, and (d) ghost cell glaucoma.
- *Cataract:* may be (a) gas-induced (usually transient), (b) silicone oil-induced (*Fig. 16.24*, also shows a superior collection of oil in the anterior chamber [hyperoleon]), and (c) vitrectomy-related (nuclear sclerosis).
- *Band keratopathy:* caused by prolonged contact between silicone oil and the endothelium.

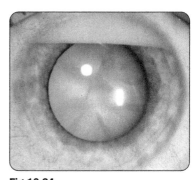

Fig 16.24

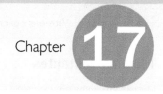

Vitreous opacities

Muscae volitantes

Muscae volitantes are extremely common minute fly- or worm-like physiological opacities best seen by the patient against a pale background. They are thought to be predominantly composed of embryological remnants in the vitreous gel.

Vitreous haemorrhage

Vitreous haemorrhage is a relatively common condition with diverse causes (*Table 17.1*).

> ### Table 17.1 Causes of vitreous haemorrhage
>
> 1. Acute posterior vitreous detachment associated either with a retinal tear (see *Fig. 16.3c*) or avulsion of a peripheral vessel (see *Fig. 16.3d*).
> 2. Proliferative retinopathies
>   - Diabetic
>   - Following retinal vein occlusion
>   - Sickle cell disease
>   - Eales disease
>   - Vasculitis
> 3. Miscellaneous retinal disorders
>   - Macroaneurysm
>   - Telangiectasia
>   - Capillary haemangioma
> 4. Trauma
>   - Blunt
>   - Penetrating
>   - Iatrogenic
> 5. Systemic
>   - Bleeding disorders
>   - Terson syndrome

- *Presentation:* varies according to the severity of the bleed and the underlying cause; mild haemorrhage causes sudden-onset blurring and floaters but may not affect visual acuity, whereas a dense bleed may result in very severe visual loss.
- *B-scan US:* initially shows a uniform appearance; once cellular aggregates develop, small focal echoes become visible; echography is used to exclude an underlying retinal detachment or prominent retinal tear.

Asteroid hyalosis

Pathogenesis: common idiopathic degenerative process, often unilateral, in which tiny calcium pyrophosphate globules collect within the vitreous gel. The prevalence increases with age; the condition is usually asymptomatic.

Diagnosis

- *Signs:* (a) numerous tiny round yellow-white particles of various sizes (*Fig. 17.1*); (b) mobile within

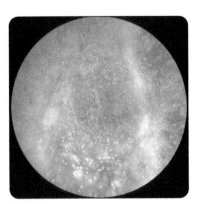

Fig 17.1

the vitreous during eye movements, but not settling inferiorly when the eye is still.

- *B-scan US:* high-amplitude echoes (*Fig. 17.2*).

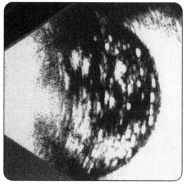

Fig 17.2

Synchisis scintillans

Pathogenesis: uncommon condition that follows a chronic vitreous haemorrhage, often in a blind eye, and usually discovered when frank haemorrhage is no longer present. The vitreous particles are derived from degraded blood cells and are composed of cholesterol.

Diagnosis: numerous flat golden-brown refractile particles; in contrast to asteroid hyalosis, they tend to sediment inferiorly when the eye is immobile.

Chapter 18

Strabismus

Amblyopia

Definition: unilateral, or rarely bilateral, subnormal best corrected VA caused by form vision deprivation and/or abnormal binocular interaction, for which there is no identifiable pathology of the eye or visual pathway.

Classification

- **Strabismic:** resulting from abnormal binocular interaction in which there is continued monocular suppression of the deviating eye.
- **Anisometropic:** caused by a difference in refractive error between the eyes.
- **Stimulus deprivation:** caused by marked vision deprivation—may be unilateral or bilateral and is caused by opacities in the media (e.g. cataract) or ptosis.
- **Ametropic:** resulting from high bilateral but symmetrical refractive error (usually hypermetropia).

Diagnosis

- In the absence of an organic lesion, a difference in best corrected VA of two Snellen lines or more (or >1 log unit) is indicative of amblyopia.
- VA in an amblyopic eye is usually better when reading single letters than letters in a row ('crowding' phenomenon).

Treatment

- It is essential to examine the fundi to diagnose any organic disease prior to commencing treatment.
- If VA does not respond to treatment, investigations (e.g. electrodiagnostics, imaging) should be considered.
- The sensitive period during which VA can be improved is usually up to about 8 years in strabismic amblyopia but may be longer for anisometropic.
- Occlusion of the normal eye is the most effective treatment, with the regimen depending on age and amblyopia density.
- The younger the patient, the more rapid the likely improvement, but the greater the risk of inducing amblyopia in the normal eye; it is essential to monitor VA in both eyes.
- In general, the better the VA at the start of treatment, the shorter the duration required.
- If there has been no improvement after 6 months of effective occlusion, further treatment is unlikely to be fruitful.
- Penalization of the normal eye with atropine is an alternative method sometimes used when compliance with occlusion is poor.

Heterophoria

Definition: heterophoria (latent squint) implies a tendency of the eyes to deviate when fusion is blocked; the 'phoria' can be either a small inward imbalance (esophoria) or an outward imbalance (exophoria).

Classification: both esophoria and exophoria can be classified by the distance at which the angle is greater: (a) convergence excess or weakness, (b) divergence excess or weakness, and (c) mixed. Slight phoria is present in most normal individuals and is overcome by the fusion reflex. When fusional amplitudes are insufficient to maintain alignment, sometimes at times of stress or poor health, the phoria is described as decompensating.

Diagnosis

- *Presentation:* symptoms of binocular discomfort (asthenopia) or double vision (diplopia).
- *Tests:* (a) cover–uncover test detects heterophoria and should be performed both for near using an accommodative target, and for distance, and (b) Maddox wing (*Fig. 18.1*) which dissociates the eyes for near fixation and measures heterophoria.

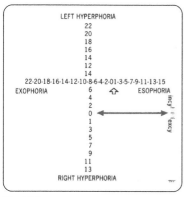

Fig 18.1

Treatment

- *Refraction:* correct significant refractive error.

- *Orthoptic treatment:* of most value in convergence weakness.
- *Symptom relief:* with temporary stick-on Fresnel prisms that may subsequently be incorporated into spectacles (maximum usually 10–12 Δ, split between the eyes).
- *Surgery:* occasionally required for large deviations.

Vergence abnormalities

Convergence insufficiency

Pathogenesis: convergence insufficiency (CI) typically affects individuals with excessive near visual demand. Accommodative insufficiency (AI) is often also present. CI is usually idiopathic and sometimes post-viral, and typically affects school-age children.

Diagnosis

- *Presentation:* with asthenopia or diplopia.
- *Signs:* (a) reduced near point of convergence independent of any heterophoria, and (b) reduced near point of accommodation in AI.

Treatment

- Orthoptic exercises aimed at normalizing the near point and maximizing fusional amplitudes.
- With good compliance, symptoms should be eliminated within a few weeks but if persistent can be treated with base-in prisms, and very occasionally surgery.
- With AI, the minimum reading correction to give clear vision is prescribed but is often difficult to discard.

Divergence insufficiency

- *Pathogenesis:* divergence paresis or paralysis is a rare condition typically associated with underlying neurological disease such as intracranial space-occupying lesions, cerebrovascular accidents, and head trauma.
- *Presentation:* at any age and may be difficult to differentiate from 6th nerve palsy, but is primarily a concomitant esodeviation with reduced or absent divergence fusional amplitudes.
- *Treatment:* difficult; prisms are the best option.

Near reflex insufficiency

- *Pathogenesis:* complete paralysis, in which no convergence or accommodation can be initiated, may be of functional origin, due to midbrain disease or may follow head trauma.
- *Signs:* (a) dual convergence and accommodation insufficiency; (b) mydriasis may be seen on attempted near fixation.
- *Treatment:* reading glasses, base-in prisms, and possibly botulinum toxin (orthoptic exercises have no effect); it is difficult to eradicate.

Spasm of the near reflex

Pathogenesis: functional condition affecting patients of all ages who are mainly female.

Diagnosis
- *Presentation:* diplopia, blurred vision, and headaches.
- *Signs:* (a) esotropia, (b) pseudomyopia, and (c) miosis. Spasm may be triggered when testing ocular movements; observation of miosis is the key to the diagnosis; refraction with and without cycloplegia confirms pseudomyopia, which must not be corrected optically.

Treatment
- *Reassurance:* with advice to discontinue any activity that triggers the response.
- *If persistent:* atropine and a full reading correction are prescribed, but it is difficult later to abandon treatment without recurrence.

Esotropia

Definition

Esotropia (manifest convergent squint) may be concomitant or incomitant; in a concomitant esotropia the variability of the angle of deviation is within 5 Δ in different horizontal gaze positions, and in an incomitant deviation the angle differs in various positions of gaze as a result of abnormal innervation or restriction. This section deals only with concomitant esotropia (classification is shown in *Table 18.1*).

Table 18.1 Classification of esotropia

1. Accommodative
   a. Refractive
      - Fully accommodative
      - Partially accommodative
   b. Non-refractive
      - With convergence excess
      - With accommodation weakness
   c. Mixed
2. Non-accommodative
   - Essential
   - Microtropia
   - Basic
   - Convergence excess
   - Convergence spasm
   - Divergence insufficiency
   - Divergence paralysis
   - Sensory
   - Consecutive
   - Acute onset
   - Cyclic

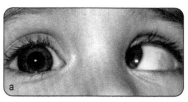

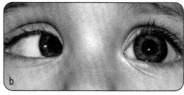

Fig 18.2

Early onset (essential) esotropia

Definition: idiopathic esotropia developing within the first 6 months of life in an otherwise normal infant with no significant refractive error and no limitation of ocular movements.

Diagnosis
- **Angle:** fairly large (>30 Δ) and stable.
- **Refraction:** normal for age (+1 to +2 D).
- **Fixation:** (a) alternates between right and left in the primary position, and (b) cross-fixating in side gaze, so that the child uses

the left eye in right gaze (*Fig. 18.2a*) and the right eye on left gaze (*Fig. 18.2b*)—may give a false impression of bilateral 6th nerve palsy.
- **Nystagmus:** usually horizontal; latent nystagmus (LN) is seen only when one eye is covered, when the fast phase beats toward the side of the fixating eye; direction of the fast phase reverses according to which eye is covered.
- **Manifest latent nystagmus:** same as LN except that it is present with both eyes open, although with increased amplitude when one is covered.
- **Asymmetry of optokinetic nystagmus**
- **Inferior oblique overaction (*Fig. 18.3*):** may be present initially or develop later.
- **Dissociated vertical deviation (*DVD*):** develops in 80% by the age of 3 years and is characterized by up-drift with excyclorotation, when the eye is covered (*Fig. 18.4*), or spontaneously during periods of visual inattention.

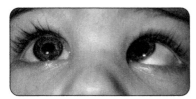

Fig 18.3

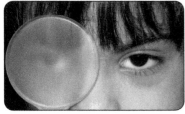

Fig 18.4

- *Differential diagnosis:*
  (a) congenital bilateral 6th nerve palsy, (b) secondary (sensory) esotropia, (c) nystagmus blockage syndrome (convergence dampens horizontal nystagmus), and (d) mechanical limitation of eye movements (e.g. Duane syndrome, Möbius syndrome, strabismus fixus).

Treatment
- *Preliminary:* correction of amblyopia and significant refractive error.
- *Initial surgery:* eyes should be aligned surgically to within 10 Δ by the age of 12 months. May involve (a) recession of both medial recti or (b) unilateral medial rectus recession with lateral rectus resection; inferior oblique overaction can be corrected at the initial operation

(e.g. disinsertion, recession, myectomy) or later if it subsequently develops (commonly at age 2 years).
- *Further surgery:* required for undercorrection, but an accommodative element should be suspected if the eyes are initially straight or almost straight after surgery and then start to reconverge; DVD may require specific surgery (e.g. superior rectus recession with or without posterior fixation sutures).
- *Amblyopia:* subsequently develops in approximately 50%, associated with unilateral fixation preference.

Accommodative esotropia

Introduction: near vision involves both accommodation and convergence. Accommodation is the process by which the eye focuses on a near target by altering the curvature of the crystalline lens. Simultaneously, the eyes converge in order to fixate bifoveally on the target. Both accommodation and convergence are quantitatively related to the proximity of the target and have a fairly constant relationship to each other; the AC/A or 'accommodative convergence to accommodation' ratio is the amount of convergence in prism dioptres per dioptre change in accommodation.

Diagnosis
- *Refractive:* AC/A ratio is normal; (a) presents at 18 months to 3 years, (b) angle varies little (<10 Δ) between distance and near, and (c) optical correction of the hypermetropia eliminates the deviation entirely in the fully

accommodative form (*Fig. 18.5*) but not entirely in partially accommodative (*Fig. 18.6*).

- **Non-refractive:** AC/A ratio is high; (a) convergence excess type (high AC/A ratio due to increased accommodative convergence; normal accommodation but increased convergence), with straight eyes for distance but esotropia for near; (b) hypoaccommodative convergence excess (high AC/A ratio due to weak accommodation necessitating increased effort, producing overconvergence), with straight eyes for distance but esotropia for near.

Treatment

- **Fully accommodative:** correction of full cycloplegic refractive error for children younger than 6 years, and the maximally tolerated subjective correction over the age of 8 years will control the deviation for both near and distance.
- **Convergence excess:** bifocals to relieve accommodation (and thereby accommodative convergence), allowing ocular alignment at near; the minimum 'add' required is prescribed, gradually reduced and eliminated by the early teens.
- **Hypoaccommodative:** bifocals are more likely to be effective when the AC/A ratio is not overly excessive; at higher levels, surgery is the better long-term solution.
- **Surgery:** aimed at restoring or improving binocular single vision (BSV) as well as addressing any cosmetic implications; it should only be considered if spectacles do not fully correct the deviation. Bilateral medial rectus recessions are performed in patients in whom the deviation for near is greater than that for distance.

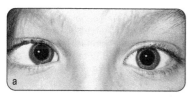
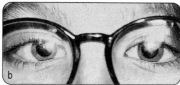

Fig 18.5

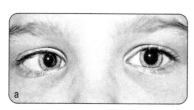
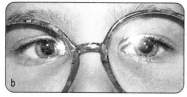

Fig 18.6

Microtropia

Definition: small-angle (<10 Δ) squint, often seen in association with other forms of strabismus; for example, a patient with fully accommodative esotropia may control with glasses to a microtropia rather than true bifoveal binocular single vision.

Diagnosis

- *Symptoms:* rare unless associated with decompensating heterophoria.
- *Angle:* very small manifest deviation that may or may not be detectable on cover testing.
- *Other signs:* (a) anisometropia, (b) amblyopia of the more ametropic eye; (c) stereopsis is present but reduced.
- *Central suppression scotoma (CSS):* in the deviating eye; 4 Δ prism test differentiates bifoveal fixation (normal BSV) and CSS in microtropia.
- *Abnormal retinal correspondence:* noncorresponding retinal elements acquire a common subjective visual direction so that fusion occurs in the presence of a small-angle manifest squint.

Treatment: correction of refractive errors and occlusion for amblyopia; most patients remain stable and symptom-free.

Other esotropias

- *Near esotropia (non-accommodative convergence excess):* (a) presentation in older children and young adults, (b) no significant refractive error, (c) esotropia for near but orthophoria or small esophoria with BSV for distance, (d) AC/A ratio normal or low, and (e) normal near point of accommodation. Treatment involves bilateral medial rectus recessions.

- *Distance esotropia:* (a) presentation in young early adult life, (b) often myopic refraction, and (c) intermittent or constant esotropia for distance but minimal or no deviation for near. Treatment is with prisms until spontaneous resolution, or surgery in persistent cases.
- *Acute (late-onset) esotropia:* (a) presentation at approximately 5 or 6 years of age with sudden onset of diplopia and esotropia; (b) eye movements are normal but an underlying 6th nerve palsy must be excluded. Treatment is aimed at re-establishing BSV to prevent suppression, using prisms, botulinum toxin, or surgery.
- *Secondary (sensory) esotropia:* caused by a unilateral reduction in VA in childhood that interferes with or abolishes fusion (e.g. cataract, optic atrophy, retinoblastoma); fundus examination is therefore essential.
- *Consecutive esotropia:* follows surgical overcorrection of an exodeviation.

Exotropia

Constant (early onset) exotropia

- *Presentation:* often at birth with a large and constant divergence; neurological anomalies are frequently present, in contrast to early onset esotropia.
- *Treatment:* lateral rectus recession and medial rectus resection.
- *Differential diagnosis:* secondary exotropia, which may conceal serious ocular pathology.

Intermittent exotropia

Classification
- **Distance:** deviation is greater for distance than near; further subdivided into 'simulated' and 'true' types.
- **Nonspecific:** deviation is the same for distance and near fixation.
- **Near:** deviation is greater for near fixation.

Diagnosis
- **Presentation:** approximately 2 years with exophoria that breaks down to exotropia (*Fig. 18.7*) under conditions of visual inattention, bright light (resulting in reflex closure of the affected eye), and fatigue or ill health.
- **Signs:** (a) straight with BSV at times, and (b) manifest exotropia with suppression at other times.

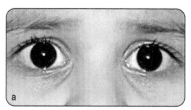

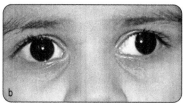

Fig 18.7

Treatment
- **Refraction:** correction of myopia may control the deviation; in some cases, an over-minus prescription may be effective.
- **Part-time occlusion:** of the deviating eye may improve control.
- **Orthoptic exercises:** for near exotropia.
- **Surgery:** if control is poor or is progressively deteriorating.

Other exotropias

- **Secondary (sensory):** caused by acquired monocular or binocular visual impairment in adulthood (*Fig. 18.8*). Treatment involves correction of the visual deficit where possible, followed by muscle surgery if still necessary.
- **Consecutive:** follows surgical correction of an esodeviation, or less commonly, spontaneously in an amblyopic eye.

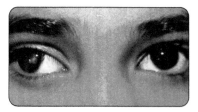

Fig 18.8

Special syndromes

Duane retraction syndrome

Pathogenesis: failure of innervation of the lateral rectus by the 6th nerve, with anomalous innervation of the lateral rectus by the 3rd nerve; involvement is often bilateral but asymmetrical.

Diagnosis

- **Primary position:** BSV (*Fig. 18.9a*), often with a face turn.
- **Signs:** (a) restricted abduction (*Fig. 18.9b*, left eye), (b) restricted adduction, although usually only partial (*Fig. 18.9c*, left eye), (c) retraction of the globe on adduction as the result of co-contraction of the medial and lateral recti, with resultant narrowing of the palpebral fissure (*Fig. 18.9c*, left eye), and (d) an upshoot or downshoot in adduction may be present.

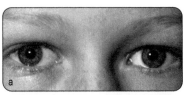
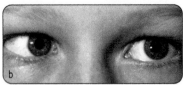
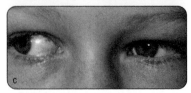

Fig 18.9

- **Huber classification:** (a) type I limitation of abduction, (b) type II limited adduction, and (c) type III both adduction and abduction are restricted.

Treatment

- **Conservative:** most do not need surgery; when amblyopia is present, it is usually the result of anisometropia rather than the strabismus.
- **Surgery:** may be indicated in young children if there is evidence of loss of BSV; in older individuals, the indication is often an uncomfortable or cosmetically unacceptable abnormal head posture (AHP).

Brown syndrome

Pathogenesis: mechanical restriction of the superior oblique muscle tendon. It is generally congenital and idiopathic but occasionally acquired following trauma or inflammation (e.g. rheumatoid arthritis) of the trochlea or tendon; involvement is usually unilateral.

Diagnosis

- **Primary position:** BSV (*Fig. 18.10a*).
- **Major signs of right Brown syndrome:** (a) limited elevation of the right eye in adduction (*Fig. 18.10b*), (b) normal right elevation in abduction, and (c) absence of right superior oblique overaction (*Fig. 18.10c*).
- **Variable signs:** (a) downshoot in adduction, (b) hypotropia in the primary position, and (c) AHP with chin elevation and ipsilateral head tilt.

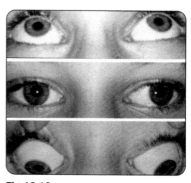
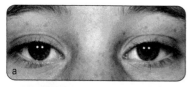

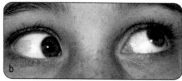

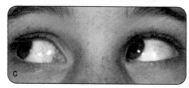

Fig 18.10

- **'V' pattern:** is significant when the difference between upgaze and downgaze is 15 Δ or more (*Fig. 18.11*); causes include inferior oblique overaction associated with 4th nerve palsy or childhood esotropias, and Brown syndrome.
- **'A' pattern:** is significant when the difference between upgaze and downgaze is 10 Δ or more (*Fig. 18.12*); causes include primary superior oblique overaction and inferior oblique underaction/palsy with subsequent superior oblique overaction.

Treatment

- **Congenital cases:** not usually required if BSV is maintained with an acceptable head position; lengthening of the superior oblique tendon is occasionally performed.
- **Acquired cases:** steroids (oral or peritrochlear injection) are sometimes used.

Alphabet patterns

- **Definition:** 'V' or 'A' pattern is present when there is a significant difference in the angle of deviation between upgaze and downgaze. It is usually due to an abnormal balance of the horizontal vectors of extraocular muscles, and can occur in both concomitant and incomitant strabismus.

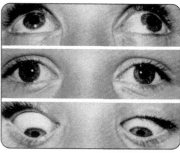

Fig 18.11

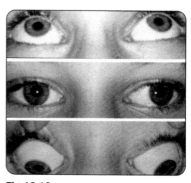

Fig 18.12

- **Treatment:** either surgery to the oblique muscles or by performing downward or upward transposition of the horizontal rectus muscles in conjunction with recessions.

Strabismus surgery

- **Aims of surgery:** to correct misalignment of the extraocular muscles including improvement of binocular function and appearance of the patient, and reduction of an AHP.
- **Types of procedure:** (a) weakening may involve recession of the muscle insertion (*Fig. 18.13*), disinsertion/ myectomy, and posterior fixation suture (e.g. Faden procedure to suture the muscle belly to the sclera posteriorly so as to decrease the pull of the muscle as the eye moves into its field of action), (b) strengthening—resection (shortening; *Fig. 18.14*), tucking (usually superior oblique), and

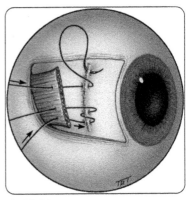

Fig 18.14

advancement nearer to the limbus of a previously recessed muscle, and (c) procedures that change the direction of muscle action (e.g. transposition for alphabet patterns).

- **Adjustable sutures:** indicated when a precise outcome is essential and when the results are likely to be unpredictable (e.g. thyroid myopathy); following surgery, slackening or tightening is carried out under topical anaesthesia (*Fig. 18.15*).
- **Botulinum toxin chemodenervation** (*Fig. 18.16*): induces temporary (3 months) paralysis of an extraocular muscle by injection of botulinum toxin under topical anaesthesia using electromyographic guidance. Indications: (a) determination of the risk of postoperative diplopia, (b) assessment of the potential for BSV in a patient with a constant manifest squint, and (c) symptom relief during recovery of a lateral rectus palsy.

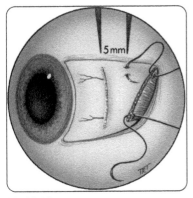

Fig 18.13

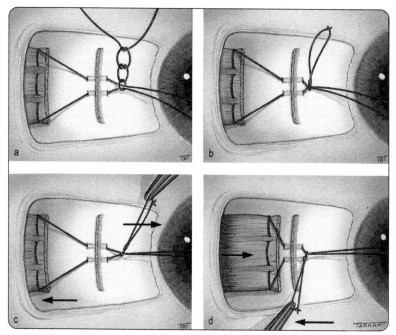

Fig 18.15

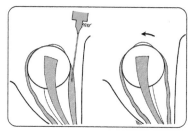

Fig 18.16

Neuro-ophthalmology

Optic nerve

Table 19.1 **Signs of optic nerve dysfunction**

- Reduced VA
- Relative afferent pupillary defect
- Dyschromatopsia: impairment of colour vision, mainly red and green
- Diminished light brightness sensitivity
- Diminished contrast sensitivity
- Visual field defects, varying with the underlying pathology

Table 19.2 **Visual field defects in optic neuropathies**

1. Central scotoma
   - Demyelination
   - Toxic and nutritional
   - Leber hereditary optic neuropathy
   - Compression
2. Enlarged blind spot
   - Papilloedema
   - Congenital anomalies
3. Respecting horizontal meridian
   - Anterior ischaemic optic neuropathy
   - Glaucoma
   - Disc drusen
4. Upper temporal defects not respecting vertical meridian
   - Tilted discs

Optic atrophy

Classification

- **Primary:** occurs without antecedent swelling of the optic nerve head. It may be caused by lesions from the retrolaminar optic nerve to the lateral geniculate body; disease anterior to the chiasm gives rise to unilateral atrophy, that of the chiasm and optic tract causes bilateral changes.
- **Secondary:** preceded by disc swelling (e.g. chronic papilloedema, anterior ischaemic optic neuropathy, papillitis).
- **Consecutive:** caused by disease of the inner retina or its blood supply (e.g. retinitis pigmentosa, central retinal artery occlusion).

Diagnosis

- **Symptoms:** varied and dependent on cause.
- **Signs:** (a) white, flat disc with clearly delineated margins in primary (*Fig. 19.1*) and consecutive atrophy, and (b) white

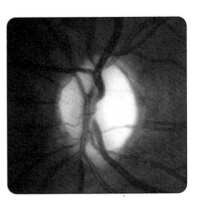

Fig 19.1

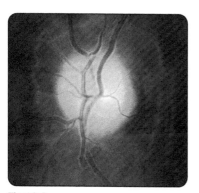

Fig 19.2

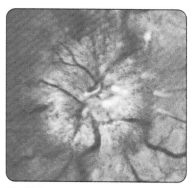

Fig 19.3

or dirty grey, slightly raised disc with poorly delineated margins and occasionally surrounding 'water marks' in secondary atrophy (*Fig. 19.2*). There is also reduction in the number of surface disc vessels in all types. In primary atrophy, changes may be sectoral depending on the lesion (e.g. temporal pallor from papillomacular bundle damage, band atrophy with sparing of the superior and inferior portions in lesions of the chiasm or optic tract).

Classification of optic neuritis

- *Ophthalmoscopic:* (a) retrobulbar neuritis, in which the optic nerve head is not primarily involved and so appears normal, (b) papillitis, characterized by disc oedema and hyperaemia, that may be associated with flame-shaped peripapillary haemorrhages (*Fig. 19.3*), and (c) neuroretinitis (see below).

- *Aetiological:* (a) demyelination (most common), (b) parainfectious, following viral infection or immunization, (c) infectious, which may be sinus-related or associated with systemic infections (e.g. syphilis, Lyme disease), and (d) other (e.g. sarcoidosis, systemic lupus erythematosus).

Demyelinating optic neuritis

Definition: demyelination is a pathological process by which nerve fibres lose their insulating myelin layer, disrupting nervous conduction within the white matter tracts of the brain, brainstem and spinal cord.

Classification: demyelinating diseases that may cause ocular problems include the following:

- *Isolated optic neuritis:* in a high proportion of cases, generalized disease subsequently develops; the overall 10-year risk of developing multiple sclerosis (MS) following an acute episode of optic neuritis is approximately 40%.

- **Multiple sclerosis:** most common by far.
- **Devic disease (neuromyelitis optica):** bilateral optic neuritis and subsequent transverse myelitis (spinal cord demyelination).

Diagnosis

- **Presentation:** in 3rd to 6th decades with (a) monocular blurring, (b) occasionally phosphenes (tiny light flashes), (c) discomfort or pain in or around the eye frequently exacerbated by ocular movements, and (d) tender globe.
- **VA:** 6/18–6/60, occasionally worse.
- **Other signs of optic nerve dysfunction:** (see above).
- **Disc appearance:** normal in the majority of cases (retrobulbar neuritis), remainder show papillitis.
- **Perimetry:** diffuse visual field depression with superimposed focal defects, typically central, altitudinal, or arcuate.
- **Course:** vision worsens over several days to 2 weeks and then begins to improve; initial recovery is fairly rapid and then there is slow improvement over months.
- **Prognosis:** 75% recover to 6/9 or better; residua include (a) abnormal colour vision and light brightness appreciation, (b) optic atrophy, and (c) a mild RAPD.

Treatment

- **Indications:** treatment may speed recovery but does not influence eventual visual outcome. It may be considered in some circumstances such as poor vision in the fellow eye or for occupational requirements.
- **Intravenous methylprednisolone:** for 3 days followed by a reducing course of oral prednisolone.
- **Immunomodulation therapy:** (e.g. interferon-beta) at the first episode of optic neuritis may reduce the risk of clinical MS in higher risk patients.

Miscellaneous optic neuritis

- **Parainfectious:** may follow various viral infections (e.g. measles, mumps, chickenpox, glandular fever), as well as immunization; prognosis is usually good and treatment is not required in the majority.
- **Sinus-related:** may be due to direct spread of infection, occlusive vasculitis, and mucocele; treatment is with antibiotics and surgical drainage.
- **Cat-scratch fever (benign lymphoreticulosis):** (see Chapter 11) typically causes neuroretinitis (see below).
- **Syphilis:** acute papillitis or neuroretinitis may occur during primary or secondary stages (see Chapter 11).
- **Lyme disease (borreliosis):** (see Chapter 11) may cause neuroretinitis and occasionally acute retrobulbar neuritis, which may be associated with neurological manifestations that can mimic MS.
- **Cryptococcal meningitis:** (see Chapter 11) may be associated with acute optic neuritis, which may be bilateral.
- **Varicella zoster virus:** may cause papillitis by spread from contiguous retinitis (e.g. acute retinal necrosis,

progressive retinal necrosis; see Chapter 11), in herpes zoster ophthalmicus or chickenpox.

- **Sarcoidosis:** optic neuritis affects a minority of patients with neurosarcoid; the optic nerve head may exhibit a lumpy appearance suggestive of granulomatous infiltration (**Fig. 19.4**), and there is often associated vitritis.
- **Autoimmune optic nerve involvement:** retrobulbar neuritis or anterior ischaemic optic neuropathy are the usual manifestations.

- **Signs of optic nerve dysfunction:** usually mild.
- **Progression of fundus signs:** (a) papillitis associated with peripapillary and macular oedema (**Fig. 19.5a**), (b) macular star develops as the disc swelling is resolving (**Fig. 19.5b**), and (c) macular star resolves with return to normal or near-normal VA in 6–12 months.

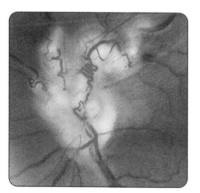

Fig 19.4

Neuroretinitis

Causes: cat-scratch fever is responsible for 60%, and approximately 25% are idiopathic (Leber idiopathic stellate neuroretinitis); other causes include syphilis, Lyme disease, mumps, and leptospirosis.

Diagnosis

- **Presentation:** gradual onset of painless unilateral visual impairment.
- **VA:** variable reduction.

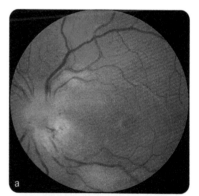

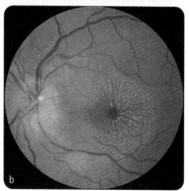

Fig 19.5

Treatment: varies according to cause; recurrent idiopathic cases may require steroids and/or other immunosuppressants.

Non-arteritic anterior ischaemic optic neuropathy

Pathogenesis: occlusion of the short posterior ciliary arteries resulting in partial or total infarction of the optic nerve head. Predispositions include (a) structural crowding of the optic nerve head so that the physiological cup is either very small or absent, and (b) cardiovascular risk factors, particularly hypertension.

Diagnosis

- *Presentation:* in 6th and 7th decades with sudden painless monocular visual loss, often altitudinal.
- *VA:* normal or only slightly reduced in approximately 30%; remainder have moderate to severe impairment.
- *Perimetry:* typically inferior altitudinal defect.
- *Signs:* (a) diffuse or sectoral hyperaemic disc swelling, often associated with a few peripapillary splinter haemorrhages (*Fig. 19.6*); (b) swelling gradually resolves and pallor ensues; involvement of the fellow eye occurs in approximately 10% of patients after 2 years.
- *Investigations:* (a) blood pressure, (b) fasting lipid profile and blood glucose; (c) it is critical to exclude occult giant cell arteritis (GCA see below).

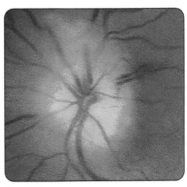

Fig 19.6

Treatment: systemic predispositions should be addressed; aspirin is frequently prescribed, but it does not appear to reduce involvement of the fellow eye.

Arteritic anterior ischaemic optic neuropathy

Pathogenesis: GCA, a granulomatous necrotizing arteritis with a predilection for large and medium-sized arteries, including the superficial temporal. The disease is strongly associated with polymyalgia rheumatica, characterized by pain and stiffness in proximal muscle groups. Rare complications of GCA include dissecting aneurysms, myocardial infarction, and stroke; 30–50% of patients develop arteritic anterior ischaemic optic neuropathy (AAION).

Diagnosis

- *Presentation of GCA:* in old age.
- *Symptoms of GCA:* (a) scalp tenderness, (b) headache, (c) jaw claudication (pain on speaking and chewing), and (d) nonspecific symptoms such as neck pain,

weight loss, fever, night sweats, malaise, and depression.

- **Superficial temporal arteritis:** thickened, tender, inflamed, and nodular arteries; absent pulsation is strongly suggestive of GCA.
- **Presentation of AAION:** (a) sudden profound unilateral visual loss (commonly light perception) that may be preceded by transient visual disturbance; (b) without treatment the fellow eye becomes

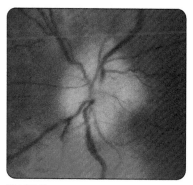

Fig 19.7

involved in 30% of cases, usually within 1 week.

- **Signs of AAION:** (a) strikingly pale oedematous disc (*Fig. 19.7*); (b) swelling resolves over 1 or 2 months and atrophy ensues.
- **Investigations:** (a) ESR is often very high (60 mm/hr or more), although normal in approximately 20%, (b) C-reactive protein is invariably raised and may be helpful when ESR is equivocal, and (c) platelet levels may be elevated.
- **Temporal artery biopsy:** should be performed urgently if GCA is

suspected; steroids (see below) should not be withheld pending biopsy.

Treatment

- **Aims:** mainly to prevent blindness of the fellow eye; very rarely, prompt treatment may result in improvement in the primary eye.
- **Regimen:** (a) intravenous methylprednisolone for 3 days followed by long-term oral prednisolone, (b) oral prednisolone alone in some circumstances, (c) antiplatelet therapy (e.g. aspirin), and (d) immunosuppressants in steroid-resistant cases or as steroid-sparing agents.

Posterior ischaemic optic neuropathy

Ischaemia of the retrolaminar portion of the optic nerve is much less common than the anterior variety; it is a diagnosis of exclusion and may be of the following types:

- **Operative posterior ischaemic optic neuropathy (PION):** develops following a variety of surgical procedures (e.g. cardiac, spinal); bilateral involvement is common and the visual prognosis often poor.
- **Arteritic PION:** associated with GCA and carries a poor visual prognosis.
- **Non-arteritic PION:** associated with the same systemic risk factors as the anterior variety apart from crowded optic discs.

Diabetic papillopathy

Pathogenesis: occurs in both type 1 and type 2 diabetics, probably due to small-vessel disease but is milder than AION.

Diagnosis

- *VA:* 6/12 or better.
- *Signs:* (a) unilateral or bilateral mild disc swelling and hyperaemia; (b) disc surface telangiectasia is common (*Fig. 19.8*).
- *Course:* usually several months.

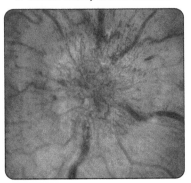

Fig 19.8

Treatment: systemic steroids are of questionable benefit.

Leber hereditary optic neuropathy

Genetics: maternally inherited mitochondrial DNA mutation that typically affects males; asymptomatic female relatives may show telangiectatic microangiopathy.

Diagnosis

- *Presentation:* between the 2nd and 4th decades with acute or subacute severe painless unilateral loss of central vision; the fellow eye is affected within weeks or months.
- *Acute signs:* (a) often subtle disc hyperaemia with obscuration

of margins (*Fig. 19.9*), (b) surface telangiectasia, (c) swelling of the peripapillary nerve fibre layer, (d) dilatation and tortuosity of posterior pole vasculature; FA shows absence of leakage; papillary light reactions may remain brisk.

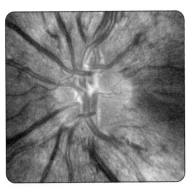

Fig 19.9

- *Course:* vessels regress, swelling resolves, and severe optic atrophy supervenes with a final VA of 6/60 or less.
- *Perimetry:* central or centrocaecal scotomas.

Treatment: generally ineffective; smoking and excessive consumption of alcohol should be discouraged.

Nutritional optic neuropathy (tobacco–alcohol amblyopia)

Pathogenesis: deficiency in protein and B vitamins after dietary neglect, particularly affecting heavy drinkers and cigar smokers; some also have defective B_{12} absorption and may develop pernicious anaemia.

Diagnosis

- **Presentation:** insidious onset of progressive, usually symmetrical, bilateral visual impairment associated with dyschromatopsia.
- **Discs:** normal at presentation in most cases, although some show subtle pallor.
- **Perimetry:** bilateral centrocaecal scotomas, easier to plot and larger with a red target.

Treatment: abstention from drinking and smoking; intramuscular hydroxocobalamin and oral multivitamins, including thiamine and folate.

Papilloedema

Pathogenesis: swelling of the optic nerve head secondary to raised intracranial pressure. It is nearly always bilateral, although may be asymmetrical. Causes of raised intracranial pressure: (a) idiopathic intracranial hypertension (pseudotumour cerebri), (b) space-occupying intracranial lesions, (c) cerebral venous sinus thrombosis, and (d) severe systemic hypertension.

Diagnosis

- **General symptoms:** (a) headache occurs early in the morning and may wake the patient from sleep; may intensify with head movement, bending, or coughing, (b) sudden nausea and vomiting, often projectile, and sometimes (c) deterioration of consciousness.
- **Visual symptoms:** (a) transient obscurations lasting a few seconds, (b) horizontal diplopia (due to stretching of one or both 6th nerves over the petrous tip),

a false localizing sign, and (c) persistent visual loss in long-standing papilloedema with secondary optic atrophy (see below).

- **Early papilloedema:** (a) mild disc hyperaemia with preservation of the optic cup, (b) indistinct peripapillary retinal nerve striations and disc margins (*Fig. 19.10a*), and (c) loss of previous spontaneous venous pulsation (also absent in 20% of normals).
- **Established papilloedema:** (a) severe disc hyperaemia, (b) moderate disc elevation with absence of the cup, (c) venous engorgement, (d) peripapillary flame haemorrhages and cotton wool spots (*Fig. 19.10b*), (e) circumferential retinal folds (Paton lines), and (f) hard exudates that typically radiate from the centre of the fovea.
- **Chronic papilloedema:** (a) severe disc elevation, (b) absence of cotton wool spots and haemorrhage (*Fig. 19.10c*), (c) optociliary shunts, and (d) drusen-like crystalline surface deposits (uncommon).
- **Atrophic papilloedema:** (a) discs are dirty grey and slightly elevated, with (b) few crossing blood vessels, and (c) indistinct margins (secondary optic atrophy; *Fig. 19.10d*).
- **Perimetry:** blind spot is enlarged in the early established stages; atrophy may be associated with constriction.
- **Investigations:** to determine the cause; MR, CT, and B-scan US show an enlarged optic nerve diameter in most cases.

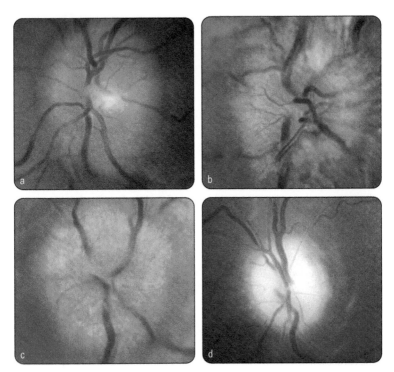

Fig 19.10

Terson syndrome

- **Definition:** combination of intraocular and subarachnoid haemorrhage secondary to rupture of an intracranial aneurysm. Intraocular haemorrhage may also occur with subdural haematoma and acute elevation of intracranial pressure from other causes.
- **Intraocular haemorrhage:** frequently bilateral and typically intraretinal and/or preretinal (subhyaloid; *Fig. 19.11*), although occasionally

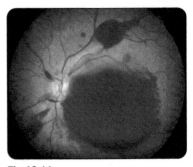

Fig 19.11

subhyaloid blood may break into the vitreous; probably caused by retinal venous stasis secondary to increased cavernous sinus pressure.

- **Prognosis:** usually good as the blood commonly resolves spontaneously within a few months; early vitrectomy may be considered for dense bilateral bleeds.

Congenital optic disc anomalies

- **Tilted optic disc:** (a) oblique entry of the optic nerve into the globe, with (b) angulation of the cup axis and elevation of the neuroretinal rim, (c) associated findings include inferonasal chorioretinal thinning (*Fig. 19.12*) and myopic astigmatic refractive error; (d) perimetry may show superotemporal defects that do not respect the vertical midline.
- **Optic disc pit:** (a) large disc, (b) round or oval pit of variable size, usually located temporally (*Fig. 19.13*); (c) perimetry may show

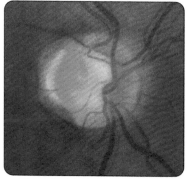

Fig 19.13

glaucoma-like defects; (d) serous macular detachment (in 50%).
- **Optic disc drusen:** (a) waxy pearl-like deposits of calcific material (*Fig. 19.14*) present in approximately 0.3% of the population, (b) difficult to detect in early childhood because they lie deep to the disc surface and may mimic papilloedema, (c) anomalous vascular patterns; (d) associations include retinitis

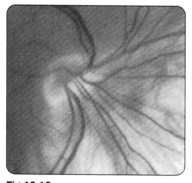

Fig 19.12

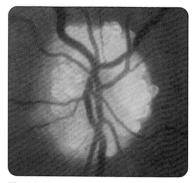

Fig 19.14

pigmentosa and angioid streaks, and (e) complications (rare) include juxtapapillary CNV and progressive but limited visual field defects; drusen are demonstrated well on B-scan US.

- **Optic disc coloboma:** unilateral or bilateral; (a) glistening white bowl-shaped excavation so that the inferior neuroretinal rim is thin or absent (*Fig. 19.15*); (b) may be associated with an adjacent choroidal and iris coloboma; (c) perimetry shows a superior defect; (d) systemic associations (uncommon) include chromosomal and CNS anomalies, and CHARGE syndrome.

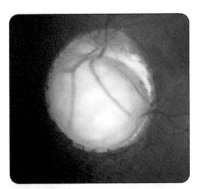

Fig 19.15

- **Morning glory anomaly:** unilateral; (a) large disc with a funnel-shaped excavation surrounded by an annulus of chorioretinal disturbance (*Fig. 19.16*), (b) white tuft of glial tissue overlies the central portion, (c) blood vessels emerge radially from the rim of the excavation, (d) serous retinal detachment (in 30%); (e) systemic associations (uncommon) include

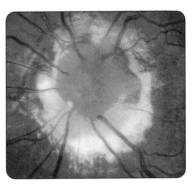

Fig 19.16

frontonasal dysplasia (mid-facial anomalies, basal encephalocele, midline brain malformations), and NF2.

- **Optic nerve hypoplasia:** may occur as an isolated anomaly in a normal eye, in a grossly malformed eye, or in association with systemic disorders, typically involving midline brain structures (e.g. de Morsier syndrome—septo-optic dysplasia— in approximately 10%). Maternal ingestion of predisposing agents (e.g. steroids, alcohol, anticonvulsants) during pregnancy has been implicated. (a) VA ranges from normal to no light perception, (b) small grey disc, (c) surrounding yellow halo of hypopigmentation (double-ring sign; *Fig. 19.17*), and (d) retinal vascular tortuosity (common).

- **Myelinated nerve fibres:** (a) white feathery streaks running within the retinal nerve fibre layer from the disc (*Fig. 19.18*); (b) ocular associations of extensive myelination include high myopia, anisometropia, and amblyopia, and (c) systemic associations include NF1.

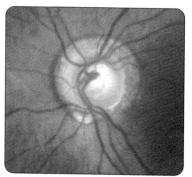

Fig 19.17

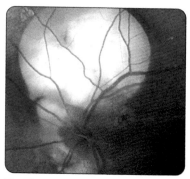

Fig 19.19

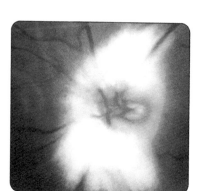

Fig 19.18

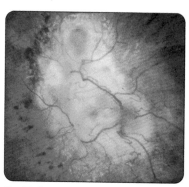

Fig 19.20

- *Aicardi syndrome:* X-L dominant condition that is lethal *in utero* in males; (a) bilateral multiple depigmented chorioretinal lacunae clustered around the disc, (b) disc may be hypoplastic, colobomatous, or pigmented (*Fig. 19.19*); (c) ocular associations include microphthalmos and iris colobomas, and (d) systemic associations a range of severe CNS and skeletal anomalies.

- *Optic disc dysplasia:* markedly deformed disc that does not conform to any recognizable category described above (*Fig. 19.20*).

Pupils

Oculosympathetic palsy (Horner syndrome)

Pathogenesis: damage to the sympathetic nervous supply of the eye, which involves three neurons (*Fig. 19.21*).

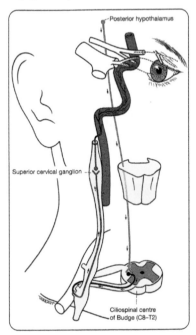

Fig 19.21

Anatomy and causes

- *First (central) neuron:* originates in the posterior hypothalamus and descends down the brainstem to terminate in the ciliospinal centre of Budge, between C8 and T2 in the spinal cord; causes of damage include brain stem disease (e.g. stroke, tumours).
- *Second (preganglionic) neuron:* passes from the ciliospinal centre to the superior cervical ganglion in the neck, where it can be damaged by apical lung disease and neck lesions including surgery.

- *Third (postganglionic) neuron:* ascends along the internal carotid artery to enter the cavernous sinus where it joins the ophthalmic division of the trigeminal nerve; sympathetic fibres reach the ciliary body and the dilator pupillae muscle via the nasociliary nerve and the long ciliary nerves; causes of damage include internal carotid artery dissection, cavernous sinus lesions, and otonasopharyngeal disease.

Diagnosis

The vast majority of cases are unilateral.

- *Mild ptosis:* (1 or 2 mm) due to weakness of Müller muscle.
- *Miosis (Fig. 19.22):* due to the unopposed action of the sphincter pupillae; miosis is accentuated in dim light since a Horner pupil will not dilate, unlike its fellow.

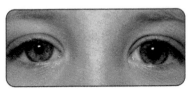

Fig 19.22

- *Hypochromic heterochromia:* in congenital or long-standing lesions.
- *Slight elevation of the inferior eyelid:* due to weakness of the inferior tarsal muscle.
- *Reduced ipsilateral sweating:* if the lesion is below the superior cervical ganglion, because the sudomotor fibres supplying the skin of the face take a

separate path along the external carotid artery.

- **Pharmacological tests:** (a) cocaine 4% is instilled into both eyes to ascertain the diagnosis—a normal pupil will dilate but a Horner pupil will not, (b) apraclonidine 0.5% or 1.0% is instilled into both eyes—Horner pupil will dilate but a normal pupil is unaffected, (c) hydroxyamphetamine 1%—will dilate both pupils in a preganglionic lesion but in a postganglionic lesion a Horner pupil will not dilate, and (d) adrenaline 0.1%—in a preganglionic lesion neither pupil will dilate, whereas in a postganglionic lesion the Horner pupil will dilate.

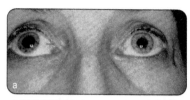
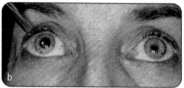
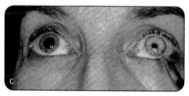

Fig 19.23

Adie pupil

Pathogenesis: denervation of the postganglionic supply to the sphincter pupillae and the ciliary muscle that may follow a viral illness. One eye is involved in 80% of cases, although the fellow eye will often be affected later; associated diminished deep tendon reflexes (Holmes–Adie syndrome) and wider autonomic dysfunction are common.

Diagnosis

- **Presentation:** early adult life, usually by noticing a dilated pupil.
- **Pupil size:** large regular pupil (*Fig. 19.23a*–right eye); in long-standing cases may become small.
- **Pupillary light reflex:** (a) direct is absent or sluggish (*Fig. 19.23b*) and is associated with vermiform movements of the pupillary

border; (b) consensual is also absent or sluggish (*Fig. 19.23c*).
- **Pupillary near reflex:** slow constriction followed by slow dilatation (tonicity).
- **Accommodation:** may manifest similar tonicity.
- **Pharmacological test:** 2.5% methacholine or 0.125% pilocarpine is instilled into both eyes—Adie pupil will constrict (denervation hypersensitivity), but not the normal pupil.

Other abnormal papillary reactions

- **Argyll Robertson pupils:** clasically caused by neurosyphilis; (a) in dim light both pupils are small and may be irregular, (b) lack of constriction to light but normal to accommodation (light-near dissociation); (c) do not dilate well in the dark.

- **Tectal (dorsal midbrain) pupils:** (a) bilateral mydriasis in dim light, which may be asymmetrical, (b) light-near dissociation, and (c) other signs of Parinaud (dorsal midbrain) syndrome.

Pituitary adenomas

Classification

- **Basophil adenoma (Fig. 19.24):** secretes adrenocorticotrophic hormone and causes Cushing disease. Bitemporal hemianopia is uncommon with secreting pituitary adenomas, which tend to present with systemic features of hypersecretion. Treatment is with surgery and medical suppression of cortisol secretion.

- **Acidophil adenoma:** causes gigantism in children and acromegaly in adults, due to excessive growth hormone. Bitemporal hemianopia (*Fig. 19.25*) and optic atrophy are relatively common. Treatment

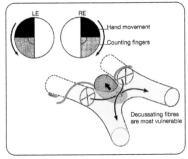

Fig 19.25

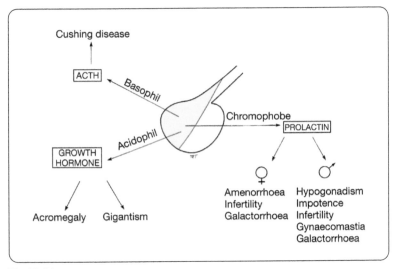

Fig 19.24

options include bromocriptine, radiotherapy, and trans-sphenoidal hypophysectomy.

- *Chromophobe adenoma:* may secrete prolactin (prolactinoma) or be nonsecreting; the most common primary intracranial tumour to produce neuro-ophthalmological features. Presentation is typically during early adult life or middle age with nonspecific headache or symptoms of endocrine disturbance. Treatment may involve bromocriptine, radiotherapy, or surgery.

Diagnosis

- *Presentation:* may not present until central vision is affected from pressure on macular fibres in the chiasm.
- *Colour desaturation:* across the vertical midline of the uniocular visual field is an early sign of chiasmal compression; can be detected simply with a red pin or pen top.
- *Optic atrophy:* present in approximately 50% of cases with field defects.
- *Field loss:* extensive loss of the temporal visual field in both eyes which can disrupt sensory fusion, decompensate a phoria, or cause problems with near vision.
- *Differential diagnosis of bitemporal field defects:* (a) dermatochalasis of the upper eyelids, (b) tilted discs, (c) optic nerve colobomas, (d) nasal retinoschisis, (e) nasal retinitis pigmentosa, and (f) functional visual loss.
- *Investigations:* MR is the key investigation, with endocrinological assessment by an appropriate specialist.

Retrochiasmal pathways

Introduction

- *Principles:* retrochiasmal pathology results in binocular visual field defects involving contralateral visual space; both eyes therefore manifest partial or total visual hemifield loss opposite the side of a retrochiasmal lesion.
- *Hemianopia:* involving the same side of visual space in both eyes is homonymous, in contradistinction to that seen in chiasmal compression, which produces heteronymous (bitemporal) hemianopia, in which opposite sides of the field are affected in each eye.
- *Incongruity:* congruity refers to how closely the extent and pattern of incomplete hemianopia in one eye matches that of the other. Almost identical field defects in either eye are therefore highly congruous, whereas mismatching right and left visual field defects are incongruous.

Optic tracts

- *Anatomy:* the optic tracts arise at the posterior aspect of the chiasm, diverging and extending posteriorly around the cerebral peduncles, to terminate in the lateral geniculate bodies.
- *Hemianopia:* caused by pathology in the anterior retrochiasmal visual pathways (e.g. the optic tracts) is characteristically incongruous, whereas that involving the posterior optic radiations shows a higher degree of congruity.
- *Optic atrophy:* may occur when the optic tracts are damaged because

the fibres in the optic tract are axons of the retinal ganglion cells.

Optic radiations

- **Anatomy:** the optic radiations extend from the lateral geniculate body to the striate cortex on the medial aspect of the occipital lobe, above and below the calcarine fissure.
- **Temporal radiations:** visual field defect consists of a contralateral, homonymous, superior quadrantanopia ('pie in the sky') because the inferior fibres of the optic radiations, which subserve the upper visual fields, first sweep anteroinferiorly into the temporal lobe as the Meyer loop (*Fig. 19.26a*).
- **Anterior parietal radiations:** visual field defect consists of a contralateral, homonymous, inferior quadrantanopia ('pie on the floor') because the superior fibres of the radiations, which subserve the inferior visual fields, proceed directly posteriorly through the parietal lobe to the occipital cortex. In general, hemianopia resulting from parietal lobe lesions tends to be relatively congruous (*Fig. 19.26b*).
- **Main radiations:** lesions deep in the parietal lobe usually cause a complete homonymous hemianopia (*Fig. 19.26c*).
- **Striate cortex:** in the striate cortex, the peripheral visual fields are represented anteriorly—this part of the occipital lobe is supplied by the posterior cerebral artery. Central macular vision is represented posteriorly, supplied by terminal

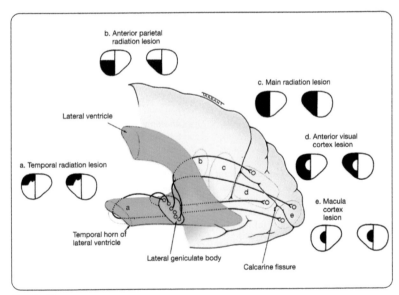

Fig 19.26

branches of both middle and posterior cerebral arteries. Occlusion of the posterior cerebral artery will therefore tend to produce a macular-sparing congruous homonymous hemianopia (*Fig. 19.26d*).

- **Damage to the tip of the occipital cortex:** as might occur from a head injury, tends to give rise to congruous homonymous central defects (*Fig. 19.26e*).

Ocular motor nerves

Third (oculomotor) nerve disease

Anatomy and causes
- **Nuclear complex:** situated in the midbrain (*Fig. 19.27*); causes of nuclear complex lesions are (a) vascular disease, (b) primary tumours, and (c) metastases. These often also involve the adjacent 4th nerve nucleus.
- **Fasciculus:** fibres passing from the nucleus; causes of nuclear and fascicular lesions are similar, with

the addition of demyelination. (a) Benedikt syndrome is characterized by ipsilateral 3rd nerve palsy and contralateral extrapyramidal signs, and (b) Weber syndrome manifests ipsilateral 3rd nerve palsy and contralateral hemiparesis.

- **Basilar part:** 'rootlets' leave the midbrain on the medial aspect of the cerebral peduncle, coalescing to form the main trunk, subsequently running lateral to and parallel with the posterior communicating artery (*Fig. 19.28*). (a) An aneurysm of the posterior communicating artery typically presents as an acute, painful 3rd nerve palsy with involvement of the pupil; (b) extradural or subdural haematoma may cause downward herniation of the temporal lobe, compressing the 3rd nerve at the tentorial edge (*Fig. 19.29*).
- **Intracavernous part:** the 3rd nerve runs in the lateral wall above the 4th nerve, dividing into superior and inferior branches which then enter the orbit (*Fig. 19.30*).

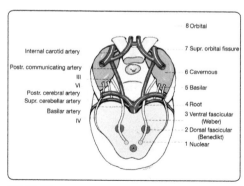

Fig 19.27

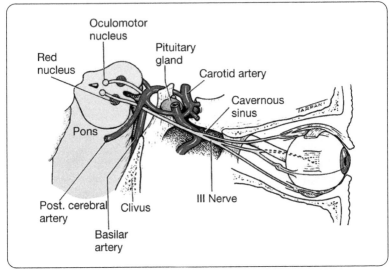

Fig 19.28

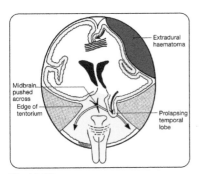

Fig 19.29

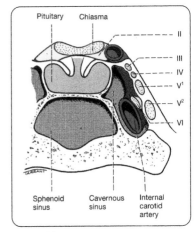

Fig 19.30

(a) Diabetes may cause a vascular paresis, which usually spares the pupil, and (b) intracavernous pathology such as aneurysm, meningioma, and carotid–cavernous fistula may all cause 3rd nerve palsy, usually associated with 4th and 6th nerve involvement because of their proximity.

- *Intraorbital part:* the superior division innervates the levator and superior rectus, the inferior division the medial rectus, inferior rectus, and inferior oblique. The branch to the inferior oblique also contains parasympathetic fibres to the sphincter pupillae and the ciliary muscle. Lesions of the superior and inferior divisions are commonly traumatic or vascular.
- *Pupillomotor fibres:* between the brainstem and the cavernous sinus, the pupillomotor fibres are superficial and are supplied by the pial vessels, whereas the main trunk of the nerve is supplied by the vasa nervorum (*Fig. 19.31*). Pupillary involvement therefore frequently differentiates a 'surgical' compressive lesion from a 'medical' lesion resulting from deeper ischaemia.
- *Causes of isolated 3rd nerve palsy:* (a) idiopathic (25%), (b) vascular (hypertension, diabetes), (c) posterior communicating artery aneurysm, (d) trauma, and (e) miscellaneous (e.g. tumours, GCA).

Diagnosis

- *Presentation:* depends on the cause.
- *Signs:* (a) profound ptosis (levator weakness; *Fig. 19.32a*), (b) abduction in the primary position (intact lateral rectus; *Fig. 19.32b*), (c) intorsion at rest (intact superior oblique), (d) normal abduction, (e) limited adduction (*Fig. 19.32c*), (f) limited elevation (*Fig. 19.32d*) and depression, and (g) mydriasis and defective accommodation.

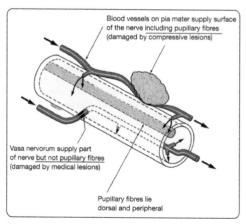

Blood vessels on pia mater supply surface of the nerve including pupillary fibres (damaged by compressive lesions)

Vasa nervorum supply part of nerve but not pupillary fibres (damaged by medical lesions)

Pupillary fibres lie dorsal and peripheral

Fig 19.31

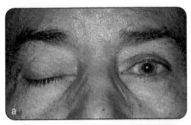
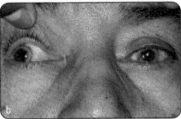
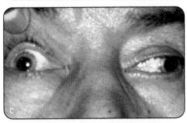
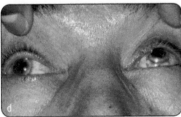

Fig 19.32

Fourth (trochlear) nerve disease

Anatomy and causes

- *Important anatomical features:*
  (a) the only cranial nerve to emerge from the dorsal aspect of the brain (*Fig. 19.33*), (b) it is a 'crossed' nerve such that it innervates the contralateral superior oblique muscle; (c) very long and slender (hence vulnerable to trauma); (d) the intracavernous part runs in the lateral wall of the sinus, inferiorly to the 3rd nerve and above the first division of the 5th nerve. The features of nuclear, fascicular, and peripheral 4th nerve palsies are clinically identical, except that nuclear palsies produce contralateral superior oblique weakness.
- *Causes of isolated 4th nerve palsy:*
  (a) congenital (common)—symptoms may not develop until decompensation in adult life (AHP on old photographs), (b) trauma (frequently bilateral lesions), and (c) vascular.

Diagnosis

- *Presentation:* vertical diplopia in the absence of ptosis, combined with a characteristic AHP, strongly suggests 4th nerve disease.
- *Signs of left 4th nerve palsy:*
  (a) left hypertropia ('left-over-right') in the primary position (*Fig. 19.34a*), (b) increase in left hypertropia on right gaze due to left inferior oblique overaction (*Fig. 19.34b*), (c) limitation of left depression on adduction (*Fig. 19.34c*), (d) normal left abduction, normal left depression, and

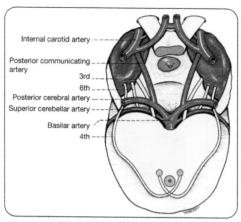

Fig 19.33

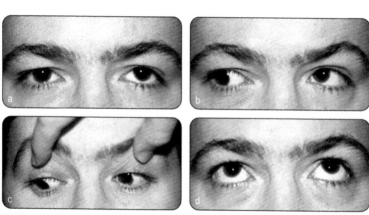

Fig 19.34

normal left elevation (*Fig. 19.34d*), and (e) AHP with contralateral head tilt, contralateral face turn, and chin depression (*Fig. 19.35*).

- *Bilateral involvement:* right hypertropia in left gaze, left hypertropia in right gaze, and a 'V' pattern esotropia.

- *Parks three-step test:* (a) Which eye is hypertropic in the primary position? Left hypertropia may be caused by weakness of one of the following: a depressor of the left eye (superior oblique or inferior rectus) or an elevator of the right eye (superior rectus or inferior

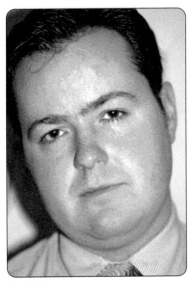

Fig 19.35

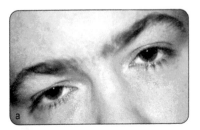

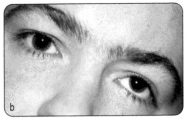

Fig 19.36

oblique); in 4th nerve palsy, the involved eye is higher. (b) Is left hypertropia greater in right gaze or left gaze? Increase on right gaze implicates either the right superior rectus or left superior oblique, and increase on left gaze implicates either the right inferior oblique or left inferior rectus; in 4th nerve palsy, the deviation is *worse* on *opposite gaze* (WOOG). (c) Bielschowsky head tilt test (3 m target); head is tilted to the right shoulder (*Fig. 19.36a*) and then to the left. Increased left hypertropia on left head tilt implicates the left superior oblique (*Fig. 19.36b*), and increase of right hypertropia on left head tilt implicates the right inferior rectus; in 4th nerve palsy, the deviation is *better* on *opposite tilt* (BOOT).

- *Double Maddox rod test:* to detect and quantify torsional abnormality.

Sixth (abducens) nerve disease

Anatomy and causes

- *Nucleus:* lies at the midlevel of the pons, closely related to the horizontal gaze centre and the fasciculus of the 7th nerve (*Fig. 19.37*). Isolated 6th nerve palsy is therefore never nuclear in origin. Nuclear lesions cause (a) ipsilateral weakness of abduction (6th nerve), (b) failure of horizontal gaze toward the side of the lesion, and (c) ipsilateral lower motor neuron facial nerve palsy.
- *Fasciculus:* leaves the brainstem at the pontomedullary junction; involvement here (vascular disease, tumours, demyelination)

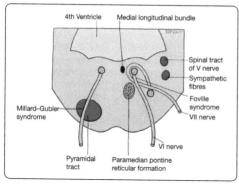

Fig 19.37

causes (a) Foville syndrome (ipsilateral lesions of 5th–8th cranial nerves, horizontal gaze centre, and central sympathetic fibres) or (b) Millard–Gubler syndrome (6th nerve, pyramidal tract causing contralateral hemiplegia, and dorsal pons).

- **Basilar part** *(Fig. 19.38):* is vulnerable to damage by acoustic neuroma (may be accompanied by hearing loss and decreased corneal sensation), nasopharyngeal tumour, basal skull fracture, or infection (Gradenigo syndrome). Raised intracranial pressure may stretch the nerve over the petrous tip to give 6th nerve palsy as a false localizing sign.

- **Intracavernous part:** runs below the 3rd and 4th nerves and the first division of the 5th nerve.

- **Intraorbital part:** enters the orbit through the superior orbital fissure within the annulus of Zinn to innervate the lateral rectus muscle.

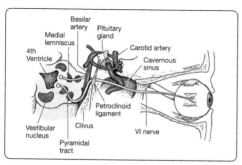

Fig 19.38

Diagnosis

- *Signs of acute left 6th nerve palsy:* (a) left esotropia in the primary position, (b) marked limitation of left abduction, and (c) compensatory face turn to the left.
- *Differential diagnosis:* (a) myasthenia gravis, (b) restrictive thyroid myopathy, (c) medial orbital wall blowout fracture with entrapment of the medial rectus, (d) orbital myositis involving the lateral rectus, (e) Duane syndrome, (f) convergence spasm, (g) divergence paralysis, and (h) acute-onset esotropia.

Supranuclear disorders of ocular motility

Horizontal gaze palsy

Anatomy

- Horizontal eye movements are generated in a common pathway from the horizontal gaze centre in the paramedian pontine reticular formation (PPRF; *Fig. 19.39*).
- From there, neurons connect to the ipsilateral 6th nerve nucleus, which innervates the lateral rectus.
- Internuclear neurons cross the midline from the 6th nerve nucleus at the level of the pons and pass up the contralateral medial longitudinal fasciculus (MLF) to synapse with motor neurons in the medial rectus subnucleus in the 3rd nerve complex that innervates the medial rectus.
- Stimulation of the PPRF on one side therefore causes a conjugate movement of the eyes to the same side, with loss of normal movement when the pathways are disrupted by disease such as demyelination, stroke, and tumours.

Diagnosis

- *PPRF lesion:* ipsilateral horizontal gaze palsy with inability to look in the direction of the lesion.
- *Left MLF lesion (internuclear ophthalmoplegia–INO):* (a) straight eyes in the primary position (*Fig. 19.40a*), (b) defective left adduction (*Fig. 19.40b*), (c) ataxic nystagmus of the right eye on right gaze, and (d) normal left gaze (*Fig. 19.40c*).
- *Bilateral INO:* (a) limitation of left adduction (*Fig. 19.41a*), (b) ataxic nystagmus of right eye on right gaze, (c) limitation of right adduction (*Fig. 19.41b*), (d) ataxic nystagmus of the left eye on left gaze, and (e) intact convergence if the lesion is discrete but may be absent if extensive (*Fig. 19.41c*).
- *Combined ipsilateral PPRF and MLF:* 'one-and-a-half syndrome' a combination of ipsilateral gaze palsy and INO.

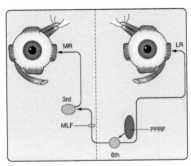

Fig 19.39

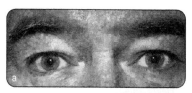
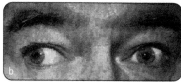
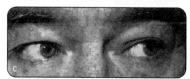

Fig 19.40

Vertical gaze palsy

Anatomy: vertical eye movements are generated from the vertical gaze centre (rostral interstitial nucleus of the MLF) in the midbrain, from where impulses pass to the subnuclei of the eye muscles controlling vertical gaze in both eyes.

Diagnosis

- *Parinaud (dorsal midbrain) syndrome:* (a) straight eyes in the primary position, (b) upgaze palsy (*Fig. 19.42a*), (c) defective convergence (*Fig. 19.42b*), (d) large pupils with light-near dissociation, (e) lid retraction (Collier sign), and (f) convergence–retraction nystagmus (see below). Causes include meningitis, pinealoma in children, demyelination in younger adults,

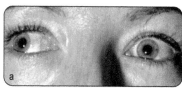
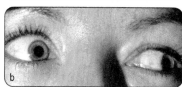
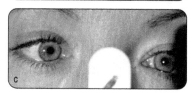

Fig 19.41

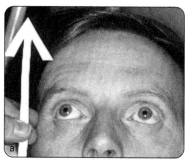
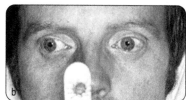

Fig 19.42

and stroke and tumours in the elderly.

- *Progressive supranuclear palsy (Steele–Richardson–Olszewski syndrome):* severe idiopathic degenerative disease presenting in old age, characterized by vertical gaze palsy (downgaze first), followed by horizontal then global gaze palsy, pseudobulbar palsy, extrapyramidal rigidity, gait ataxia, and dementia.

Nystagmus

Introduction

Definition: repetitive involuntary to-and-fro oscillation of the eyes, which may be physiological or pathological. In pathological nystagmus, each cycle of movement is usually initiated by an involuntary defoveating drift of the eye away from the object of interest, followed by a returning refixation saccadic movement.

Characteristics: can be documented using the scheme shown in *Figure 19.43*.

- *Plane:* horizontal, vertical, torsional, or nonspecific.
- *Amplitude:* fine or coarse.
- *Frequency:* high, moderate, or low.
- *Direction:* described in terms of the direction of the fast component.
- *Jerk nystagmus:* is saccadic with a slow defoveating 'drift' movement and a fast corrective refoveating saccadic movement. Jerk nystagmus can be divided into gaze-evoked and gaze-paretic; the latter is slow and usually indicates brain stem damage.
- *Pendular nystagmus:* equal velocity in both directions (nonsaccadic).

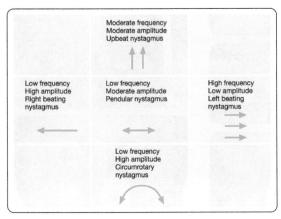

Fig 19.43

Physiological nystagmus

- **End point:** fine jerk nystagmus when the eyes are in extreme positions of gaze.
- **Optokinetic (OKN):** jerk nystagmus induced by moving repetitive targets (e.g. OKN tape or drum) across the visual field; the slow phase is a pursuit movement in which the eyes follow the target, whereas the fast phase is a saccadic movement in the opposite direction as the eyes fixate on the next target.
- **Vestibular:** jerk nystagmus caused by altered input from the vestibular nuclei to the horizontal gaze centres. It may be demonstrated by caloric stimulation: (a) cold water into the right ear elicits left jerk nystagmus (i.e., fast phase to the left), and (b) warm water into the right ear elicits right jerk nystagmus (mnemonic is 'COWS'—cold-opposite, warm-same).

Motor imbalance nystagmus

Motor imbalance nystagmus is the result of primary defects in efferent mechanisms.
- **Primary congenital nystagmus:** presentation approximately 2 or 3 months of age, with variable inheritance modes; (a) low-amplitude pendular nystagmus in the primary position, converting to jerk nystagmus on side gaze, (b) horizontal plane, (c) may be dampened by convergence and is not present during sleep; (d) there is usually a null point—a position of gaze in which nystagmus is minimal, and an AHP may be adopted to take advantage of this; in contrast to acquired nystagmus, oscillopsia is absent.
- **Spasmus nutans:** rare condition presenting between 3 and 18 months. There is unilateral or bilateral small-amplitude high-frequency horizontal nystagmus associated with head nodding; can be idiopathic (spontaneously resolves) or due to anterior visual pathway pathology including glioma.
- **Periodic alternating nystagmus:** conjugate horizontal jerk nystagmus interspersed with a 4- to 20-sec interlude after which the direction reverses; 1- to 3-min cycle in total; causes include isolated congenital, cerebellar disease, ataxia telangiectasia, and drugs (e.g. phenytoin).
- **Convergence–retraction nystagmus:** (a) induced by rotating OKN tape or drum downwards, when on the upward refixation saccade, the eyes move toward each other in a rhythmic convergence movement due to co-contraction of the medial recti; (b) associated retraction of the globe; causes include lesions of the pretectal area (Parinaud syndrome) such as pinealoma and vascular accidents.
- **Downbeat nystagmus:** vertical nystagmus with the fast phase downwards; causes include lesions of the craniocervical junction at the foramen magnum (e.g. Arnold–Chiari malformation), drugs, Wernicke encephalopathy, demyelination, and hydrocephalus.
- **Upbeat nystagmus:** vertical nystagmus with the fast phase upwards; causes include posterior fossa lesions, drugs, and Wernicke encephalopathy.

- *See-saw nystagmus of Maddox:* pendular in which one eye elevates and intorts while the other depresses and extorts; the eyes then reverse direction; causes include parasellar tumours (often associated with bitemporal hemianopia), syringobulbia, and brainstem stroke.

Sensory deprivation nystagmus

Sensory deprivation (ocular) nystagmus is caused by severe bilateral impairment of central vision before the age of approximately 2 years (e.g. congenital cataract). The nystagmus is horizontal and pendular and can often be dampened by convergence. Compensatory AHP may be adopted to move the eyes into a null point and decrease the amplitude.

Surgery for nystagmus

Surgery for nystagmus may be considered if there is an AHP with a null position or for congenital motor/sensory nystagmus without a null point.

- *To mimic a null point:* muscles are moved in order to duplicate the tension in each judged to be present when the face is turned into the null point; for example, with a null point in left gaze (i.e., with a right head turn), the right medial rectus is recessed (weakened) and the right lateral rectus resected (strengthened), and left lateral rectus is weakened and the left medial rectus strengthened.
- *Surgery for congenital motor/sensory nystagmus:* involves large recessions on the four horizontal recti to reduce

the amplitude, but should be contemplated only when the wave form and characteristics of the nystagmus have been determined by eye movement studies.

Nystagmoid movements

- *Definition:* movements resemble nystagmus, but the initial defoveating movement is a pathological saccadic intrusion.
- *Ocular flutter and opsoclonus:* saccadic oscillations with no intersaccadic interval; in ocular flutter, oscillations are purely horizontal, and in opsoclonus they are multiplanar; causes include viral encephalitis, myoclonic encephalopathy in infants ('dancing eyes and dancing feet'), transient (idiopathic) in healthy neonates, and drug-induced.
- *Ocular bobbing:* rapid, conjugate, downward eye movements with a slow drift up to the primary position; causes include pontine lesions (usually haemorrhage), cerebellar lesions compressing the pons, and metabolic encephalopathy.

Ocular myopathies

Myasthenia gravis

Pathogenesis: autoimmune disease in which antibodies mediate damage to acetylcholine receptors in striated muscle. The resultant impairment of neuromuscular conduction causes weakness and fatigue of skeletal musculature but not of cardiac and involuntary muscles. The disease affects females twice as commonly as males. Involvement can be predominantly ocular or systemic (including the eyes).

Diagnosis

- *Presentation:* in 3rd decade, most frequently with ptosis or diplopia; generalized involvement may cause fatigue, often worse toward the end of the day or brought on by exercise.
- *Systemic features:* (a) fatigue of the limbs, face (lack of expression and ptosis—myopathic facies; *Fig. 19.44*), and eyes, (b) bulbar (medulla oblongata) problems (dysphagia, dysarthria), and (c) respiratory difficulty (rare).
- *Ocular features:* involvement occurs in 90% and is the presenting feature in 60%; (a) ptosis (may be precipitated by prolonged upgaze; *Fig. 19.45*), (b) diplopia—frequently vertical, although any of the extraocular muscles may be affected, (c) nystagmoid movements, (d) bizarre defects of ocular motility (e.g. mimicking INO); (e) Cogan twitch sign is a brief upshoot of the eyelid as the eyes

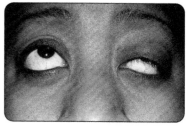

Fig 19.45

saccade from depression to the primary position.

- *Ice pack test:* ptosis usually improves after an ice pack is placed on the lid for 2 min because cold improves neuromuscular transmission; test is negative in non-myasthenic ptosis.
- *Edrophonium test:* edrophonium is a short-acting anticholinesterase agent that increases the amount of acetylcholine available at the neuromuscular junction, resulting in transient improvement in myasthenic features; objectivity can be improved by using a Hess test. Sensitivity is approximately 85% in ocular and 95% in systemic myasthenia; uncommon complications include bradycardia, loss of consciousness, and even death.
- *Serum acetylcholine receptor antibody levels:* elevated in up to 90% of patients with systemic disease and 50% of ocular cases.
- *Anti-muscle-specific kinase (MuSK) antibodies:* may be elevated.
- *Single-fibre electromyography:* highly sensitive and specific.
- *Thoracic MR or CT:* to detect thymoma, present in 10% of cases.

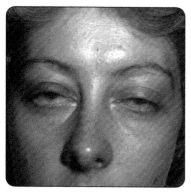

Fig 19.44

Treatment
- *Options:* (a) anticholinesterase drugs (e.g. pyridostigmine, neostigmine), (b) steroids, (c) other immunosuppressants (azathioprine, ciclosporin), (d) plasma exchange, (e) intravenous immunoglobulins, and (f) thymectomy (usually not helpful in pure ocular myasthenia).
- *Botulinum toxin injection and/or muscle surgery:* sometimes used for patients with stable ocular deviations.

Myotonic dystrophy

Genetics: AD inheritance. Two types: (a) classic—DM1, caused by a mutation in gene DMPK on chromosome 19—this form is considered below; and (b) DM2, characterized by proximal muscle myopathy, fewer systemic features, and a better long-term prognosis.

Diagnosis
- *Presentation:* in 3rd to 6th decades with weakness of the hands and difficulty walking.
- *Systemic features:* (a) difficulty in releasing grip, (b) muscle wasting and weakness, (c) mournful facial expression with bilateral facial wasting (*Fig. 19.46*), (d) slurred speech, (e) frontal baldness (males), and (f) intellectual decline.
- *Ophthalmic features:* (a) early onset cataract, (b) ptosis, (c) external ophthalmoplegia (uncommon), (d) light-near dissociation, (e) mild pigmentary retinopathy, (f) bilateral optic atrophy (uncommon), and (g) low IOP.

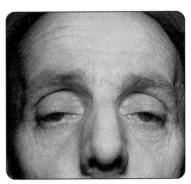

Fig 19.46

- *Investigations:* electromyography shows myotonic and myopathic potentials; serum creatine kinase is elevated.

Treatment: exercise and prevention of contractures.

Chronic progressive external ophthalmoplegia

Definition: Chronic progressive external ophthalmoplegia (CPEO) comprises a group of mitochondrial cytopathies characterized by ptosis and slowly progressive bilateral ocular immobility, with a range of causative mitochondrial DNA abnormalities. The clinical features of CPEO may occur in isolation or associated with a systemic condition such as Kearns–Sayre syndrome.

Diagnosis
- *Presentation:* in young adulthood with bilateral ptosis, which may be asymmetrical (*Fig. 19.47a*), followed by limitation of upgaze.
- *External ophthalmoplegia:* unremitting progressive course of bilateral symmetrical involvement (*Figs. 19.47b* and *19.47c*)—

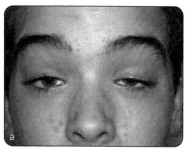

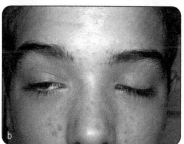

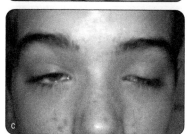

Fig 19.47

diplopia is rare; inadequate convergence may affect reading.

- **Kearns–Sayre syndrome:** (a) cerebellar ataxia, (b) cardiac conduction abnormalities, (c) fatigue and proximal muscle weakness, (d) occasionally deafness, diabetes, short stature, renal disease, and dementia; (e) fundus typically shows a

'salt-and-pepper' pigmentary retinopathy most striking at the macula.

- **Lumbar puncture:** elevation of cerebrospinal fluid protein.
- **ECG:** cardiac conduction defects.
- **Histology:** affected muscles in CPEO show 'ragged red fibres' due to intramuscular accumulation of abnormal mitochondria.

Neurofibromatosis

Genetics

The two main types are NF1 and NF2. NF1 (von Recklinghousen disease) is a disorder that primarily affects cell growth of neural tissues. Inheritance is AD (gene locus on 17q11) with irregular penetrance and variable expressivity, although approximately 50% have new mutations. NF2 is AD (gene on 22q12).

NF1

- **Systemic features:** (a) intracranial tumours (e.g. meningioma, glioma), (b) neurofibromas of peripheral and autonomic nerves, (c) skeletal abnormalities (e.g. short stature, mild macrocephaly, facial hemiatrophy (*Fig. 19.48*), absence of the greater wing of the sphenoid bone, scoliosis), (d) dermal abnormalities (café-au-lait macules (*Fig. 19.49*), neurofibromas (*Fig. 19.50*), axillary and inguinal freckles), and (e) other features (malignancies, hypertension, mental handicap).
- **Orbital lesions:** (a) optic nerve glioma in 15%, (b) other tumours (e.g. neurilemmoma, plexiform

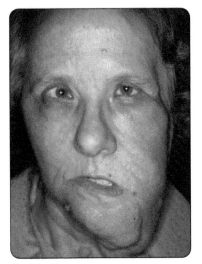

Fig 19.48

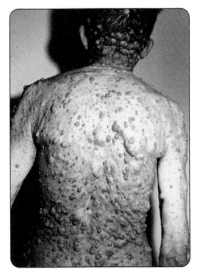

Fig 19.50

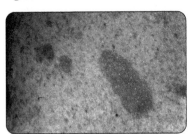

Fig 19.49

neurofibroma, meningioma), and
(c) spheno-orbital encephalocele
due to absence of the greater
wing of the sphenoid.

- *Eyelid:* neurofibromas (nodular
  or plexiform); may cause a
  mechanical ptosis.
- *Iris:* (a) Lisch nodules in 95% (*Fig.
  19.51*), (b) congenital ectropion
  uveae (uncommon; *Fig. 19.52*),
  and (c) rarely mammillations (*Fig.
  19.53*).

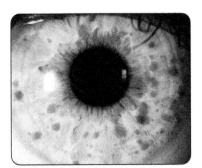

Fig 19.51

- *Prominent corneal nerves:*
  uncommon.
- *Glaucoma:* (rare) is usually
  unilateral and congenital; 50%
  have associated facial
  hemiatrophy.
- *Fundus:* choroidal naevi (common)
  with increased risk of choroidal

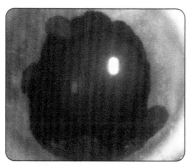

Fig 19.52

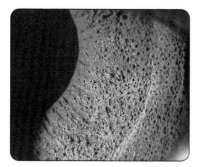

Fig 19.53

melanoma, and retinal astrocytomas (rare).

NF2

- *Neurological features:* bilateral acoustic neuromas (*Fig. 19.54*), usually presenting in the late teens or early 20s with hearing loss, tinnitus, or imbalance.
- *Cataract:* affects approximately two-thirds of patients, and usually develops prior to the age of 30 years.

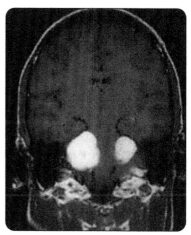

Fig 19.54

- *Fundus:* combined hamartomas of the retina and RPE, and perifoveal epiretinal membranes.
- *Other uncommon ocular features:* motility abnormalities, optic nerve sheath meningioma, optic nerve glioma, unilateral Lisch nodules, and an abnormal electro-retinogram.

Migraine

Definition: recurrent attacks of headache and/or other symptoms, widely variable in intensity, duration, and frequency.

Diagnosis
- *Common migraine (migraine without aura):* headache with autonomic dysfunction (e.g. pallor and nausea), but without neurological or ophthalmic features. Premonitory features (e.g. mood change) may occur; headache is pounding or

throbbing, spreads to involve half or more of the head and lasts from hours to a day or more. The patient is frequently photophobic and phonophobic.

- **Classic migraine (migraine with aura):** an attack is heralded by a visual aura (e.g. scotomata, bright or dark spots, zigzag 'fortification spectra'), typically lasting 10–30 min and followed by a headache that is usually hemicranial, opposite the hemianopia, and which may be severe and accompanied by nausea and photophobia. The headache may, however, be absent or trivial, and there is considerable variation between attacks even in the same individual.
- **Visual aura without headache (migraine sine migraine):** fairly common.
- **Cluster headache (migrainous neuralgia):** typically affects men during the 4th and 5th decades and is characterized by an excruciating unilateral oculotemporal headache 10 min to 2 hr in duration occurring almost every day, not infrequently at approximately 2 a.m., accompanied by various autonomic phenomena (e.g. lacrimation, conjunctival injection, rhinorrhoea); may cause a transient or permanent postganglionic Horner syndrome.
- **Focal migraine:** transient dysphasia, hemisensory symptoms or focal weakness in addition to other symptoms of migraine.
- **Retinal migraine:** acute unilateral transient visual loss, that should be investigated as retinal

embolization until proved otherwise.
- **Ophthalmoplegic migraine:** rare, and typically starts before the age of 10 years; characterized by a recurrent transient 3rd nerve palsy that begins after the headache.
- **Familial hemiplegic migraine:** may have failure of full recovery of focal neurological features after an attack of migraine subsides.
- **Basilar migraine:** occurs in children and is characterized by a typical migrainous aura associated with numbness and tingling of the lips and extremities, together with other neurological phenomena.

Treatment
- **General measures:** elimination of precipitants (e.g. chocolate, cheese, long intervals without food).
- **Prophylaxis:** involves beta-adrenergic blockers, calcium channel blockers, amitriptyline, clonidine, pizotifen, and low-dose aspirin.
- **Treatment of an acute attack:** simple analgesics and an anti-emetic; drugs for refractory patients include sumatriptan and ergotamine.

Neuralgias

The following conditions should be considered in the differential diagnosis of ocular or periocular pain in the absence of apparent physical disease:
- **Herpes zoster ophthalmicus:** presents with pain 2–3 days before the onset of the characteristic vesicular rash; very occasionally no rash will form (zoster sine herpete).

- *Trigeminal neuralgia:* brief attacks of severe pain that start in the distribution of one of the divisions of the trigeminal nerve; facial sensation is normal.
- *Raeder paratrigeminal syndrome:* affects middle-aged men and is characterized by severe unilateral headache with periocular pain in the distribution of the first division of the trigeminal nerve, associated with ipsilateral Horner syndrome; may last from hours to weeks.
- *Carotid dissection:* headache with peri- or retrobulbar pain; there may be other features such as Horner syndrome.
- *Occipital neuralgia:* attacks of pain that begin in the occipital region and then spread to the eye, temple, and face.

Facial spasm

Essential blepharospasm

Definition: distressing idiopathic condition typically presenting in women (3:1) in the 6th decade. In severe cases, blepharospasm is disabling because it may temporarily render the patient functionally blind.

Diagnosis
- Bilateral involuntary spasm of the orbicularis oculi and upper facial muscles (*Fig. 19.55*) with no other neurological signs.
- Spasms may be precipitated by a variety of factors, notably stress and anxiety.

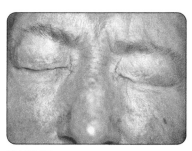

Fig 19.55

Treatment
- *Exclude:* reflex blepharospasm (e.g. ocular surface disease) and extrapyramidal disease (e.g. parkinsonism).
- *Botulinum toxin injection:* along the upper and lower eyelid and eyebrow affords temporary relief in most patients and is typically repeated every 3 or 4 months. Side effects include ptosis and other abnormalities of lid position, and occasionally diplopia due to extraocular muscle paralysis; these are virtually always temporary.

Hemifacial spasm

Diagnosis
- Brief episodes of unilateral spasm of the orbicularis oculi that spreads along the distribution of the facial nerve (*Fig. 19.56*); presents in the 5th and 6th decades.

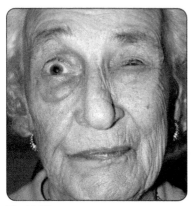

Fig 19.56

- May be idiopathic or the result of irritation at any region from the facial nucleus to the peripheral nerve; occasionally seen months or years after a Bell palsy.
- Neuroimaging should be performed to exclude a compressive aetiology.

Treatment: similar to that of essential blepharospasm.

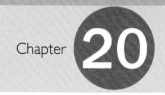
Ocular side effects of systemic medication

Cornea

Vortex keratopathy (cornea verticillata)

- *Signs:* (a) fine greyish or golden-brown opacities in the inferior corneal epithelium, (b) progressing to a whorl-like pattern that originates from a point below the pupil and swirls outwards, sparing the limbus (*Fig. 20.1*); usually reversible on cessation of medication. Vision is not impaired, but some patients may experience haloes.

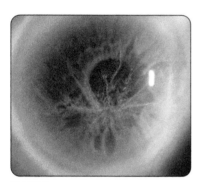

Fig 20.1

- *Causes:* quinolone antimalarials (chloroquine, hydroxychloroquine) and amiodarone.

Chlorpromazine

Long-term therapy may cause subtle and visually innocuous yellowish-brown granular deposits in the endothelium, Descemet's membrane, and deep stroma.

Argyrosis

Keratopathy in argyrosis (silver deposition) is characterized by greyish-brown granular deposits in Descemet's membrane (*Fig. 20.2*); conjunctival involvement may also occur (*Fig. 20.3*).

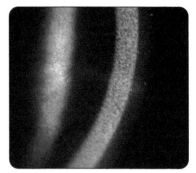

Fig 20.2

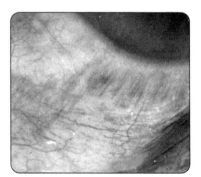

Fig 20.3

Chrysiasis

Chrysiasis describes the deposition of gold in tissues after prolonged administration (chrysotherapy), usually in the treatment of rheumatoid arthritis. Keratopathy is characterized by asymptomatic dust-like or glittering purple granules scattered throughout the epithelium and stroma.

Amantadine

Soon after commencement of therapy, some patients develop reversible diffuse white punctate opacities sometimes associated with epithelial oedema.

Lens

Steroids

Both systemic and topical steroids are cataractogenic. The relationship between dose and duration of systemic administration and cataract formation is unclear. Opacities are initially posterior subcapsular (*Fig. 20.4*) and later anterior subcapsular; early opacities may sometimes regress if therapy is discontinued, but progression commonly occurs despite withdrawal.

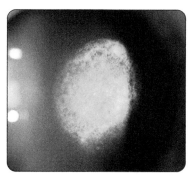

Fig 20.4

Other drugs

- **Chlorpromazine:** fine stellate yellowish-brown granules on the anterior lens capsule within the pupillary area (*Fig. 20.5*) develop in 50% of patients who have received a cumulative dose of 1000 g. The deposits persist despite discontinuation of therapy, but are visually innocuous.

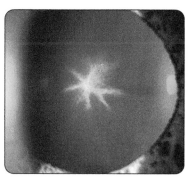

Fig 20.5

- **Busulphan:** occasionally causes lens opacities.
- **Gold:** innocuous anterior capsular deposits in approximately 50% of patients treated for more than 3 years.
- **Allopurinol:** increases the risk of cataract formation in elderly patients with large cumulative doses.

Uveitis

Rifabutin

- Acute anterior uveitis, typically unilateral and frequently associated with hypopyon; associated vitritis may be mistaken for endoph-thalmitis. Treatment involves withdrawal of the drug or reduction of dose.

- Drugs that inhibit metabolism of rifabutin (e.g. clarithromycin, fluconazole) increase the risk of uveitis.

Cidofovir

- Acute anterior uveitis with few cells but a marked fibrinous exudate may develop following several intravenous infusions; vitritis is common and hypopyon may occur with long-term administration.
- Treatment with topical steroids and mydriatics is usually successful, avoiding the need to discontinue therapy.

Retina

Antimalarials

- **Pathogenesis of toxicity:** antimalarials are melanotropic drugs that become concentrated in melanin-containing structures of the eye, such as the RPE and choroid. Administration of chloroquine in normal doses is rarely associated with retinal damage, but the risk increases significantly when the cumulative dose exceeds 300 g. Hydroxychloroquine is much safer than chloroquine, and if the daily dose does not exceed 400 mg, the risk of retinotoxicity is negligible.
- **Premaculopathy:** (a) VA is normal; (b) scotoma to a red target located between 4° and 9° from fixation; (c) a subtle colour vision defect may be present on specialized testing.

- **Early maculopathy:** (a) VA 6/9–6/12, with (b) a subtle 'bull's-eye' macular lesion (*Fig. 20.6*) that may progress even if the drug is stopped.
- **Moderate maculopathy:** (a) VA 6/18–6/24, and (b) obvious 'bull's-eye' maculopathy.
- **Severe maculopathy:** (a) VA 6/36–6/60, and (b) widespread RPE atrophy surrounding the fovea.
- **End-stage maculopathy:** (a) VA CF–PL, (b) marked RPE atrophy, retinal arteriolar attenuation (*Fig. 20.7*), and peripheral pigment clumping.

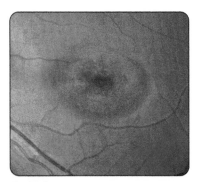

Fig 20.6

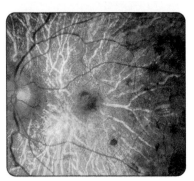

Fig 20.7

Phenothiazines

- **Thioridazine:** doses exceeding 800 mg/day for just a few weeks may be sufficient to cause reduced VA and impairment of dark adaptation. Progression of retinotoxicity is as follows: (a) 'salt-and-pepper' pigmentary disturbance at the mid-periphery and posterior pole, (b) plaque-like pigmentation, and (c) loss of the RPE and choriocapillaris (*Fig. 20.8*).
- **Chlorpromazine:** retinotoxicity may occur with large doses over a prolonged period; it is characterized by nonspecific pigmentary granularity and clumping.

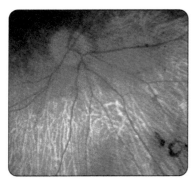

Fig 20.8

Drug-induced crystalline maculopathies

- **Tamoxifen:** retinotoxicity may rarely develop, usually in patients on high doses. (a) Fine yellow crystalline deposits in the inner retina, and (b) punctate grey lesions in the outer retina and RPE (*Fig. 20.9*). Visual impairment is thought to be caused

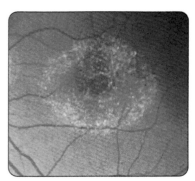

Fig 20.9

by maculopathy associated with foveolar cyst formation.
- **Canthaxanthin:** long-term use may cause the deposition of innocuous glistening yellow inner retinal deposits in a doughnut shape at the posterior pole (*Fig. 20.10*).
- **Methoxyflurane:** can be associated with calcium oxalate crystals scattered throughout the retina, which may later be associated with RPE hyperplasia at the posterior pole (*Fig. 20.11*).

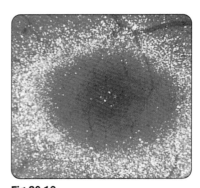

Fig 20.10

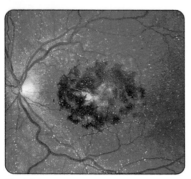

Fig 20.11

- *Nitrofurantoin:* long-term use may result in slight visual impairment associated with glistening retinal deposits.

Other drugs

- *Interferon-alpha:* retinopathy (cotton wool spots and intraretinal haemorrhages) develops in some patients but usually resolves spontaneously with cessation of therapy.
- *Desferrioxamine:* retinotoxicity typically presents with rapid visual loss; the fundi may be normal, but within several weeks mottled pigmentary changes develop.
- *Nicotinic acid:* rarely patients on high doses develop cystoid maculopathy suggestive of cystoid macular oedema, but without leakage on FA.

Optic nerve

Ethambutol

- *Incidence of toxicity:* optic neuropathy is dose- and duration-dependent; up to 6% at a daily dose of 25 mg/kg, typically within 3–6 months of starting treatment.
- *Presentation:* sudden visual impairment, with normal or slightly swollen optic discs and associated splinter haemorrhages.
- *Signs:* (a) central scotoma, (b) decreased VA, (c) blue-yellow dyschromatopsia, and (d) constriction of peripheral fields with red-green dyschromatopsia.
- *Prognosis:* usually good following drug discontinuation.
- *Screening:* every 4 weeks for doses higher than 15 mg/kg and every 3–6 months for lower doses.

Amiodarone

- *Incidence of toxicity:* optic neuropathy, probably demyelinating, is rare and not dose-related, affecting approximately 1% of patients during the initial years of therapy.
- *Presentation:* insidious unilateral or bilateral visual impairment associated with disc swelling.
- *Prognosis:* variable; drug cessation may not result in improvement.
- *Screening:* not appropriate but patients must be warned to report visual symptoms.

Vigabatrin

- *Pathogenesis of optic neuropathy:* probably idiosyncratic rather than dose-related.
- *Presentation:* concentric or binasal field defects months or years after starting treatment.
- *Fundus:* usually normal; occasional changes include peripheral atrophy, nasal disc atrophy, arteriolar

narrowing, altered macular reflex, and surface wrinkling.
- **Perimetry:** recommended prior to starting treatment, then every 6 months for 3 years, and subsequently annually.

Topiramate

- **Ocular toxicity:** ciliochoroidal effusion leading to acute angle-closure glaucoma, with associated myopia.

- **Presentation:** blurred vision and sometimes haloes, ocular pain, and redness, usually within 1 month of starting treatment.
- **Signs:** shallowing of the anterior chamber and raised IOP.
- **Prognosis:** good provided the complication is recognized.

Trauma

Eyelid trauma

Periocular haematoma

- A 'black eye,' consisting of a haematoma (focal collection of blood) and/or periocular ecchymosis (diffuse bruising) and oedema, is a very common result of blunt injury and is generally innocuous.
- It is important to exclude serious associated damage to the eyeball or orbital structures, particularly occult orbital roof fracture (subconjunctival haemorrhage without a visible posterior limit may be an indicator), and basal skull fracture (may give bilateral ring haematoma—'panda eyes'; *Fig. 21.1*).

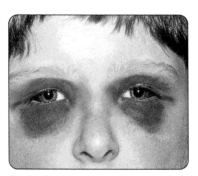

Fig 21.1

Laceration

Repair should be by direct closure whenever possible, because this affords the best functional and cosmetic result.

- **Marginal lacerations:** sutured with perfect alignment to prevent notching.
- **Extensive tissue loss:** may require a major reconstructive procedure as following tumour resection.
- **Canalicular lacerations** (*Fig. 21.2*): should be repaired within 24 hr with bicanalicular (e.g. Crawford) or monocanalicular (e.g. Mini Monoka) silicone stenting.

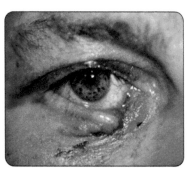

Fig 21.2

Blow-out orbital floor fracture

Pathogenesis: sudden increase in orbital pressure due to an impacting object (*Fig. 21.3*). The fracture most frequently involves the relatively weaker floor of the orbit along the thin bone covering the infraorbital canal. Occasionally, the orbital wall,

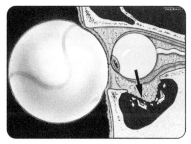

Fig 21.3

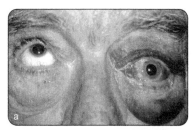

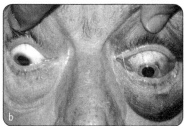

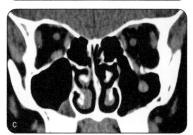

Fig 21.4

the rim, and/or adjacent facial bones may be fractured.

Diagnosis

- *Periorbital:* (a) ecchymosis, (b) oedema, and (c) occasionally subcutaneous emphysema.
- *Infraorbital nerve anaesthesia:* (lower lid, cheek, side of nose, upper lip, upper teeth, gums) is common.
- *Mechanisms of diplopia:* (a) restriction due to haemorrhage and oedema, (b) mechanical entrapment of extraocular muscle or adjacent connective tissue within the fracture, with diplopia typically occurring in both up- (*Fig. 21.4a*) and downgaze (*Fig. 21.4b*), and (c) direct injury to an extraocular muscle (negative forced duction test).
- *Enophthalmos:* in severe fracture.
- *Globe damage:* uncommon but should be excluded.
- *CT:* with coronal views for fracture evaluation (*Fig. 21.4c*).
- *Hess test:* for monitoring diplopia.

Initial treatment

- *Oral antibiotics:* no nose blowing because infected sinus contents may be forced into the orbit.
- *Ice packs and nasal decongestants:* for swelling.
- *Systemic steroids:* occasionally required for severe oedema, especially if there is optic nerve compromise.

Subsequent treatment

- **Aims:** prevention of permanent diplopia and/or cosmetically unacceptable enophthalmos.
- **Surgery not required:** (a) fractures involving up to one-third of the orbital floor, (b) little or no herniation, (c) no significant enophthalmos, and (d) improving diplopia.
- **Surgery within 2 weeks:** (a) fractures with entrapment of orbital contents, (b) enophthalmos greater than 2 mm, and (c) significant diplopia.
- **Urgent surgery:** (a) early marked enophthalmos, and (b) 'white-eyed' fracture subgroup with acute trap-door incarceration of herniated tissue. This requires urgent repair to avoid permanent neuromuscular damage; patients are typically younger than 18 years of age with little visible external soft tissue injury, and CT signs may be subtle.
- **Surgical technique:** (a) transconjunctival or subciliary approach, (b) removal of entrapped orbital contents, and (c) defect is covered with a synthetic patch (e.g. silicone; Fig. 21.5).

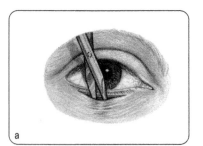
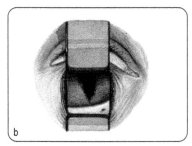
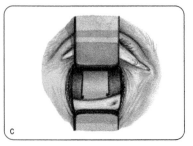
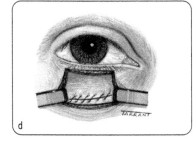

Fig 21.5

Trauma to the globe

Definitions

- **Closed injury:** commonly due to blunt trauma; the corneosclera is intact.
- **Open injury:** full-thickness wound of the corneoscleral envelope.
- **Rupture:** full-thickness wound caused by blunt trauma; the globe gives way at its weakest point, which may not be at the site of impact.
- **Laceration:** full-thickness defect in the eye wall produced by a tearing injury, usually due to a direct impact.
- **Incised injury:** caused by a sharp object such as glass or a knife.
- **Penetrating injury:** single full-thickness wound, usually caused by a sharp object, without an exit wound; may be associated with an intraocular foreign body.
- **Perforating injury:** full-thickness entry and exit wounds, usually caused by a missile.

Imaging

- **Plain radiographs:** may be taken when a foreign body is suspected.
- **CT:** superior to plain radiographs in detection and localization of foreign bodies.
- **MR:** more accurate than CT in assessment of the globe such as detection of an occult posterior rupture, although not for bony structures. MR should never be performed if a ferrous foreign body is suspected.
- **US:** may identify an intraocular foreign body, globe rupture, suprachoroidal haemorrhage, and retinal detachment.

Blunt trauma

- **Corneal abrasion:** breach of the epithelium, demonstrated by fluorescein staining (*Fig. 21.6*).
- **Corneal oedema:** folds in Descemet membrane and stromal thickening (*Fig. 21.7*).
- **Hyphaema:** blood in the anterior chamber with a horizontal 'fluid level' pattern (*Fig. 21.8*).
- **Pupillary damage:** (a) compression of the pupillary margin against the lens results in imprinting of pigment (Vossius ring; *Fig. 21.9*), (b) damage to the iris sphincter may cause

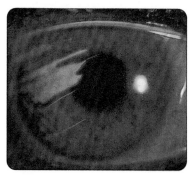

Fig 21.6

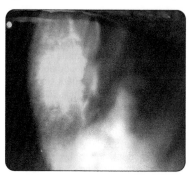

Fig 21.7

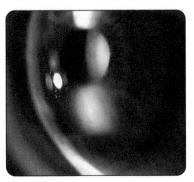

Fig 21.8

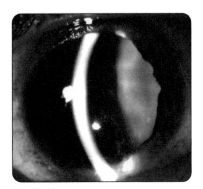

Fig 21.10

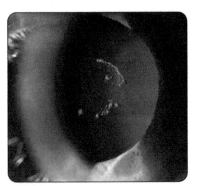

Fig 21.9

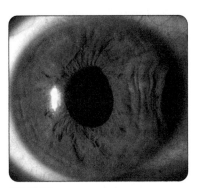

Fig 21.11

mydriasis, and (c) radial tears in the pupillary margin (*Fig. 21.10*).

- *Iridodialysis:* dehiscence of the iris from the ciliary body at its root. The pupil is typically D-shaped and the dialysis is seen as a dark biconvex area near the limbus (*Fig. 21.11*).
- *Angle recession:* tear involving the face of the ciliary body that carries a risk of late glaucoma.
- *IOP:* (a) elevation (hyphaema, inflammation), and (b) hypotony (temporary cessation of aqueous secretion—'ciliary shock').

- *Lens damage:* (a) flower-shaped 'rosette' opacity (*Fig. 21.12*), (b) tearing of the zonular fibres may lead to subluxation; complete dislocation is rare and may be into the vitreous or anterior chamber (*Fig. 21.13*).
- *Globe rupture:* usually anterior, with prolapse of iris and vitreous (*Fig. 21.14*), but may be masked by subconjunctival haemorrhage; an occult posterior rupture should be suspected if the anterior chamber is unusually deep and IOP is low.

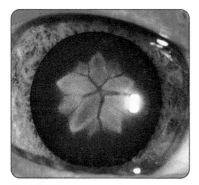

Fig 21.12

- **Vitreous haemorrhage:** often in association with posterior vitreous detachment.
- **Commotio retinae:** concussion of the sensory retina resulting in cloudy swelling that gives the involved area a grey appearance. If the macula is involved, a 'cherry-red spot' may be seen at the fovea (*Fig. 21.15*). Prognosis is dependent on severity and may include progressive pigmentary degeneration and macular hole formation (*Fig. 21.16*).

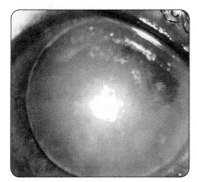

Fig 21.13

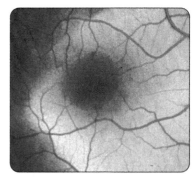

Fig 21.15

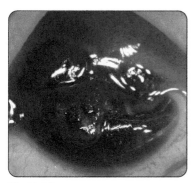

Fig 21.14

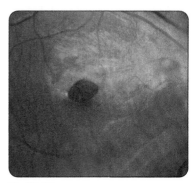

Fig 21.16

- **Choroidal rupture:** (a) a fresh rupture may be partially obscured by subretinal haemorrhage (*Fig. 21.17*); (b) following absorption of blood, a white crescentic vertical streak of exposed sclera concentric with the optic disc becomes visible (*Fig. 21.18*). The visual prognosis is poor if the fovea is involved; an uncommon late complication is choroidal neovascularization.
- **Retinal breaks and RD:** trauma is responsible for approximately 10% of RD and is the most common cause in children. A dialysis (break at the ora serrata) is commonly caused by impact-related traction of the gel along the posterior aspect of the vitreous base; it may be associated with avulsion of the vitreous base giving rise to a 'bucket-handle' appearance (*Fig. 21.19*); equatorial breaks and macular holes are less common.

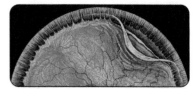

Fig 21.19

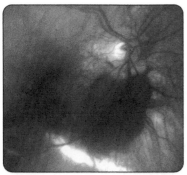

Fig 21.17

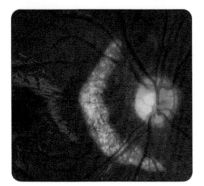

Fig 21.18

- **Traumatic optic neuropathy:** presents with sudden visual loss that cannot be explained by other pathology. Vision is often very poor from the outset, with only perception of light in 50%. Typically, the only objective finding is an APD, with disc pallor developing subsequently. Some spontaneous improvement occurs in up to half of indirect injury cases, but if there is initially no light perception the prognosis is very poor. No clear benefit has been demonstrated for any form of treatment, but steroids, optic nerve decompression, or fenestration may be useful in some cases.
- **Optic nerve avulsion:** rare and typically occurs when an object intrudes between the globe and the orbital wall, displacing the eye. Fundus examination shows a striking cavity where the optic nerve head has retracted from its dural sheath (*Fig. 21.20*).

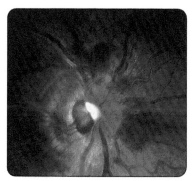

Fig 21.20

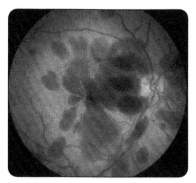

Fig 21.21

Shaken baby syndrome (non-accidental head injury)

Pathogenesis: physical abuse occurring in children typically younger than age 2 years caused principally by violent shaking; brainstem traction injury causes apnoea, consequent hypoxia leading to raised intracranial pressure and ischaemia. Mortality is more than 25%, and it is responsible for up to 50% of deaths from child abuse.

Diagnosis
- *Presentation:* irritability, lethargy, and vomiting; often misdiagnosed because the history of injury is withheld.
- *Systemic features:* impact head injuries (bruising, skull fractures, subdural and subarachnoid haemorrhage), and rib and long bone fractures.
- *Ocular features:* (a) periocular bruising, (b) subconjunctival haemorrhage, (c) APD, (d) poor visual responses, and (e) retinal haemorrhages, typically involving multiple layers (*Fig. 21.21*); visual loss occurs in 20%, mainly due to cerebral damage.

Penetrating trauma

Causes: penetrating injuries are more common in males than in females (3:1); 50% are aged 15–34 years. The most frequent causes are assault, domestic and occupational accidents, and sport.

Treatment
- *Corneal wounds:* (a) small self-sealing shelving wounds with a formed anterior chamber (*Fig. 21.22*) may not require suturing because they will usually heal spontaneously or with a bandage contact lens; prophylactic topical antibiotics are essential, and topical steroid and a mydriatic may be needed for traumatic iritis; (b) large wounds should be sutured urgently; devitalized incarcerated iris should be abscised (*Fig. 21.23*), but healthy iris reposited.
- *Lens damage:* corneal/scleral lacerations are sutured, following

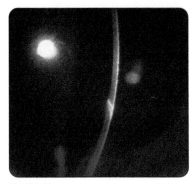

Fig 21.22

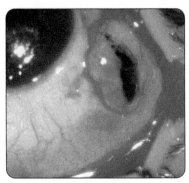

Fig 21.24

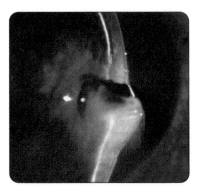

Fig 21.23

which the lens is removed. Implantation of an IOL is generally associated with a favourable visual outcome and a low rate of complications.

- *Anterior sclera laceration (Fig. 21.24):* every attempt should be made to reposit viable uveal tissue and cut prolapsed vitreous flush with the wound in order to

reduce the risk of tractional retinal detachment.

- *Posterior scleral laceration:* frequently associated with retinal damage. Primary repair of the sclera should be the initial priority, with subsequent vitreoretinal assessment.
- *Tractional RD:* requires pars plana vitrectomy.

Superficial foreign bodies

- *Subtarsal:* small foreign bodies such as particles of steel, coal, or sand often impact on the corneal or conjunctival surface and sometimes adhere to the superior tarsal conjunctiva (*Fig. 21.25*), from where the cornea is abraded with every blink—a pathognomonic pattern of linear corneal abrasions is usual. Removal with a cotton bud is usually easy.
- *Corneal (Fig. 21.26):* ferrous foreign bodies of even a few hours' duration often result in rust staining ('rust ring'). There is a risk of secondary bacterial keratitis, which is probably

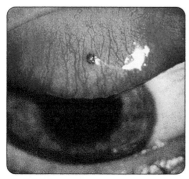

Fig 21.25

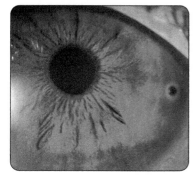

Fig 21.26

higher with organic particles and stone fragments. The foreign body is removed under slit-lamp visualization using a sterile needle (e.g. 26 gauge), following which antibiotic ointment is instilled together with a cycloplegic and/or typical NSAIDs to promote comfort. A residual 'rust ring' is easiest to remove with a sterile burr, if available.

Intraocular foreign bodies

Introduction: an intraocular foreign body (IOFB) may traumatize the eye: (a) mechanically (e.g. cataract, retinal haemorrhages, retinal tears), (b) by introducing infection (especially stone and organic foreign bodies), and (c) by exerting other toxic effects on the intraocular structures. A ferrous IOFB undergoes dissociation resulting in the deposition of iron in the intraocular epithelial structures (siderosis). An IOFB with a high copper content induces a violent endophthalmitis-like picture. An alloy with lower copper content such as brass results in chalcosis in which dissociated copper becomes deposited intraocularly, giving similar ocular features to Wilson's disease.

Diagnosis
- *Accurate history:* to determine the likelihood and origin of an IOFB.
- *Examination:* to confirm presence and location; if the posterior segment view is poor, associated signs such as damage to anterior segment structures may be critical.
- *Gonioscopy:* may reveal an IOFB lodged in the anterior chamber angle (*Fig. 21.27*).
- *Siderosis:* (a) radial iron deposits on the anterior lens capsule, (b) reddish-brown staining of the iris (*Fig. 21.28*), sometimes with heterochromia iridis; (c) complications include secondary glaucoma and pigmentary retinopathy, followed by atrophy of the retina and RPE (*Fig. 21.29*) with severe visual loss.

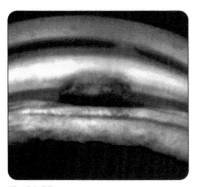

Fig 21.27

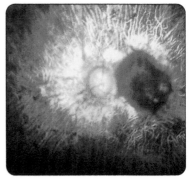

Fig 21.29

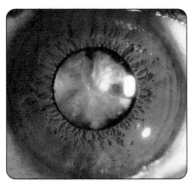

Fig 21.28

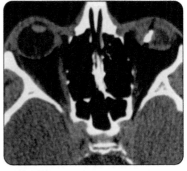

Fig 21.30

- *Chalcosis:* (a) Kayser–Fleischer ring, (b) anterior 'sunflower' cataract, and (c) golden retinal plaques. Because copper is less retinotoxic than iron, degenerative retinopathy does not develop, and visual function may be preserved.
- *CT:* axial (*Fig. 21.30*) and coronal cuts used to detect and localize a metallic IOFB.

- *B-scan US:* often very helpful, although care should be taken not to exert pressure on an open eye.
- *MR: contraindicated* in the context of a ferrous IOFB.

Treatment
- *Magnetic removal:* of ferrous IOFB involves the creation of an adjacent sclerotomy, with application of a magnet followed by cryotherapy and scleral

buckling to a retinal break as necessary.
- *Forceps removal:* for nonmagnetic IOFB or ferrous IOFB that cannot be safely removed with a magnet.
- *Prophylaxis against infection:* critical (see below).

Enucleation

- *Primary enucleation:* only for very severe injuries, with no prospect of retention of vision and when it is impossible to repair the sclera.
- *Secondary enucleation:* following primary repair if the eye is severely and irreversibly damaged, particularly if it is also unsightly and uncomfortable. It has been recommended that enucleation should be performed within 10 days of the original injury in order to prevent the very remote possibility of sympathetic ophthalmitis (see Chapter 11), but objective evidence for this is lacking.

Bacterial endophthalmitis

Risk factors: endophthalmitis develops in approximately 8% of cases of penetrating trauma with retained foreign body. Risk factors include (a) delay in primary repair, (b) retained IOFB, and (c) position and extent of the laceration. Clinical signs are the same as for acute postoperative endophthalmitis (see Chapter 9).

Treatment
- *Prophylaxis:* (a) oral fluoroquinolone antibiotics (ciprofloxacin, moxifloxacin) for open globe injuries, together with topical antibiotic, steroid, and cycloplegic, (b) prompt removal and culture of retained IOFBs,

and (c) intravitreal antibiotics for high-risk cases such as agricultural injuries.
- *Treatment of established cases:* same as that of acute postoperative bacterial endophthalmitis (see Chapter 9).

Chemical injuries

Introduction: alkalis tend to penetrate more deeply than acids because the latter coagulate surface proteins, forming a protective barrier. Pathological effects include necrosis of the conjunctival and corneal epithelium with disruption, occlusion of the limbal vasculature and loss of limbal stem cells, and damage to internal tissues following anterior chamber penetration; hypotony and phthisis may ensue in severe cases.

Diagnosis
- *History:* delayed until after initial treatment as below.
- *Grading (Roper-Hall system):* aids the planning of later treatment and gives an indication of prognosis; (a) grade 1—clear cornea (epithelial damage only) and no limbal ischaemia (excellent prognosis), (b) grade 2—hazy cornea but with visible iris details and less than one-third limbal ischaemia (good prognosis), (c) grade 3—total loss of corneal epithelium, stromal haze obscuring iris details, and between one-third and half limbal ischaemia (guarded prognosis; *Fig. 21.31*), and (d) grade 4—opaque cornea and more than half limbal ischaemia (very poor prognosis; *Fig. 21.32*).

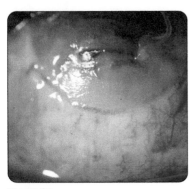

Fig 21.31

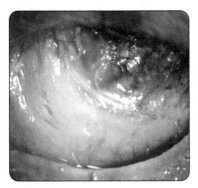

Fig 21.32

Treatment

- *Immediate emergency treatment:* (a) copious irrigation with normal saline or Ringer solution (tap water to avoid delay) for 15–30 min or until pH is neutral, (b) double-eversion of the upper eyelid, and (c) debridement of contaminating debris and necrotic areas of epithelium.
- *Treatment of mild (grade 1 and 2) injuries:* topical antibiotic ointment for approximately 1 week, with topical steroid and cycloplegic if necessary.
- *Treatment of moderate–severe injuries:* (a) topical steroid, initially 4–8 times daily then tailed off after 7–10 days and replaced by topical NSAID, cycloplagic, antibiotic, ascorbic and citric acid, and acetylcysteine, (b) systemic ascorbic acid and tetracycline (for corneal melting), (c) lysis of developing symblepharon with a sterile glass rod or damp cotton bud, and (d) monitoring of IOP.
- *Early surgery:* in severe cases to maintain corneal integrity (e.g. advancement of Tenon capsule to re-establish limbal vascularity, limbal stem cell transplantation, amniotic membrane grafting, gluing or keratoplasty for actual or impending perforation).
- *Late surgery:* (e.g. division of conjunctival bands, conjunctival or other mucous membrane grafts, correction of eyelid deformities, keratoplasty, keratoprosthesis).

Index

Printed and bound by CPI Group (UK) Ltd, Croydon, CR0 4YY

03/10/2024

01040451-0001